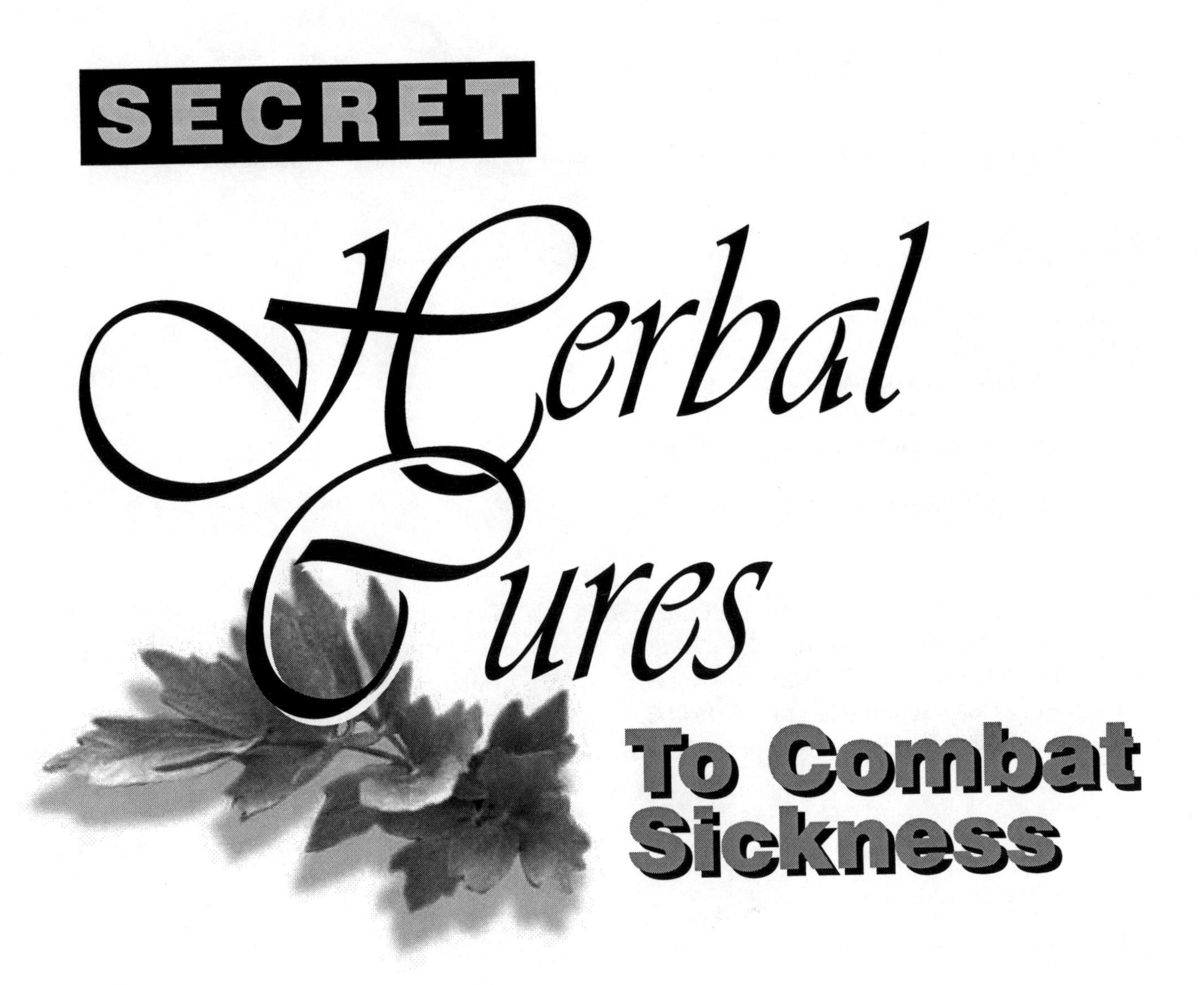

SECRET Herbal Cures To Combat Sickness

LOMBARDI

Published by Doctors Health Press, a division of Lombardi Publishing Corporation.

Written by: David Juan, M.D.

Editorial: Jeff Jurmain, M.A.

Managing Editor: Meghan Jackson, B.A.

Book Design: Audrey O'Handley

Cover Design: Jay Eckert

Secret Herbal Cures to Combat Sickness is published by Doctors Health Press, a division of Lombardi Publishing Corporation. In the U.S.: 28 State Street, Suite 1100, Boston, MA 02109-1775; in Canada: P.O. Box 428, Kleinburg, Ontario, L0J 1C0.

Secret Herbal Cures to Combat Sickness

ISBN# 0-9734125-8-5

Printed in Canada.

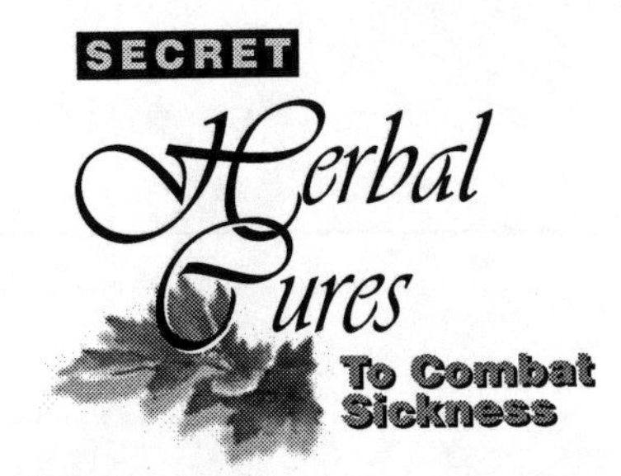

Table of Contents

PART THREE

INDEX OF HERBS 149

PART FOUR

MENTIONABLE NUTRACEUTICALS 209

APPENDIX

HERBS UNAPPROVED BY GERMANY'S COMMISSION E 227

YOUR HERBAL MEDICINE DIARY 231

FOUR COMMON MYTHS 239

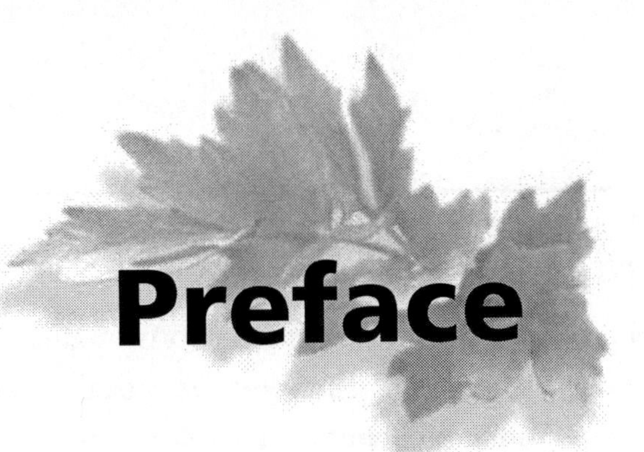

Preface

Introduction

Herbal products are widely used in North America. Of the hundreds throught to play a role in medicine, these are the most popular herbal products: ginkgo biloba, St. John's wort, ginseng, garlic, echinacea/goldenseal, saw palmetto, kava-kava, pycnogeno/grapeseed extract, cranberry, valerian, evening primrose, bilberry, and milk thistle. It is estimated that about 25% to 45% of adults have used one or more herbal product(s) to treat a medical illness within the past year. Why are herbal products so popular? There are several reasons including:

- Herbal products are "natural" and therefore safer than drugs;
- Herbal products may offer health benefits unmatched by drugs;
- Herbal products have more "science" behind them than drugs; and
- Herbal products offer equal health benefits, but with fewer side effects.

According to the World Health Organization, herbal medicines can be broken down into three categories:

1. Phytomedicine (*phyto* is the Greek word for "plant") sold as over-the-counter products in various dosage forms such as tablets, capsules, and liquids for oral use.
2. Dietary supplements containing herbal ingredients (also called "nutraceuticals") available in various dosage forms.
3. Herbal medicines consisting of crude, semi-processed, or processed medicinal plants. These are primarily used in developing countries.

In Germany and France, herbal medicines have been used as prescription drugs for more than three decades. In terms of the size of the herbal medicine or nutraceutical market in the U.S. and Europe, it is estimated to be somewhere between $80 billion and $250 billion.

Herbs: Food or Drug?

Even though we consider herbal products to be either foods or dietary supplements, we should really think of all herbal products as drugs in the truest sense of the word. This is because, as with drugs, herbal products contain complex chemicals and have dose-related side effects as with all drugs. Plus, drugs and herbs are closely related – it's estimated that up to 45% of drugs used today have botanical origins. Let's look at a few examples:

- Aspirin (salicylic acid) comes from the bark of the white willow tree and meadow-sweet plant.
- Atropine, used for the treatment of irregular heartbeats, is made from from belladonna leaves.
- Colchicine is used in the treatment of gout and comes from autumn crocus.
- Digoxin (Lanoxin), the most widely prescribed heart medication for heart failure and irregular heartbeat, comes from foxglove, a poisonous plant. Dr. William Withering published his clinical trials in 1785 in a book entitled: *An Account of the Foxglove and Some of Its Medical uses.*
- The asthma treatment ephedrine comes, not shockingly, from the ephedra plant.
- Morphine and codeine are commonly used narcotics made from the opium poppy.
- Pacitaxel (Taxol), used in the treatment of ovarian cancer, comes from the yew tree.
- Quinine, a drug that is meant to treat malaria, originate, in chinchona bark.
- Vinblastine (Velban) and vincristine (Oncovin) are anticancer drugs from periwinkle.

Lessons from Japan

In Japan, herbal products have been used for centuries. In fact, the majority of Japanese doctors not only routinely (80% of the time) prescribe herbal products for their patients, but also consider herbal products to be their treatment of choice for certain medical conditions. Therefore, given this long and rich experience with the medical use of herbal products, there are many lessons that could be learned by North American consumers and the medical community (including physicians, pharmacists, dietitians, and nurses).

There are seven medical conditions in which most Japanese physicians would recommend the use of herbal products as the primary form of treatment:

1. **Herbs combined with drugs (prescribed or over-the-counter) to reduce side effects.**

   It is widely known that chemotherapy for cancer is associated with many side effects, including nausea, vomiting, loss of appetite, hair loss, anemia, and kidney or heart damage. The addition of herbal products may reduce these side effects and in some cases also enhance the chance of remission.

2. **Herbs combined with drugs (prescribed or over-the-counter) to increase effectiveness.**

   There are many cases in which the addition of a herbal product enhances the effectiveness of traditional drug. For example, by using a ginseng formula, physicians were able to reduce the dosage of prednisolone, a steroid drug used to treat lupus, and therefore the many side effects associated with steroid use.

3. **Herbs for patients with allergies or adverse side effects to standard medical treatment.**

   Nonsteroidal anti-inflammatory drugs (NSAIDs) are used for the treatment of arthritis. These include Aspirin and ibuprofen. Yet many people develop gastrointestinal complaints from these drugs. There are herbal products which can relief arthritic pain just as well as NSAIDs without these side effects. Antidepressants are commonly prescribed drugs for even mild depression. However, the price of taking these types of drugs often includes weight gain, fatigue, loss of libido, or emotional "high." There are herbal products, which could relieve mild depression (i.e. St. John's wort) just as well as standard antidepressants without any of these aforementioned side effects.

4. **Herbs to treat subjective symptoms.**

   There are many symptoms, which do not fit any particular diagnosis – menopausal discomforts and chronic fatigue, to name a couple. Many herbal products have been shown effective in relieving these non-specific symptoms.

5. **Herbs to treat psychosomatic and psychiatric illnesses.**

   Herbal products have been used for decades in the treatment of many psychosomatic and psychiatric symptoms. Of particular interest are the many Chinese and Japanese herbal products, which neither overstimulate nor depress the central nervous system. Moreover, they do not produce the side effects commonly associated with antidepressants and psychiatric drugs such as drowsiness, fatigue, and tremors, nor do they trigger manic behavior, hallucinations, or nightmares.

6. **Herbs to boost the immune system.**

   Herbal products could boost your immune system. There are many diseases in which the immune system does not work properly such as in rheumatoid arthritis, lupus, asthma, and various allergic conditions.

7. **Herbs to treat diseases in older individuals.**

   As one gets older, the number of complaints increase as do the number of drugs that are taken. The chance of drug interactions as well as side effects increases with the number of drugs taken. Thus, there is a distinct advantage in taking herbal products for these conditions and avoiding both drug interactions as well as the known drug side effects.

How is *Secret Herbal Cures to Combat Sickness* Different from Other Books?

✔ **More medically oriented**

Unlike many books on herbal medicine written by non-physicians, this one has been put together with advice from me, a practicing physician with special interests in rational therapeutics using traditional drugs or herbal products. In my clinics, I see that many of my patients simply are medically ignorant in terms of some of the common symptoms associated with their condition or illness. It is extremely important to be knowledgeable of the key symptoms associated with each condition, not only for your own benefit, but also for those individuals you love or care about. Therefore, in *Secret Herbal Cures*, I have intentionally emphasized the common symptoms associated with each medical condition. As in daily life, knowing what the problem is means you are half-way to solving it. The same is true for any medical condition.

✔ **More up-to-date**

Secret Herbal Cures provides you with the most up-to-date information available in medical literature. In fact, I spent hours searching the Internet for the latest clinical studies on every herbal product mentioned in this book. I strongly feel that an informed consumer is vital in this information-laden age with so much misinformation and so many false claims out there. I strongly encourage you to keep yourself updated with high quality information sources such as subscribing to my monthly ***Vitamin Doctor*** newsletter.

✔ **More comprehensive**

Unlike some books on herbal medicine in which the authors cover only each herbal product, in *Secret Herbal Cures,* I try to cover common medical conditions as well as key herbal products. In Part Two, I cover more than 70 medical conditions. Then, in Part Three, I go deeper to describe in detail more than 75 herbal products (although a few are supplements not derived from plants).

I see a lot of drug-induced side effects in my practice. Therefore, I am particularly sensitive to such adverse reactions as drug interactions. In Part Three, I discuss these under the subheads "Considerations" and "Side Effects" for each herbal product.

✔ **More authoritative, unbiased and better documented**

I have taught in medical schools and have written dozens of peer-reviewed articles on nutrition and drugs effects in medical journals. Moreover, I have conducted many nutritional research studies in the past. Right at this moment, I am conducting human research on the effects of two micronutrients on memory, Type II diabetes, and physical stamina. With my academic and scientific background, I undertake the writing of *Secret Herbal Cures* with not only a wealth of medical knowledge, but also with a healthy skepticism of any published information. Therefore, in Part Two of *Secret Herbal Cures* I emphasize the "gold standard" of scientific proof of effectiveness of any herbal product, namely, the placebo-controlled, double-blinded studies. Since I am a scientist at heart, I also mention "negative" data in which certain herbal products have shown not to be effective for certain medical conditions. Moreover, unlike some books on herbal medicine in which every single animal study is cited as if the animal data invariably applies to human conditions (which, by the way, is often not the case), I rarely mention animal studies as "proof" of effectiveness of any herbal product.

Acknowledgments

The creation of any book always involves the cooperation and efforts of many individuals and *Secret Herbal Cures* is no exception. Thank you to the team behind this book: Jeff Jurmain, M.A.; Chris Robinson; Meghan Jackson; Audrey O'Handley; and Stephanie Raymond. Finally, I thank my wife, Shirley and daughters, Emily, Rosaline, and Karen for pitching in to allow me the time and space, let alone the use of the computer, needed to produce *Secret Herbal Cures*.

NOTES

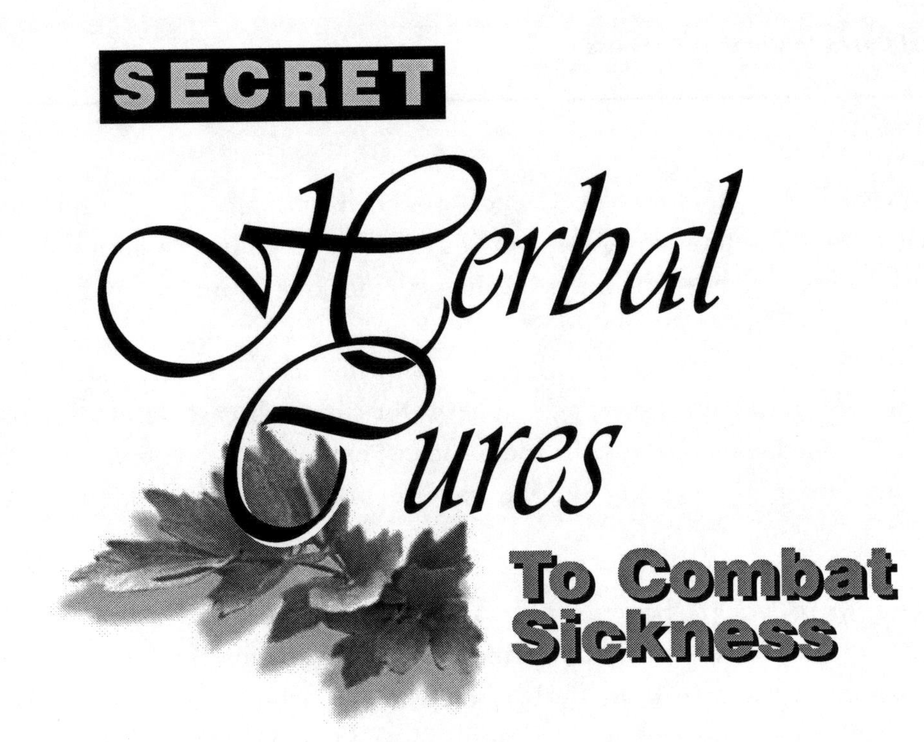

Part One

UNLOCKING THE DOOR TO SECRET HERBAL CURES

There's no question about it—some of the most powerful substances in the entire world can be found anywhere from the forests of Paraguay to the herb garden just beyond the porch in your own backyard. Herbs have been the magic healing cure for our entire human history. Records of herbal medicines in China can be found as far back as 5,000 years ago. Egyptian history dating from 2,800 BC lists mint, marjoram, and juniper as medicines. Hippocrates, the "father of medicine," taught his students the miracle of herbs for curing disease and easing pain. Or how about "Ayurvedic" medicine, that rose in India somewhere between 3,000 and 5,000 years ago? It is still going strong by focusing on the balance of life energies rather than individual symptoms.

These days, we're looking back to these ancient beliefs, and more and more people are understanding the role herbs can play in medicine. In fact, one-third of all Americans use herbal supplements. Many turn to herbal remedies to avoid the harmful side effects of prescription drugs; some are looking to simplify their lives and get back to a natural way of living; and many others are looking to cure their diseases and relieve their symptoms when no doctor seemed able help.

No matter what your motivation, *Secret Herbal Cures to Combat Sickness* is the essential book for your herbal medicine library.

Secret Herbal Cures to Combat Sickness focuses on herbal remedies, from the commonly known to the completely obscure. You get an in-depth, analysis of what each herb is proven to do, and any caution you should use with it at the same time—eliminating the need to guess and wonder which ones really have been tested and which ones truly are recognized by the medical world. More and more herbs are being recognized every year. Skipping the guesswork means you can choose the herbal cure that's both right and safe for what ails you.

In this groundbreaking book, we debunk herbal cure myths and reveal the truth. We present interesting and informative studies, then cut through the muddle and give you the straight facts on herbal remedies.

Whatever your ailment, whatever your concern, *Secret Herbal Cures to Combat Sickness* is the key you need to open the door to a world of natural health for you and your family.

Feel better and live longer – *Secret Herbal Cures to Combat Sickness* can show you how!

USING HERBAL CURES SAFELY

There's an old myth that we need to get straight before we even think about taking a herb in an effort to combat an illness. It's important to understand that just because something is "natural" does not necessarily mean it's safe to use. For example, as many people are well aware, certain types of mushrooms are extremely toxic—they're 100% natural, but they're also deadly.

We don't want to scare anyone away from taking herbal cures; we just want you and your family to be safe. There are some herbs that should never be taken if you suffer a particular condition, because they run the risk of disrupting any medication you might be taking, or exacerbating a blood pressure problem, or a cholesterol problem, or any number of issues that are affecting your health.

It is becoming more and more clear that people are using herbal remedies without speaking to a healthcare provider. In many cases, this is fine. To address this fact, *Secret Herbal Cures to Combat Sickness* has tried to identify those conditions and herbs that always need to be discussed with a doctor, no questions asked. Not a lot of consumer books take this approach, and information like this is usually stuffed into dense medical textbooks that doctors have on the shelves of their office. This book did take this approach, because of the fact that many of us are conducting our own research into the alternative medicine world. And the safety of herbs is very important. In the following pages are herbs that have been found to work, those that are thought to work, and in some cases those that have only a loose link to being effective. In any case, we've said so.

So here's the warning: Please look carefully into any herbal remedy before starting treatment. It is never a bad idea to talk to your doctor, your pharmacist, and read any enclosed literature that comes with any herbal product you buy. Because many herbs have not been adequately tested, their effect on people can be somewhat unknown – or at least, unproved. Keep your doctor in the loop.

This book is a great starting ground – it tells you what herbs make good treatments for some of the most common ailments. In Part Two of this book, we recommend a variety of herbal cures for diseases and conditions from which you might be suffering. Finding the herbal cure that's right for you is a two-part search: one, it's understanding the variety of treatments available; two, it's a trial-and-error process of testing a variety of cures and finding the one that fits your needs, lifestyle, budget, and quality of life. To help your understanding of herbs, we've compiled health and safety information on a number of herbal cures, some common and some that you may not have ever heard about before. In Part Three of this book, we touch on who should take extra caution when considering specific herbal treatments, what the common uses are for over a vast number of herbs, and listed side effects (including dangerous ones) as well as drug interactions that you must watch for and be wary of.

For the safety of both mother and child, it is critical to note that pregnant women should take herbs only under the specific direction of a knowledgeable physician, midwife, or healer. We also note this fact throughout Part Three.

Similarly, not all herbal remedies are safe for children. Again, please consult your health-care practitioner before giving any medication, including a herbal one, to your child.

Unless you are a skilled botanist, it is not safe to gather wild-growing herbs. One percent of all plants are poisonous—and many look just like other plants to the unknowing eye.

Never exceed the recommended dose of any herbal cure—many of the dangerous side effects of certain herbs are only seen after consumption of large doses. Also note that there is always the potential for an allergic reaction to any herbal treatment. It's best to start with a small dose and "work your way up" to the recommended dose, just to make sure you don't have an allergy.

The recommended dose of any particular herb is often slightly flexible. The amount needed for the desired effect varies from person to person, due to weight, height, age, health, and physical condition etc. It may take a little bit of trial and error to determine the perfect dose to cure what ails you. If you are taking other medications for a condition, any interactions between those drugs and a herb may dictate the dosage for you.

Most herbal remedies are also to be taken for only a short period of time, although some are more preventative and therefore are safe to be taken on a regular basis. This is where your health-care provider and merchant are most helpful—in determining the dosage and length of treatment that is right for you. **Never exceed a recommended dose.**

Herbs taken on a daily or regular basis are best taken on a full stomach, to help avoid common side effects like nausea, upset stomach, or diarrhea.

Be careful taking herbs with sedative properties before driving or working, and don't take herbs with stimulant properties before bed. A bit of common sense will go a long way.

Of course, with any matter related to your health, caution is always advised. As the saying goes, "better to be safe than sorry!"

HOW DOES HERBAL MEDICINE WORK?

We've already talked briefly about how herbal medicines contain "active compounds" and "healing powers," but we'd like to tell you a little bit more about how herbal cures actually work.

Herbal remedies are not magic. In fact, herbal medicine has a lot more to do with chemistry than wizardry. Just like any pharmaceutical, commercial drug, herbal cures work because of their chemical composition. It is the chemistry involved that makes herbal cures *seem* like magic. Herbs, like any other medicine, have profound effects on our heart, lung, kidney, liver, nervous system, gastrointestinal tract, and other organs. How they work isn't folklore—it's science! They can mimic the actions of other, more well-known drugs created by massive pharmaceutical companies.

Herbs range from mild, like peppermint, to extremely potent, like the poppy, just like prescription drugs do. Taking herbal cures should be done as carefully and consciously as you would any prescription medication. Choosing the herbs that are right for you is relatively easy in this modern world, as scientific studies have been thoroughly conducted on more than 5,000 traditional herbal medicines.

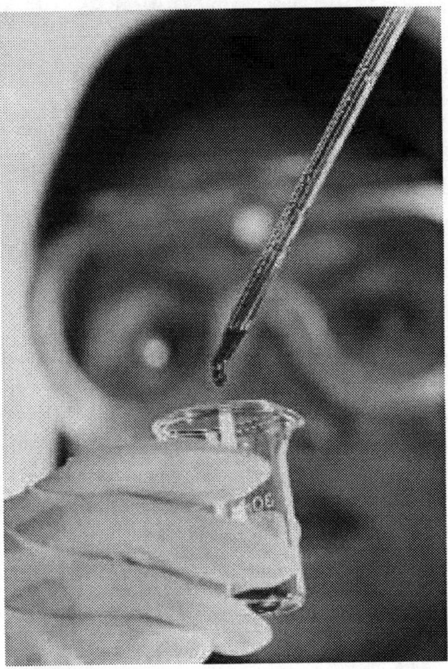

Such clinical and laboratory tests have determined that herbal medicine works because of the active, chemical compounds herbs contain. Decades, and indeed centuries, of research have classified the active properties and ingredients of herbs so we have a greater understanding of exactly what herbs do in our bodies than any of our ancestors had before. By understanding the activity of these chemical compounds, we've come a long way in transforming herbal medicine from the stories of tribal healers into a viable medical discipline that is revolutionizing health care as we know it today.

Ongoing research has identified many categories of the active properties of herbal medicines. The following are the 25 most common categories of herbal medicines:

1. *Adaptogenic*—adaptogens affect the adrenal glands. They trigger the "fight or flight" mechanism of human's reaction to stress or other stimuli. Just as the word "adaptogenic" implies, these herbs help us *adapt*.

   Examples include Ginseng, Ashwagandha, Cat's Claw, Licorice, and Gotu Kola.

2. *Alterative*—these herbs *alter* how our bodies function. For example, in a diseased state, our bodies often function below what is considered "normal." Alterative herbs help restore the balance of our health, minds, and bodies.

   Examples include Devil's Claw, Garlic, Cayenne, St. John's Wort, and Black Cohosh.

3. *Anthelmintic*—if you or a family member is suffering from parasites, like intestinal worms, you'll seriously want to look into the anthelmintic family of herbs. These herbs destroy or eliminate parasites.

   An example is Garlic.

4. *Anti-inflammatory*—these herbs reduce swelling and inflammation and help relieve pain.

   Examples include Goldenseal, Licorice, St. John's wort, White Willow, Yarrow, Black Cohosh, and Evening Primrose.

5. *Antimicrobial*—these herbs strengthen the body's immune system and help destroy or fight microorganisms and germs that cause disease.

   Examples include Echinacea, Sage, Lavender, Peppermint, and Tea Tree Oil.

6. *Antiseptic*—these herbs help prevent infection in wounds, lesions, burns, and abrasions.

   Examples include Basil, Chamomile, and Saw Palmetto.

7. *Antispasmodic*—these herbs help reduce and soothe muscle *spasms* and cramping.

   Examples include Valerian, Peppermint, Yarrow, Black Cohosh, Sage, and Lavender.

8. *Astringent*—these herbs help reduce inflammation, prevent infection, and reduce irritation.

   Examples include Goldenseal, Lavender, Bilberry, and Cinnamon.

9. *Antitussive*—"antitussive" is a formal way of saying "cough suppressing." Specifically, these herbs are used for dry coughs.

   Examples include Licorice, Echinacea, Slippery Elm, and Plantain.

10. *Antipyretic*—these herbs help reduce fever.

    Examples include Rosemary, Yarrow, Licorice, and Ginger.

11. *Bitter*—these herbs stimulate our nervous system and gastrointestinal tract and have a detoxifying effect.

    Examples include Goldenseal, Dandelion, and Artichoke.

12. *Carminative*—these herbs stimulate the digestive system.

    Examples include Valerian, Basil, and Fennel.

13. *Demulcent*—these herbs soothe inflamed or irritated internal tissues throughout the body.

    Examples include Aloe, Plantain, Mullein, and Slippery Elm.

14. *Diuretic*—diuretic herbs increase urine production and elimination of toxic substances by the kidney. They are important for detoxification.

    Examples include Nettle, Parsley, Saw Palmetto, and Cranberry.

15. *Emmenagogue*—these herbs are important for the female reproductive system. Specifically, they stimulate menstrual flow.

    Examples include Black Cohosh, Blue Cohosh, Vitex, and Sage.

16. *Expectorant*—these herbs help *expel* fluid and mucus from the sinuses, bronchial tubes, and lungs.

    Examples include Garlic, Mullein, Peppermint, and Horseradish.

17. *Hepatic*—hepatics affect the liver. They increase bile, help in detoxification, and stimulate proper digestion.

    Examples include Dandelion, Milk Thistle, Dandelion, Fennel, Phyllanthus, and Red Peony.

18. *Hypnotic*—these herbs help induce sleep and relaxation and calm nerves.

    Examples include Valerian, St. John's Wort, Green Tea, Chamomile, and Kava.

19. *Hypotensive*—hypotensive herbs lower and regulate blood pressure.

    Examples include Garlic, Valerian, Hawthorne, Yarrow, and Olive Leaf.

20. *Laxative*—these herbs help eliminate waste from the digestive tract. They work in three ways: they provide bulk, stimulate bile production, and activate the contractions of the muscles in the digestive system.

    Examples include Senna, Psyllium, and Goldenseal.

21. *Nervine*—these herbs affect the *nerves*. They calm the nervous system and help you cope with anxiety and stress.

    Examples include St. John's Wort, Vervain, Valerian, and Black Cohosh.

22. *Sedative*—these herbs facilitate sleep and relaxation. They calm the nerves and reduce stress.

    Examples include Valerian, Corydalis, Kava, and Lavender.

23. *Stimulant*—these herbs have the opposite effect of sedatives. They stimulate and speed up the psychological, physical, and metabolic processes in our body.

    Examples include Ginseng, Astragalus, Evening Primrose, and Echinacea.

24. *Tonic*—tonics strengthen, enliven, and nurture the various systems in our body.

    Examples include Black Cohosh, Nettle, and Sage.

25. *Vasodilator*—these herbs *dilate* the blood vessels, helping with inflammation and heart conditions.

    Examples include Garlic and Ginseng.

HERBAL CURES ARE HERE TO STAY!

While some people think of herbal cures as folklore, archaic, or some new-age fad, many more are embracing the healing powers nature has to offer through herbal medicines. If one thing's for certain, it's that herbal cures are here to stay.

Here's why:

- Herbal cures have fewer side effects than prescription medications;
- Herbal cures have thousands of years of testimonials behind their efficacy, while pharmaceuticals often have less than 20 years of clinical testing;
- Herbal cures are readily accessible and reasonably priced;
- Herbal cures help people take an active role in preventing and even curing their own health concerns; and
- Herbal cures WORK!

Contrary to some closed-minded individuals' opinions, herbal remedies are not just for "hippies," "witches," or "radical vegetarians." Herbal remedies are being used by people just like you and me – regular people that want to live healthier and longer lives.

Need proof that herbs really are as curative as prescription medicine? Consider this: many of today's popular prescription drugs and over-the-counter medications are actually manmade versions of herbal cures. Plant- and herb-based medicine has played a pivotal role in the development of Western medicine as we know it today. Natural cures that have been used for thousands of years have been "modernized" by making pharmaceutical copies of what Mother Nature herself created. Why? Because it's more profitable to use a synthetic version than the "real" thing. As you know, in today's society, money talks. In addition, because natural products cannot be patented, it's actually in a company's best interest to make a commercial, synthetic version of a herbal cure, just for the sole reason that it can be patented. That patent is what big pharma drives for, and it's that patent which gives them a guaranteed seven-or-so year money making venture where nobody else can copy them.

Still, today's consumers are smarter, more educated, and more concerned about their health and well being than they ever have been before. People are questioning their doctors' advice about popping pills and looking into alternative treatments that are better for their bodies, minds, and the world in which they live.

The interest we see today in herbal remedies is not isolated to North America, either. It is indeed a global phenomenon to return to natural health treatments and a balanced coexistence between man and nature.

Many people are now looking to take an active role in their own health – we're steering away from clinical settings with hands-off physicians and drug treatments and returning to a more personal, individualized, natural way of healing ourselves, in a partnership with today's health-care practitioners. In fact, many physicians are ignorant of herbal medicine because they were trained in the art of pharmaceuticals and surgery and have simply not been made aware of nature's healing power. That is because herbal medicine is only slowly being accepted into mainstream medicine, but will always likely remain on the fringes. Thus, an educated consumer can help make physicians and the medical community in general more aware of how herbs can play a role in medicine.

The curative power of herbs has been witnessed by men and women since the very beginning of civilization. In fact, nearly 80% of the global population still uses traditional medicine as its primary health care system. This means that we, who have depended on Western medicine for decades, are actually in the minority of the world population. Truth be told, almost every culture is more accepting of natural, herbal remedies than we are here in North America. These days, doubting the powerful effects of herbal cures is, in reality, a rather outdated way of thinking.

Now, it is very important to understand that we are not recommending that you completely abandon your practice of going to a family physician for your annual check-ups or seeing a specialist for your specific health care concerns. Our philosophy is that a combination of complementary or holistic approaches, including Western medicine, herbal medicine, holistic healing, and Eastern medicine, is the best way to prevent or treat a disease, symptom, or disorder.

Learn all you can about any medical treatment that you are considering, from chamomile tea to chemotherapy, you'll be better off and healthier in the long run by being well informed about all of the therapies available to you and your family.

Don't take anything for granted when it comes to your health. Discuss what you learn in this book or any other resource with your primary health care provider, your family, your friends, and your neighborhood pharmacist. A community, educated approach to health – that includes you – is the most powerful cure in the world.

HOW TO USE THIS BOOK

Secret Herbal Cures To Combat Sickness is laid out in such a way that you can retrieve information in a couple of different ways. After the Introduction are the main thrusts of the book – Parts Two and Three where you will find the herbal information.

When Looking Up a Condition:

Let's take "hypertension" as an example, if you will.

- First, look up hypertension in the "Table of Contents" and turn to its page in the book.
- Once there you will find an opening paragraph in *italics* that discusses the condition. You will find information on symptoms, causes, what exactly it is, how prevalent it is in society, etc.
- With an understanding of what causes hypertension, and what part of the body (or what system) it affects, you look down to the area under "Herbs To Try."
- Under that heading will be a list of herbs (and in this book the number will vary from as few as one or two to maybe 10). Using this example, hypertension has six.
- Each herb has a short paragraph with it describing why it is effective. Included are any clinical studies that have looked at the herb in relation to either the condition or symptoms of that condition.
- Often a herb has not been fully evaluated by scientists for its effectiveness, but it is still believed to possibly work. It is always mentioned whether this is the case.
- Based on this information, you can see which herbs are available for treating hypertension, and even still which have the best shot of working most effectively for you.
- Underneath "Herbs to Try" you will often find another small list called "Other Nutraceuticals That May Work." This list includes mostly non-herbal treatments that

have also either been proven or hinted at being effective. They are not the focus of this book for the most part, but are also listed so you know all the natural remedies at your disposal. (Consequently, at the back of this book there is a rundown of all the nutraceuticals mentioned in the preceding pages, and a description of each.)

When Looking Up a Herb

- You may do this at the start, or after you look up a condition. Say you find that "Hawthorn" is a useful herb to treat hypertension and you want to know more. Turn to the "Index of Herbs" that serves as Part Three and scroll down alphabetically to the herb you are interested in.

- There are a few items in the Index that are not herbs – this is because some other supplements were mentioned in the book as being effective for particular conditions. They are there so you are informed of them, and occasionally because there is a lack of herbs for that illness.

- Each herb is broken up into five subheadings: Overview, Benefits, Considerations, Side Effects, and Dosage.

- In "Overview" you will find a description of the plant where applicable, and a little bit about what part of the plant is generally used in medicine. Often it will discuss the particular ingredient within a herb's root or its leaves that provides the medicinal effect.

- In "Benefits" you are told what the herb is used to treat. This may include both what it's been clinically tested for treating, what it's been traditionally used for, and what it *may* be effective in relieving.

- In "Considerations" you will find a couple of things. This is an important section. You will find out what drugs or other supplements that the herb may react with – the ones you should not be taking if you choose this herb. (i.e. hawthorn may react negatively if you are taking calcium channel blockers… thus you should use caution.) It will talk about illnesses and conditions – if you have a certain medical condition, or if a woman is pregnant or lactating, it will mention whether or not that herb should be taken. It may often say consult a doctor because there isn't enough evidence into a herb's side effects.

- In "Side Effects" you will find out any negative effects that are known to occur with a herb. Often there are none; more often there are some possibilities. Note that just because nausea, diarrhea, bloating, or stomachache are listed as side effects, they are not universal and everyone will not experience them. They are only what has been linked to being a *possibility*. It could have been that one study in 1999 found 10 out of 85 people came down with a headache. Thus, that becomes a side effect.

- Finally, in "Dosage" you will find exactly that. It describes what forms that herb can be taken (i.e. capsules, tea, tincture) and what the typical recommended dose is for a day. Also, it may describe how long you should take it, and whether it will take a few weeks for you to see any positive changes. It's very important to know that this is only a guideline. You should supplement this knowledge by reading all literature you receive with a herb or any other natural remedy. Read the package. Consult your doctor. It's unwise to begin any course of herbal treatment on your own. And never, ever, exceed a recommended dose!

NOTES

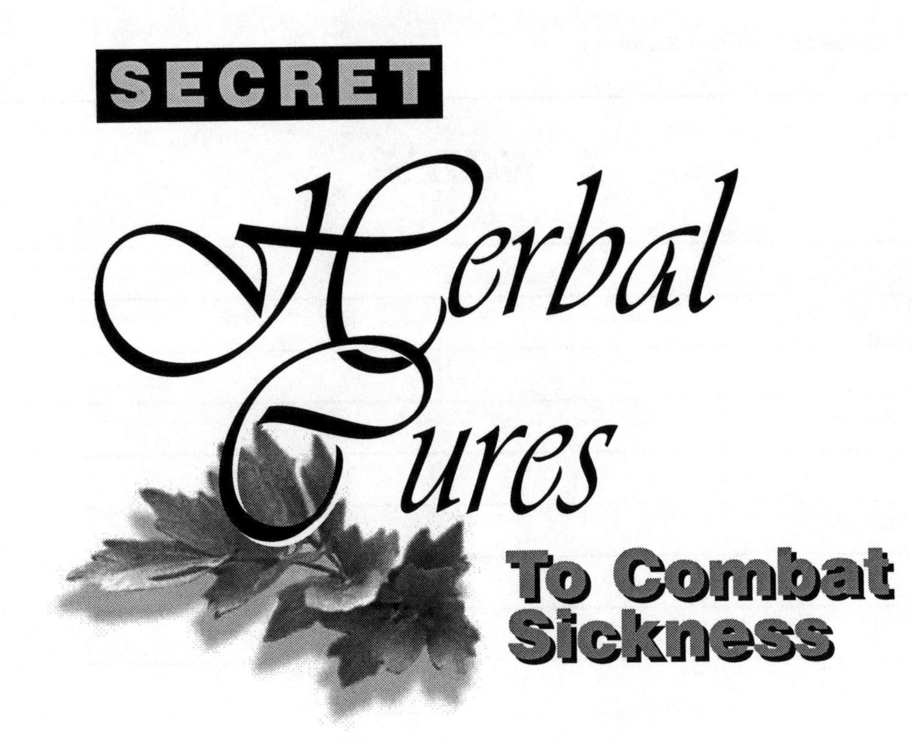

Part Two

YOUR SECRET HERBAL CURES REVEALED

NOTES

Acid Reflux

Acid reflux (or "gastroesophageal reflux disease") is a painful and uncomfortable condition of growing prevalence in North America. It is characterized by chest pain and indigestion, and occurs because stomach acid and stomach/intestine contents are "refluxing" or moving up the esophagus, causing inflammation and pain. It can become so painful that it feels as though your chest is on fire. If the sphincter in your lower esophagus weakens or relaxes abnormally, then stomach acid can back up and cause difficult swallowing and heartburn (its more common name). It is usually felt after eating, especially when lying down or bending over. Most people try to deal with the discomfort by changing their habits, their diet (less spicy food, coffee, alcohol, and citric acid) and maybe buying some antacids. There are herbal treatments, though, that exist for this condition. They work as anti-inflammatories to alleviate the discomfort and burning, but they also act to lubricate the esophagus and therefore protect its delicate lining.

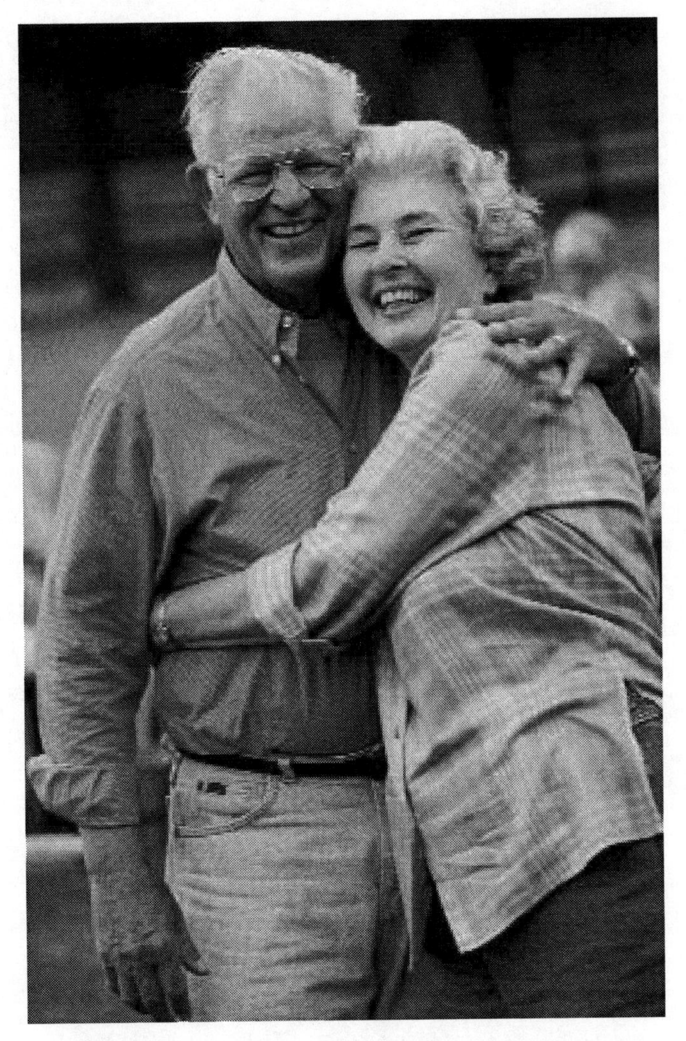

Most people try to deal with the discomfort of acid reflux by changing their habits, their diet, and maybe buying some antacids.

HERBS TO TRY:

Licorice: In particular, "deglycyrrhizinated licorice" (or DGL) can be useful in stomach ulcers and acid reflux. Many people are recommended this extract. Unlike regular licorice root, which has been linked to high blood pressure, this type has an ingredient – glycyrrhizin – removed. Chewable DGL has proven useful in healing stomach, duodenal and even canker sores [*Gut* 1985;26:599-602... *Lancet* 1982;ii:817... *J Assoc Physicians India* 1989;37:647]. Two double-blind trials found that a drug very similar to a main ingredient of licorice was effective against acid reflux [*Curr Med Res Opin* 1978;5:637-44... *Scand J Gastroenterol* 1986;21:1098-104]. In fact, one of them found it was 50% faster in curing acid reflux than placebo, and was 82% successful. This is about as close as medical studies have come to proving this type of licorice helps with the esophagus and movement of stomach acid. One trial showed that this same combination of drugs is as effective as "cimetidine" – the common drug used to treated acid reflux [*Gut* 1990;31:351-4]. Could licorice be your answer?

Aloe Vera: The herb commonly found in skin creams can also be of help when taken internally. The gel extract may stop your stomach from secreting acid, as its anti-inflammatory traits can soothe an inflamed esophagus that would let the acid seep through. Make sure you're using a purified gel extract or capsules and not the bitter aloe latex or juice, which is a strong laxative. Since it is normally used as a cream, there is little substantial evidence into how it can help you internally. But in some preliminary research, Japanese investigators gave juice to 18 patients with peptic ulcers. All but one found relief. Other trials in Japan show that certain ingredients in aloe vera help limit the secretion of stomach juices and the formation of lesions.

Chamomile: This herb has shown an ability to stop inflammation and even act an as antispasmodic. It is commonly prepared as tea, two to three teaspoons of flowers in boiling water. Clinical studies are lacking into its affect on heartburn, but what is known is that drinking the tea can relieve esophageal irritation because of its soothing nature on all gastrointestinal tissues.

Notable Herbs

Deglycyrrhizinated licorice

Aloe Vera

Chamomile

Other Nutraceuticals That May Work:

Calcium carbonate

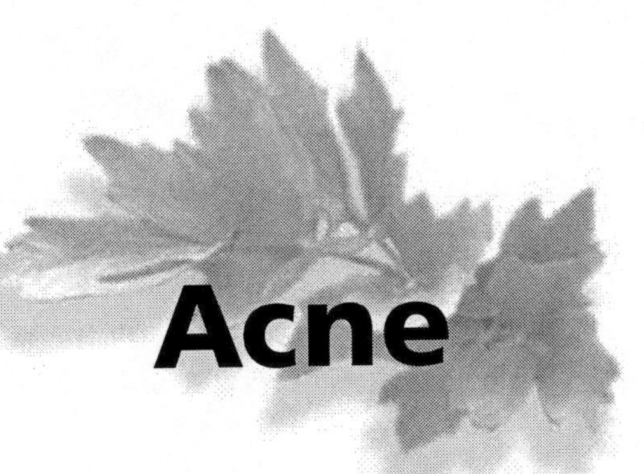

Acne

Acne is a widely used, and often improperly used, term for a variety of skin disorders caused by clogged pores and pustules. An overproduction of oil, irritated hair follicles in the skin, or a buildup of bacteria will also lead to acne. Specifically, the hair follicles of the face get plugged with oil and dead skin cells. It's thought that hormones, bacteria, heredity, stress, and some medications play a role in the overproduction of oil. The symptoms of acne include infamous whiteheads and blackheads, pimples, cysts, nodules, and pustules that occur on the face, neck, chest, back, shoulders, and arms. It's probably the most pervasive condition in health, affecting 80% of people at least once. Some have acne well into their 40s and 50s. Many people with severe acne also are troubled by depression and anxiety. Herbal treatments work to clear the skin from the inside and on the outside. They also assist in reducing pain and inflammation.

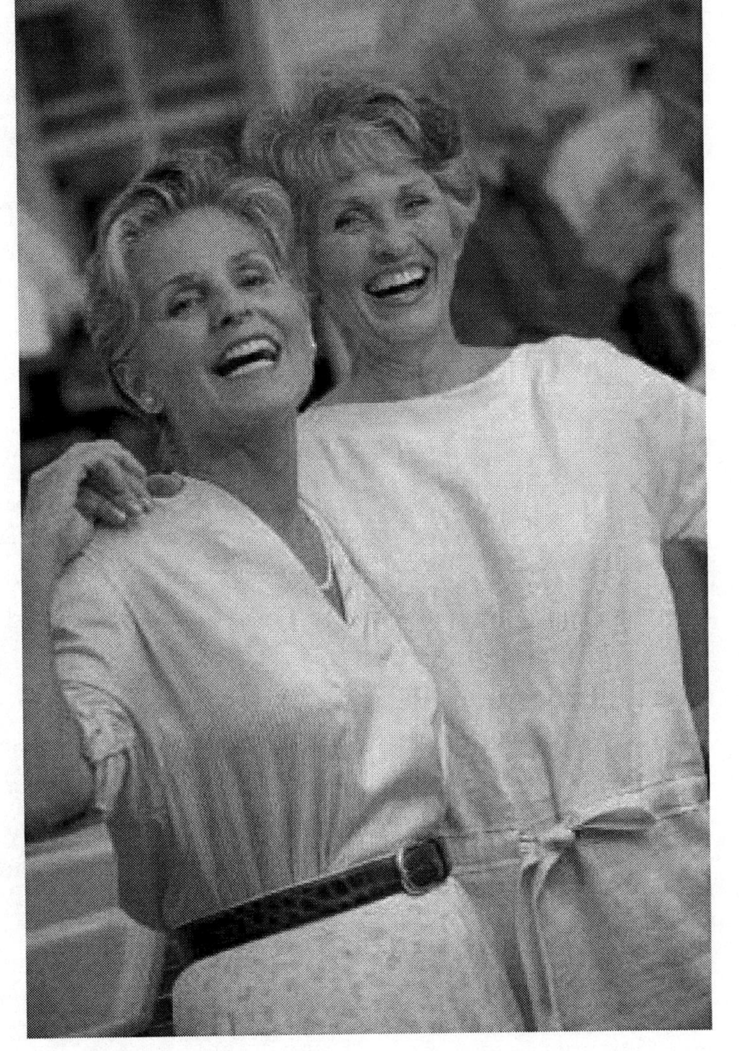

Acne is probably the most pervasive condition in health, affecting 80% of people at least once. Some have acne well into their 40s and 50s.

HERBS TO TRY:

Arnica: Dried flower heads are reputed to treat acne. In tincture form, they may prevent and reduce skin inflammation. This herb is only used on the skin, in cream form with a maximum of 15% arnica oil. This perennial plant with yellow-orange flowers similar to daisies is thought to improve acne because of its anti-inflammatory qualities, but unfortunately there are no studies that have been done to document its effectiveness. Thus it remains a widely known, but not backed-up herb to combat acne.

Tea Tree Oil: The anti-bacterial effects of tea tree oil may help cure your acne. The essential oil from this Australian tree has proven antimicrobial properties. Thus, the study that backs up tea tree oil comes from Down Under: in 124 people with mild to moderate acne, a gel with five percent tea tree oil was nearly as effective in treating acne as a five percent benzoyl peroxide lotion (a common over-the-counter medicine). It did surpass the drug, however, in that tea tree had fewer side effects, such as dryness, itching, and redness. [*Med J Aust* 153:455-8, 1990] The oil can be dabbed onto the acne, or the cream can be applied.

Lavender: Few studies exist into herbal acne remedies, possibly because researchers are preoccupied in testing Accutane, a widely used drug that has been linked to depression and even suicide. Thus, no expert evidence exists to suggest that lavender essential oil works for acne, but herbalists maintain that lavender can be an effective treatment. They say to dab this antimicrobial, anti-inflammatory astringent on individual pimples and wait for results.

Dandelion: That yellow weed lawn-lovers spend half the summer trying to remove from between blades of grass may actually play a role in relieving acne symptoms. Follow this path for a moment: if your liver is backed up, or sluggish, and can't clear hormones quickly enough, this can aggravate acne. Keeping a normal level of reproductive and adrenal hormones is one key to alleviate acne in older people. This is all to say, the dandelion has been shown to stimulate the liver into increasing the flow of bile: thus cleansing it. Two studies in Europe have found dandelion successful in treating people who have diseases caused by inadequate bile *secretion. [Australian Journal Medical Herbalism* 1991;3(4)] Dandelion, as a "liver tonic" may then be able to quell one of the biggest causes of adult acne: too many hormones.

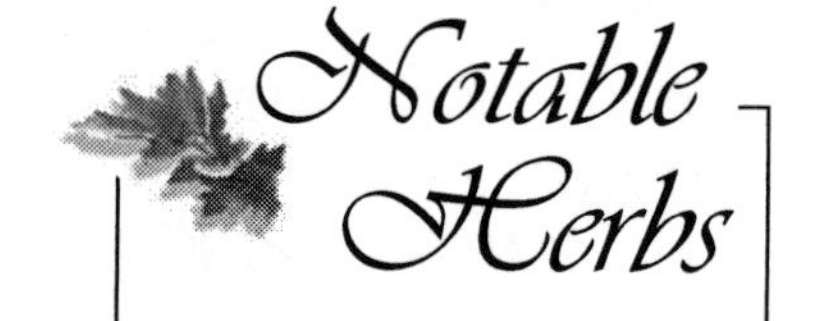

Arnica

Tea Tree

Lavender

Dandelion

Other Nutraceuticals That May Work:

Vitamin A

Vitamin C

Zinc

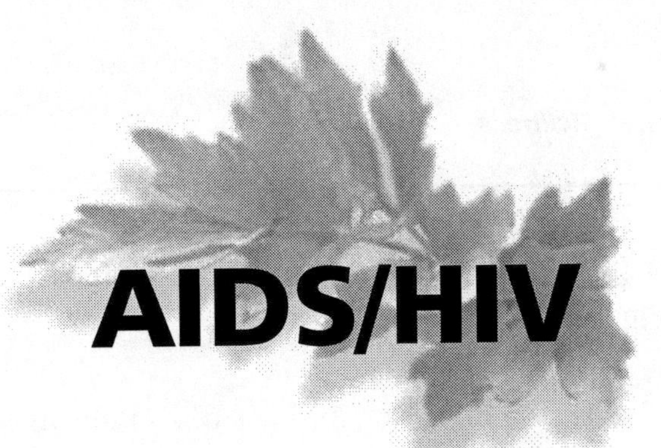

AIDS/HIV

Most everyone knows about these two acronyms, related immunodeficiency viruses that cause a dramatic weakening of the immune system. AIDS is a chronic illness caused by HIV – it disrupts your ability to fight off viruses, bacteria, and fungi. This leaves your critical internal systems susceptible to all sorts of infections such as meningitis and pneumonia that other people can more easily deal with. AIDS and HIV can result in serious infections and, as has been well documented, death. The virus affects the central nervous system specifically. It is a global epidemic, and in the U.S. it affects nearly one million people. Emerging strains of HIV that may resist the powerful "antiretroviral" drugs that have arisen since 1995 to reduce complications now threaten any positive news surrounding the disease. With uncertainties about drugs, perhaps herbal remedies can be useful – they can help restore a balance to the immune system. It is extremely important to consult your doctor before taking any complementary approaches to this disease, and know that there is no firm evidence backing any protective effects of herbs over AIDS.

HERBS TO TRY:

Garlic: This aromatic herb has been examined in the treatment of HIV. It is a botanical medicine used by many people who have HIV – in fact, it has been reported that garlic is the most frequently used botanical medicine among infected patients who utilize complementary and alternative medicine. Over half chose garlic ["Alternative Medicine Care Outcomes in AIDS" study, Bastyr University, 1995-1997]. About half of those who undergo antiretroviral therapy take garlic supplements. Garlic appears to lower lipids and glucose in the body, which might play a role in hypertensive AIDS patients. Many of garlic's qualities in the treatment of hypertension may be relevant in managing potent drug therapy in HIV subjects.

Aloe Vera: Preliminary evidence exists showing that aloe vera – and in particular, its ingredient "acemannan" – can act as an immune booster and thus could be of use in treating AIDS. In test-tube studies, acemannan showed action against HIV. At best, acemannan could reduce a patient's need for AZT, a common drug used that comes with unpleasant side effects. The American Foundation for AIDS Research said that acemannan hasn't been toxic in pilot trials on humans. Thus, it's safe to use.

Boxwood: The leaves and stem of this plant were tested in a double-blind study on patients with HIV. At a dose of 990 mg a day, they found – by measuring cell counts – that boxwood could help prevent the progression of the HIV infection. Boxwood also has shown no direct side effects. [*Phytomedicine* 1998;5(1):1–10]

Licorice: In test tubes, and then in clinical trials, licorice's main ingredient, "glycyrrhizin," has shown some positive effect on AIDS. It should be noted that glycyrrhizin was isolated from licorice and injected into patients for this effect. [*Antivir Res* 1989;11:255–62.] As for taking licorice supplements orally, there is only minor evidence. A small study showed that it may be a safe, effective treatment for HIV, although it needs to be substantiated far beyond these results. [*Int Conf AIDS* 1993;9:234] Prolonged use of licorice should come with caution because it has been linked to hypertension.

Asian Ginseng: A relatively confusing study did find that this type of ginseng, an immune booster, had positive effects against HIV and even helped the major AIDS drug, AZT, combat the illness as well. [*Int Conf AIDS* 1994;10:215]

Echinacea: Interesting to note, but a controversial note at that, this common supplement may just play a role in HIV infection. What began as a disappointing connection – echinacea actually seemed to provoke the virus to spread in the test tube – took a turn in 1998 when oral supplements of the herb seemed to fight the infection. A double-blind study found that echinacea boosted immune activity against HIV. [*Int Conf AIDS* 1998;12:582]

Cat's Claw: This vine, native to South America, derives its name from the claw-like hook that it forms. It is commonly used to boost the immune system in fighting diseases. Certain alkaloids are primarily thought to produce the medicinal benefits. There is little clinical evidence to support this herb, but some reports say that HIV patients have increased levels of helper T cells, reduced viral loads, and higher vitality when taking cat's claw. What is known is the cat's claw is high in oxindole alkaloids, which have been proven to stimulate the immune system. [US Patent no. 5,302,611, April 12, 1994] It isn't known whether this is enough to have an effect on disease.

Other hopeful herbs include: St. John's wort; Shiitake mushrooms, Bupleurum, Skullcap, Turmeric, and Tea tree oil.

Notable Herbs

Garlic

Aloe Vera

Boxwood

Licorice

Ginseng

Echinacea

Cat's Claw

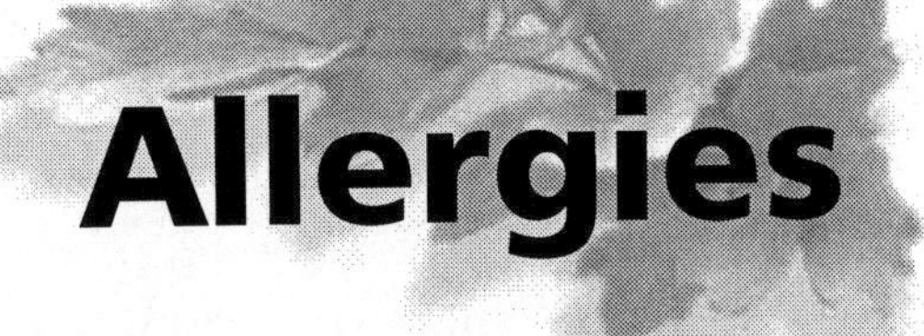

Allergies

An allergy is a sensitivity or reaction caused by exposure to an environmental or ingested antigen. There can be many symptoms, including sneezing, swelling, headaches, and sinus congestion... and seemingly harmless symptoms can become quite serious in a short period of time. At the very worst of the list are fatal allergies to such substances as bee stings or peanuts. And at the other end of the spectrum, seasonal allergies (which of course can be very miserable themselves) pop up when the body's histamines overreact to tree pollen, dust, or ragweed and incorrectly consider them a threat. Allergies can be split up into four categories: environmental, respiratory, skin and food, and drugs. Allergy medications offer antihistamines, meaning they try to inhibit your histamines from going overboard and causing your allergy symptoms. Herbal remedies also have an anti-histamine or anti-inflammatory effect, and work by reducing symptoms, rather than protecting the allergy sufferer from the reaction itself. As usual, not a great amount of testing has been performed on herbal remedies for allergies, but there are some purported to work for the 50 million or so Americans who suffer from annual allergies.

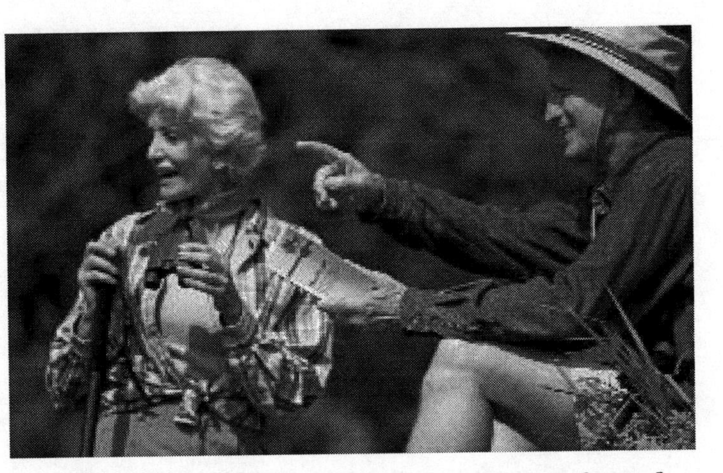

Not a great amount of testing has been performed on herbal remedies for allergies, but there are some purported to work for the 50 million or so Americans who suffer annual allergies.

HERBS TO TRY:

Butterbur: A major clinical journal has found this herb, native to northern temperate regions, effective in reducing allergy symptoms such as runny nose, itchy nose, watery eyes, and sneezing. Butterbur is also known as butterdock, bog rhubarb, and butterfly dock. It seems the leaves and roots of butterbur have what are called "petasines" that inhibit certain components of anti-inflammatory activity seen when someone is sensitive to allergens. The *British Medical Journal* found that butterbur could be as effective as the prescription antihistamine "Zyrtec." Those who used the herb also showed less drowsiness, which is a big side effect of allergy drugs. [*BMJ* 2002;324:144–146]. *Caution: Avoid any butterbur extracts that have "unsaturated pyrrolizidine alkaloids" as these may be toxic to your liver and kidneys and could even cause cancer.*

Nettle: It's thought that this perennial plant has ingredients that attach to your histamines to prevent them from hitting the cells of your body during an allergic reaction. Nettle also contains "quercetin" – a flavonoid that works against histamine production. It is a strong anti-inflammatory that may help those in particular with rhinitis (inflammation in the mucus membrane of the nose). Thus, nettle may be a natural decongestant. One double-blind study in 1990 found that "stinging nettle" helped relieve sneezing, eye irritation, and other allergy symptoms because of its ability to reduce inflammation. After only a week, nearly 60% of study participants had reduced allergic symptoms. [*Planta Medica*, 1990, vol. 56]

Licorice: Although it appears that no studies have tried to clinically prove its usefulness, it has been widely suggested that licorice root can help prevent allergy symptoms. In particular, it is glycyrrhizin, the active ingredient that counters symptoms because of its anti-inflammatory properties. Licorice also thins mucus and soothes the respiratory tract, reducing irritation usually brought on by allergies.

Peppermint: By drinking tea that contains peppermint oil, allergy sufferers may help relieve nasal inflammation, a.k.a. congestion. In particular, it is the ingredient menthol that helps do this, as well as ease your breathing. As it stands, this oil is found in many over-the-counter cough remedies and decongestants. Commonly thought of as an effective remedy for upset stomach, peppermint also has proven to be a powerful tool in the struggle against allergies. There isn't much scientific evidence into this one either, except for a 2001 study into rats that found when given a peppermint leaf extract, their nasal blockage was significantly reduced. [*Biological and Pharmaceutical Bulletin* 2001;24(1):92-95] It may work for you.

Note... Ephedra May Be Dangerous: If you are somehow getting your hands on ephedra to combat allergy symptoms, you should stop. This Chinese herb has roots in medicine that stem from centuries past, among them the treatment of allergy, hay fever, and the common cold. But this "herbal ecstasy" may in fact increase your risk of seizure, stroke, and heart attack. In late December 2003, the FDA decided to ban ephedra because of "unacceptable health risks" found by researchers at the University of California at San Francisco.

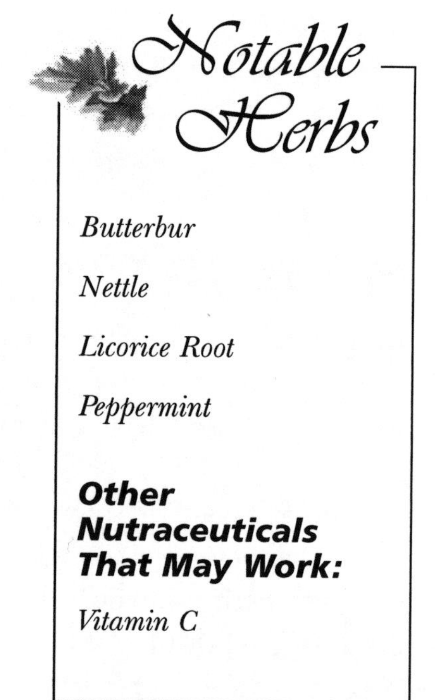

Alzheimer's Disease/Dementia

Alzheimer's disease afflicts the most powerful part of your body, the mind, and gradually leads to mental deterioration and dementia. There is unfortunately no recovery for those who have this degenerative disease of the brain. What happens is that the disease attacks nerve cells in the brain – this means a person is no longer in charge of their emotions, their movement, and their memory. It is one of the most frustrating and sad illnesses around. This long-term disorder affects a large number of people over the age of 65, and is the fourth leading cause of death in adults. With the aging population increasing in number, many think Alzheimer's could become an epidemic. Herbs that help people with this disease center around boosting memory and improving brain functioning. Much research is currently being conducted in this area.

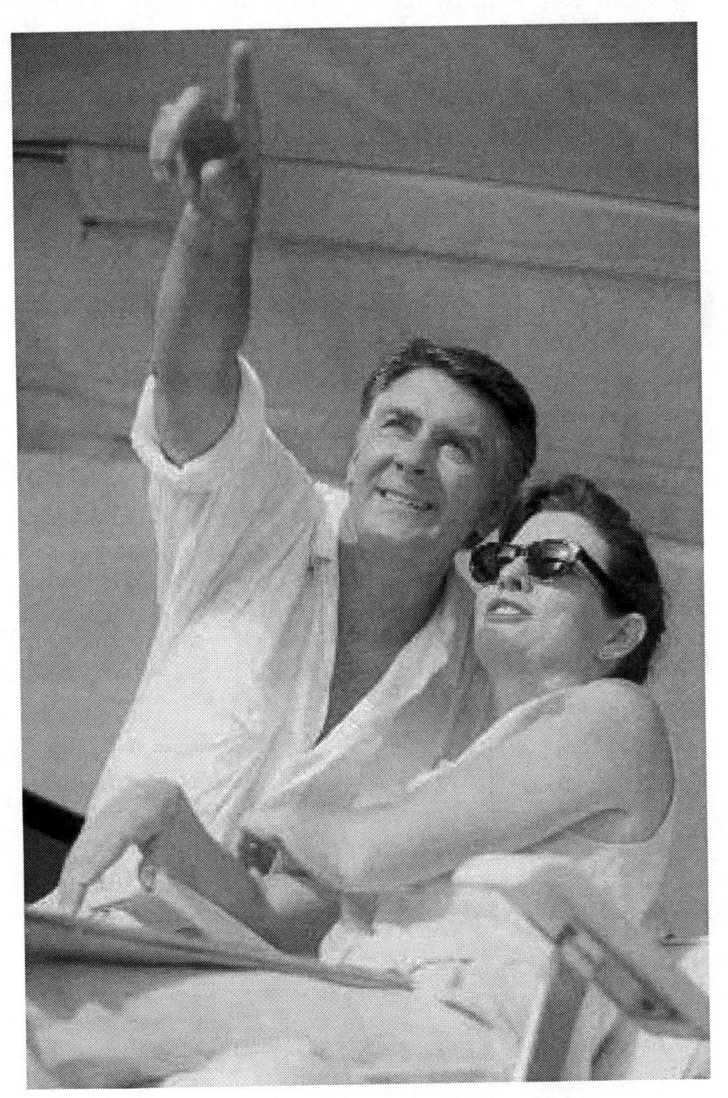

Herbs that help people with this disease center around boosting memory and improving brain functioning.

HERBS TO TRY:

Ginkgo Biloba: This Chinese herb has long been known for its link to memory boosting. It is a very common herb that acts as an antioxidant and may increase blood circulation to the brain. Many studies have looked into ginkgo's effect on memory, and they have reported mixed results. One double-blind study found that in 48 healthy, older patients, six weeks of ginkgo treatment led to significant improvements in memory. [*Hum Psychopharmacol* 2002;17:267-77] Several others have reported similar results. At the same time, another study the same year found it ineffective in improving memory. [*JAMA* 2002;288:835-40] The last word: ginkgo biloba is a promising supplement in improving memory in age-associated memory decline and perhaps in mild Alzheimer's disease.

Sage: A recent study has reported that people with mild to moderate Alzheimer's may benefit from the herb sage. The four-month study involved 30 people between 65 and 85 years of age with Alzheimer's disease. Those taking sage showed significant improvements in cognition after the four months, with benefits starting to show at one month of treatment. Those not taking sage were more agitated, suggesting the herb may also help with mood – an important point for a disease that is so frustrating. [*J Clin. Pharm. Therapeutics* 2003;28:53-59]

Huperzine A: This is a purified chemical from a Chinese moss, used for years in the treatment of schizophrenia, inflammation, and memory loss. In a Chinese publication in 2002, researchers reported that patients with mild to moderate Alzheimer's experienced improvement in memory, behavior, daily living, and mood when they took this supplement.

Turmeric: The spice that contains curcumin, which is responsible for the yellow colour in curry dishes, has properties that may benefit Alzheimer's patients. Evidence suggests that curcumin naturally protects brain cells against the disease. [*J Nat Prod* 2002 Sep;65(9):1227-31] The only truly tested evidence appears to be in mice that experienced significant reductions in oxidative damage and inflammation when they were given curcumin. [*J Neurosci* 2001;21:8370-7] Food for thought: in India, elderly residents who eat large amounts of curry have the lowest incidence of Alzheimer's in the world.

Notable Herbs

Gingko Biloba

Sage

Huperzine A

Turmeric

Other Nutraceuticals That May Work:

Vitamin E

Vitamin B-12

L-Carnitine

Angina (Chest Pain)

Occurring because your heart is in need of more oxygen than is available in the blood supply, angina is a recurring pain or discomfort that hits your chest. Chest pain in itself is one of the most common reasons behind telephone calls to paramedics. About four million people in the U.S. walk into doctor's offices complaining of angina. Where does it come from? Physical exertion, stress, heavy meals, alcohol, cigarettes, or extreme temperature all may have triggered it. Or, it could signal something a little more troublesome, such as coronary heart disease, for which chest pain is a common symptom. Angina occurs when blood vessels to the heart get blocked or are narrowed. Not all chest pain is angina – the one that is will feel like a squeezing pain in the chest under the breast bone that goes away after a few minutes by resting. If it is recurring, it is important to get it checked out in case it is in any way related to your cardiovascular system.

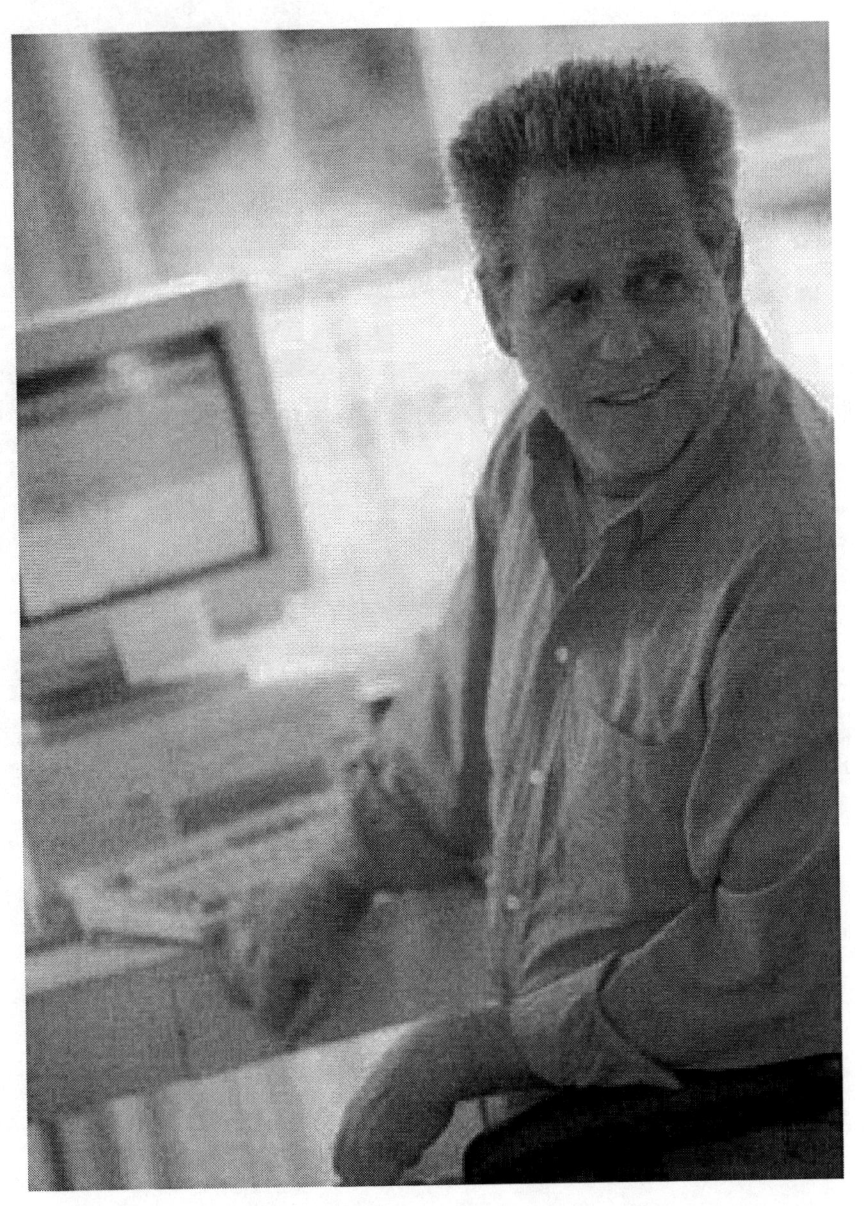

Chest pain in itself is one of the most common reasons behind telephone calls to paramedics.

HERBS TO TRY

It's important to establish with your doctor what may be causing your angina and try herbal remedies to deal with it.

It may be heartburn – See the **Acid Reflux** chapter.

It may be anxiety – See the **Anxiety** chapter.

It may be linked to hypertension – See the **High Blood Pressure** chapter.

It may be atherosclerosis – See the **Arteriosclerosis** chapter.

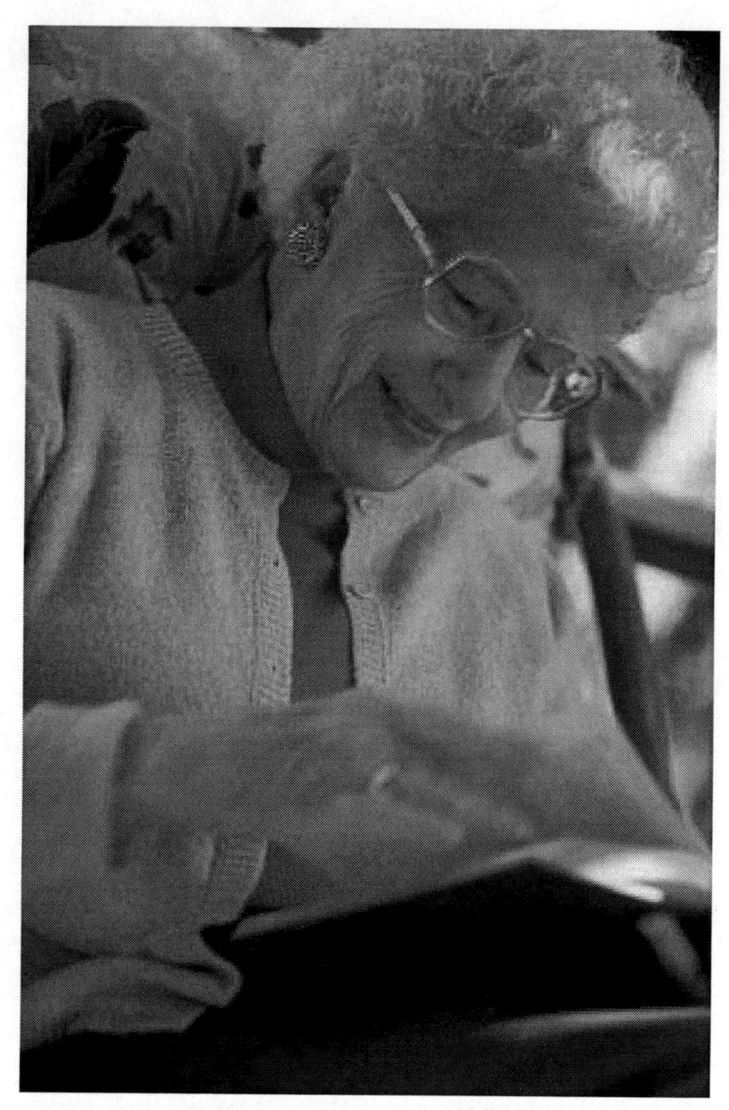

It's important to establish with your doctor what may be causing your angina.

Anxiety

Anxiety affects everyone from time to time. The fear and other emotions triggered by anxiety often also have physical effects. Anxiety can also be an ongoing psychiatric disorder that affects a person's quality of life by limiting their ability to function on a social and an employment basis. In fact, anxiety can be broken up into three categories. Social anxiety, thought to affect about eight percent of the population, means people are nervous in public places, feel they are being constantly watched, and often only feel normal alone behind a closed door. Panic disorder affects about five percent of the population, and can include heart palpitations, hyperventilation, fainting, pain, and fright. And generalized anxiety disorder affects about three percent, and involves extreme thoughts and dwelling, panicking, allowing the mind to take over in a fever of "what ifs?" Other common symptoms include: muscle tension, trembling, dizziness, sweating, irritability, and insomnia. For all, herbal treatments are often sedatives or relaxing agents to help put the mind at ease. Because in the end, it's all about the mind.

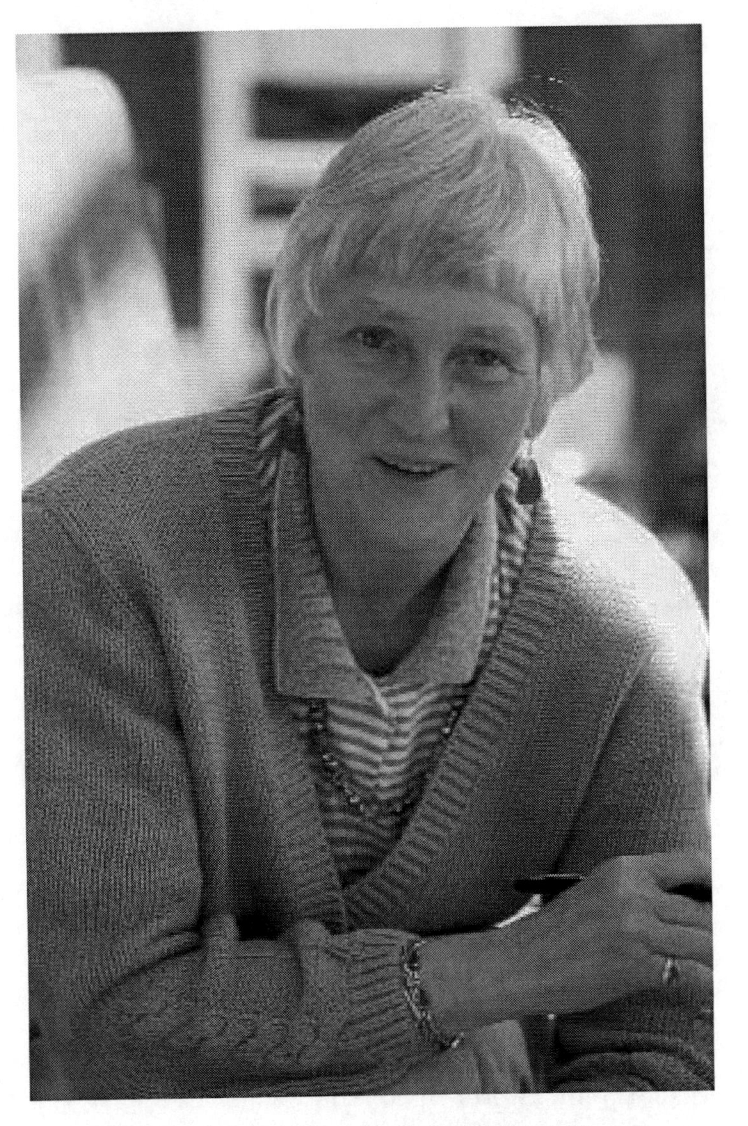

Anxiety can be an ongoing psychiatric disorder that affects a person's quality of life by limiting their ability to function on a social and an employment basis.

HERBS TO TRY:

Kava: This herb is widely used in Europe for anxiety and tension. It's thought to work as well as the prescription drugs "Xanax" and "Valium." In the South Pacific it's been used for centuries to promote relaxation. Many studies have examined this herb's ability to reduce anxiety, and many have found very favorable results. One looked at a kava special extract, WS1490, which was found to be superior to placebo in every category, and was well-tolerated by patients even after they had been taking drug treatments. [*Psychopharmacology* 2001 Sep;157(3):277-83] A review of seven clinical trials into kava found that all evidence implied that the herb is superior to placebo, and is a safe treatment option for anxiety. [Cochrane Database Syst Rev. 2002;(2):CD003383].

Valerian: It is a bit of a mystery why this age-old remedy for insomnia and anxiety works – one theory has it that the herb binds itself to brain receptors and there, inserts its sedating, calming effects. It is thought to calm nerves, balance mood swings, and reduce stressful situations. A study that looked at valerian and kava found that both reduced stress on participants far more than placebo. The results indicate that valerian could be beneficial in reducing the body's reactive tendencies during stressful situations that are brought on by anxiety. [*Phytother Res*. 2002 Feb;16(1):23-7]

Chamomile Tea: This herbal tea is meant to be soothing and act as a sedative, limiting the effects of anxiety and panic. There are no studies into humans that back this up, although studies involving test tubes have found that chamomile has compounds that exert a calming action. [*Planta Med* 1995;61:213–16] On animals, a study found chamomile beneficial in reducing anxiety. [*Biol Pharm Bull* 1996;19:1244–46] Despite a lack of solid evidence, drinking a few cups of chamomile tea when feeling anxious is an inexpensive and easy way to try and deal with it.

St. John's Wort: Here's a supplement that is being extensively studied for its health benefits and for any potential interactions with drugs. It is an effective treatment for mild depression, and thus it's assumed since anxiety is part of depression that St. John's wort can be of benefit here as well. It's a controversial herb to say the least. Some studies draw links to an affect on depression, other studies report conflicting results. One study specifically into anxiety, found that St. John's wort helped reduce mild cases. [*Pharm Acta Helv* 1997;72:153–57] You should typically consult your doctor before beginning herbal treatment – for this one, it is without question.

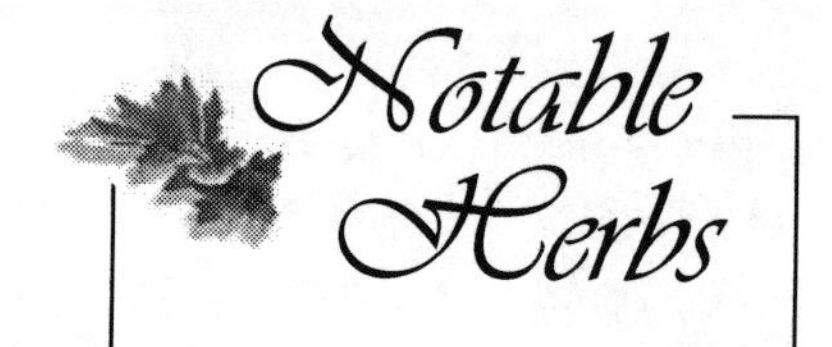

Kava

Valerian

Chamomile

St. John's Wort

Other Nutraceuticals That May Work:

5-HTP

Multivitamin/mineral

Melatonin

Arteriosclerosis (Artherosclerosis)

"Arteriosclerosis" is a complicated way of saying "hardening of the arteries." It results from calcium, cholesterol, or other build-up on the lining of the arteries. It can lead to heart attack, heart disease, poor circulation, blood clots, and stroke. Artherosclerosis is restricted or tightened blood vessels that lead to the heart, brain, arms and legs, and is caused by the same sort of build-up. About one million Americans die each year from artherosclerosis. The first is caused mostly by an overstock of calcium and the second by more fatty substances. Common symptoms include: pain and cramps at the site, ulcer and muscle wasting. Herbal medicines work as anti-inflammatories, protect the vascular system, remove plaque, and stimulate circulation.

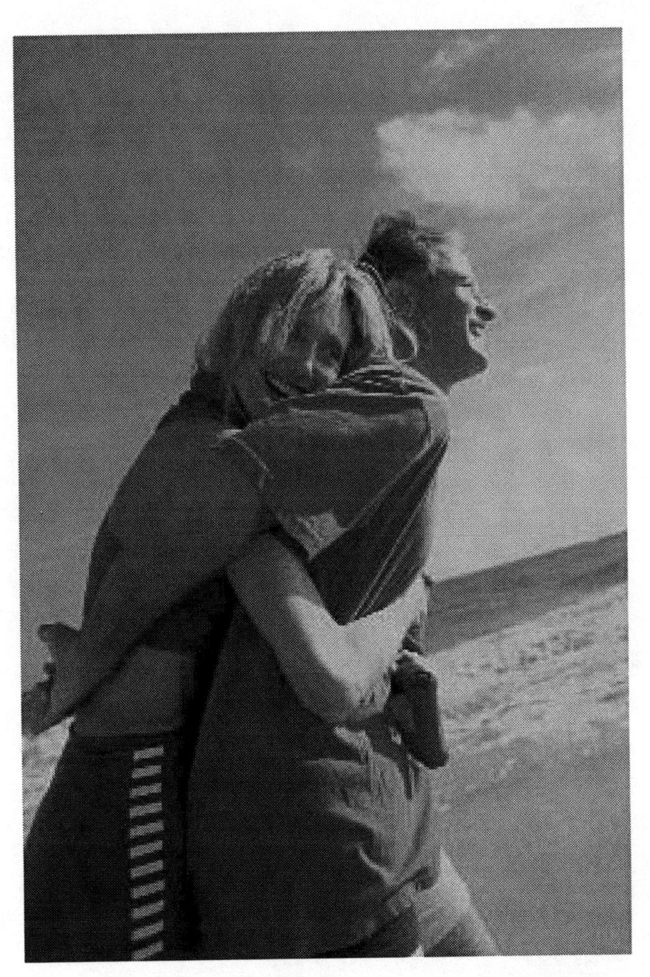

Hawthorn is one of the most prescribed natural remedies in Europe. Herbalists have used it for hundreds of years to help relieve chest pain.

HERBS TO TRY:

Hawthorn: High in flavonoids, hawthorn may work by widening the arteries and thus improving the flow of blood – an action otherwise known as "dilation." This theory was backed up by the results of one study out of Germany [*Arzneirminelforschung* 1995;45: 842-845]. Because of these cardiovascular health benefits, hawthorn is one of the most prescribed natural remedies in Europe. Herbalists have used it for hundreds of years to help relieve chest pain. Hawthorne is usually seen as a small shrub, and because of its thorns it is a member of the rose family. Its berries, flowers, and dried leaves all show benefits to the heart. While German studies have proven its benefits on the heart, no major study has looked into the issue on North American soil.

Soy Protein: Soy has isoflavones whose effects reduce the risk of arteriosclerosis. The FDA has reported that it accepts soy protein, at 25 grams a day when taken within a diet low in saturated fat and cholesterol, as a legitimate way to reduce the risk of heart disease.

Garlic: This herb is well known for its cardiovascular and circulation-improving traits. A major journal by the American Heart Association reported that garlic can maintain the elasticity of aging blood vessels, which tend to lose their ability to stretch with time. [*Circulation* 1997;96(8):2649-2655] Garlic helps widen blood vessels as a result of relaxing the muscles that surround the walls, which is why it's a major herb for hypertension. Garlic has gone through a tremendous number of tests, including one for "intermittent claudication," which is restricted blood flow in the leg. In the double-blind trial, those who received garlic powder were able to walk significantly farther than others; the herb allowed greater blood flow to the leg and reduced pain. [*Clin Investig 1993;71: pp.383-6*]

Green Tea: Although much of the research is preliminary, there is evidence that green tea can fight against arteriosclerosis. When there is oxidative damage to LDL cholesterol in the blood, the risk for arteriosclerosis becomes greater. In this respect, green tea increases the body's antioxidant activity, which then protects against the artery-thinning disease, as a Japanese study found out in 2000. [*Ann Epidemiol* 2000;10:401–8]

Omega-3 Fatty Acids: There's a bundle of evidence into the health benefits of this supplement. For this chapter, it is believed that increasing the amount of omega-3 in your system helps prevent cardiovascular complications – including slowing the growth of an arteriosclerotic plaque. The American Heart Association recommends, on the basis of this cardiovascular evidence, that everyone should have two servings of fish a week. You can also find these fatty acids in flaxseed and walnuts – and their respective oils. [*Circulation* 2002;106(21):2747-2757]

Notable Herbs

Hawthorn

Soy Protein

Garlic

Green Tea

Omega-3

Other Nutraceuticals That May Work:

Vitamin E

Vitamin C

Coenzyme Q_{10}

Selenium

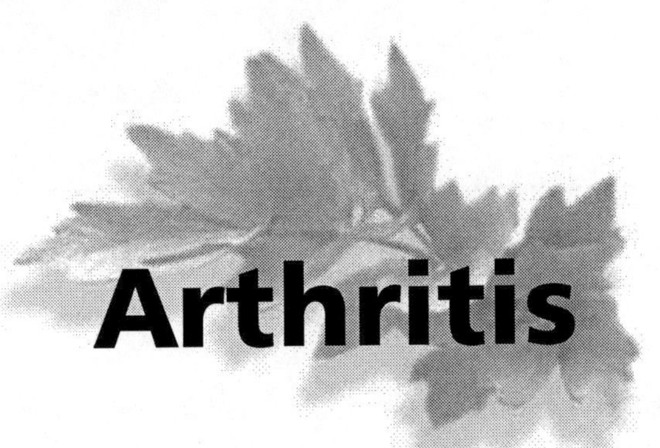

Arthritis

The Greek words arthron (joint) and itis (inflammation) form the word used to describe the leading cause of disability in North American adults, limiting everyday activities for millions of people. This also makes it one of the most prevalent diseases in society. One of the myths is that it strikes later in life, but the truth is that it can set in at any point in an adult life depending on how joints are used. The truth is also that arthritis is on the rise, and afflicts about one in three Americans (according to the Arthritis Foundation, 2002). Most people are familiar with this frustrating, painful condition characterized by inflamed joints usually in the extremities. The disease causes your joints to feel painful, stiff, and swollen and what makes it so crippling is that these symptoms are chronic. Arthritis is an umbrella term for many joint disorders, including the two most prevalent kinds: osteoarthritis and rheumatoid arthritis. The former often strikes the hips, knees, feet, hands, and back, and is characterized by deteriorated cartilage. Rheumatoid is an autoimmune disease that is chronic and inflammation of joints can spread to inflame many other tissues and organs as well. Most herbal supplements will aim to suppress inflammation, bring down any swelling, and of course relieve pain as much as possible.

HERBS TO TRY:

Cayenne: Also known as capsaicin, this cream (sold over the counter) is meant to provide short-term relief of arthritis. One of its primary ingredients is found in chili peppers—it's what makes them hot—and can lessen pain when put on the skin. Capsaicin works by decreasing the level of substance P, which is a neuropeptide that communicates pain sensations. With fewer impulses sent via substance P, you feel less pain. It needs to be applied three or four times a day. One study found that just a 0.025% capsaicin cream worked significantly better than normal cream for osteoarthritis of the knee. [*Seminars in Arthritis and Rheumatism* 1994;23:Suppl 3:25-33]. In another study, 100 arthritic patients received capsaicin cream or placebo – those taking the chili pepper ingredient had significantly more relief from pain, 80% of them experienced pain reduction after two weeks. [*Clin Ther*. 1991;13(3):383-95]

Boswellia: This Ayurvedic herb can defend against inflammation and restore blood vessels in connective tissue. Used in arthritis, this herb causes no side effects while providing reasonable pain relief for sore joints. The boswellic acid, in particular, is thought to reduce inflammation. A review of unpublished studies into this herb found that double-blind trials, deduced that it was effective in relieving rheumatoid arthritis symptoms. [*Phytomed* 3(1): 67–70, 1996]. A number of scientific studies have confirmed the effectiveness of Boswellin. In a study of 175 people with arthritis, four weeks of boswellia treatment helped 122 of them reduce pain and stiffness. It also seemed particularly effective in lowering back pain. [www.wholehealthmd.com]

Ginger: Among the best studied herbs for arthritis, researchers have found that ginger root may inhibit prostaglandins and leukotrienes, which are involved in inflammation and pain. Thus, the spice is an anti-inflammatory. It's been found to reduce knee pain in arthritis patients when standing or walking, as well as enhance the quality of life better than placebo. Patients receiving ginger extract had fewer gastrointestinal side effects and needed far fewer pain killers. [*Arthritis Rheum* 2001;44(11):2531-8] Ginger may work by slicing substance P levels. Some believe an oral dose of two to four grams of dry ginger per day is a good idea; or a half-inch of sliced ginger root.

Turmeric: What makes curry yellow may also treat osteoarthritic pain and inflammation. Turmeric is part of the ginger family and has proven in animal studies to reduce inflammation, a belief held for centuries in India. The spice, taken internally, may work in this way by inhibiting the production of prostaglandins, which are inflammatory chemicals. Some doctors use the this broad-leafed shrub specifically for rheumatoid arthritis. Its main ingredient is curcumin, which is said to reduce inflammation by lowering histamine levels. The Arthritis Foundation reports that one small human study reduced pain by using a concoction of turmeric, boswellia, and zinc in osteoarthritis patients. Although never studied on its own in humans, turmeric should still be considered mildly effective.

Cod liver oil: Taking these pills has long been thought to help reduce the level of enzymes that cause arthritic damage. As reported by the BBC, a study in early 2004 out of Cardiff University (U.K.) found that cod liver oil may help prevent arthritis – 86% of arthritic patients taking this oil showed significantly reduced enzyme levels that cause cartilage damage compared to just 26% on placebo. Since gout is a form of arthritis and both are linked to inflammation, cod liver oil's anti-inflammatory action may be useful in gout.

TWHF: This Chinese herb with one of the most awkward names — Tripterygium wilfordii Hook F — has been found to possess anti-inflammatory and immunosuppressive traits. Its main ingredient, triptolide, is said to have these properties and has been shown to protect neurons from injury and thus pain. [*J Neuroimmunol.* 2004 Mar;148(1-2):24-31] TWHF has been used for over 2,000 years in Chinese medicine. Western medicine has finally recognized it for the treatment of rheumatoid arthritis and leprosy. Researchers believe it is promising and should be studied for autoimmune diseases and all kinds of inflammation.

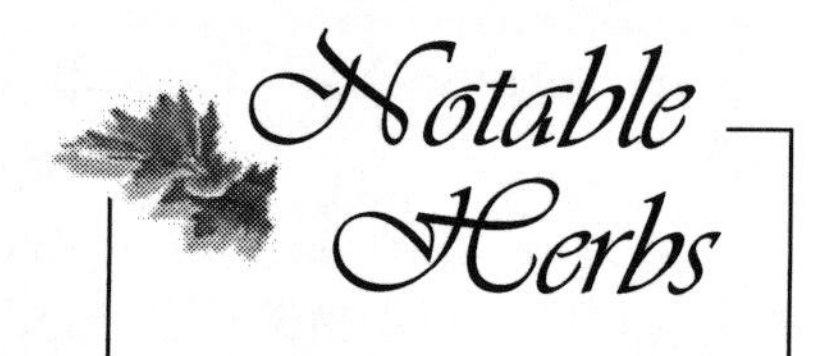

Cayenne
Boswellia
Ginger
Turmeric
TWHF

Other Nutraceuticals That May Work:

S-adenosylmethionine
Glucosamine
Folic Acid
Cod Liver Oil

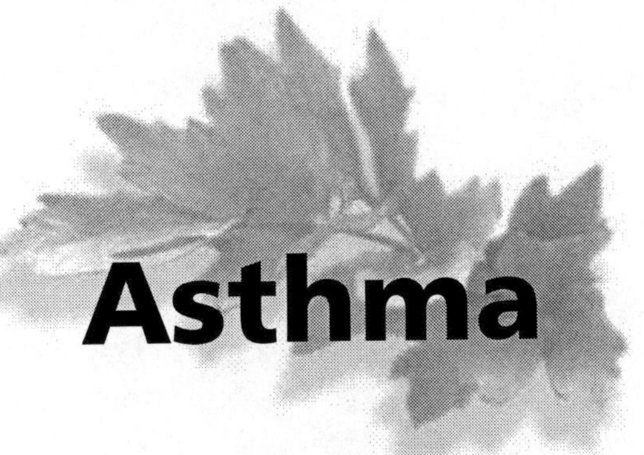

Asthma

Asthma affects children and adults. It is a bronchial disorder that causes an obstruction to the airways, ranging from very mild to very severe. When an asthma attack strikes, muscles that surround the lungs spasm and constrict, blocking air from being exhaled. Symptoms include coughing, shortness of breath, tightness in the chest, and wheezing. Causes include allergic antigens, smoking households, bronchitis, aspirin use, and respiratory infections. Some experts believe the number of asthma cases is climbing toward epidemic-like quantities. This rising trend has people looking at possible environmental factors such as pollution, global warming, toxins, and food additives. In any event, herbal remedies act to open the airways, and can take the form of anti-histamines, anti-inflammatories, and cough suppressants. There are few that have clinical evidence backing them, and in addition to the two described below, nettle and omega-3 oils may be of potential help to asthma sufferers.

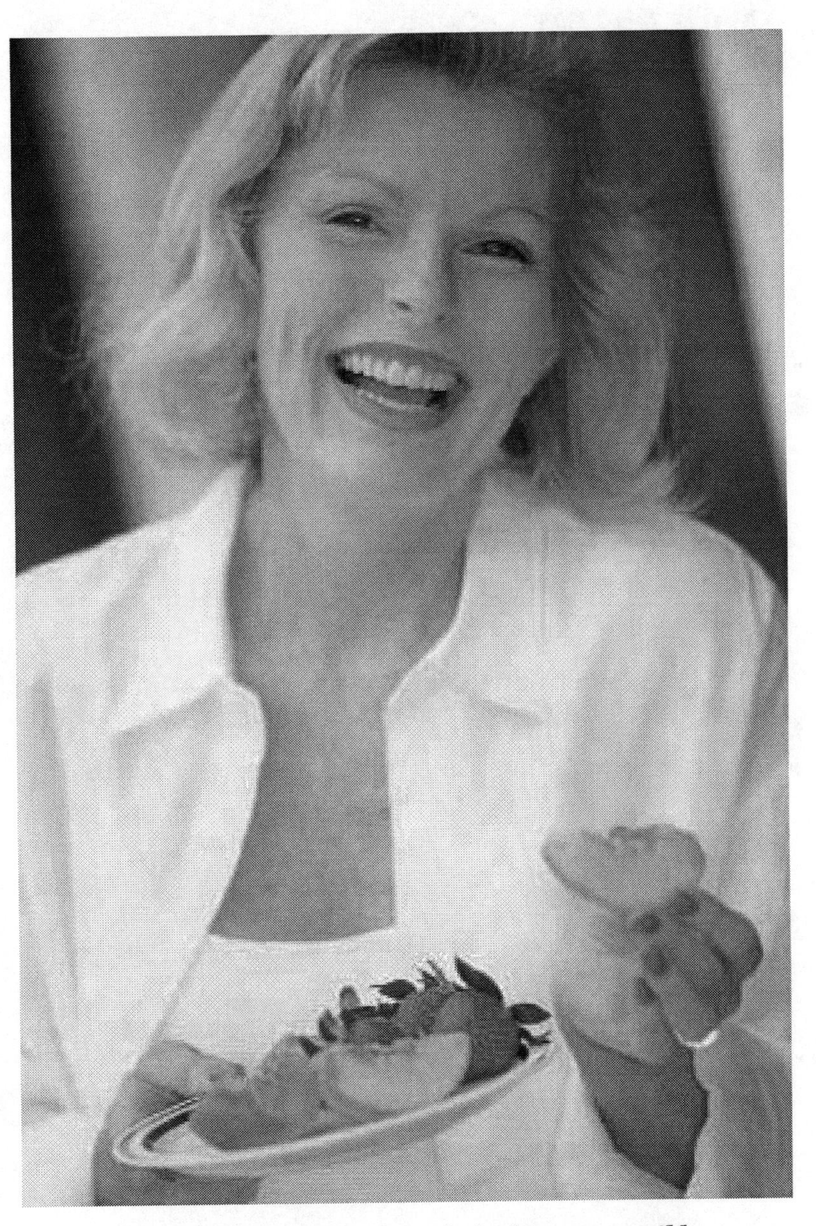

This rising trend has people looking at possible environmental factors such as pollution, global warming, toxins, and food additives.

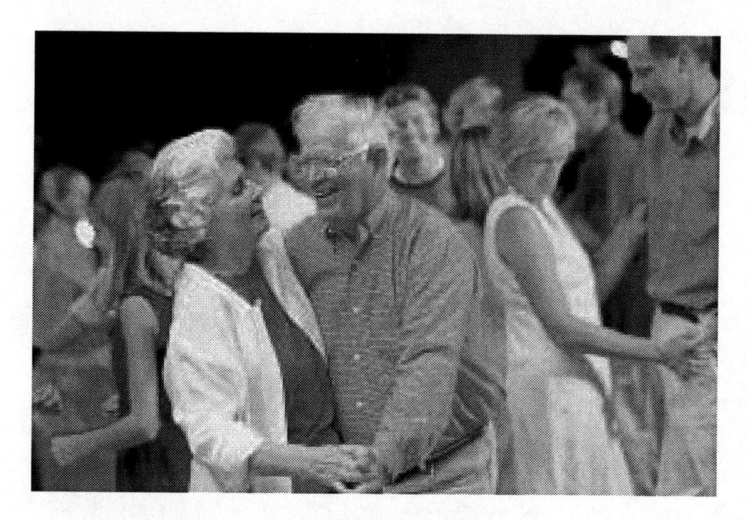

One trial found that tylophora led to moderate or complete asthma relief.

HERBS TO TRY:

Tylophora: Some mixed results exist for this Indian climbing plant and its effect on asthma. Traditionally, people in India have used tylophora to help cure bronchial asthma and bronchitis. There is some evidence behind it. One trial found that the herb's leaf, when swallowed for six days led to moderate or complete asthma relief. [*J Allergy* 1969;43:145–50] Another found similar success using powder from the leaves. [*J Indian Med Assoc* 1978;71:172–6] This isn't the end-all cure, though, because it has been found, at least in one double-blind trial, to have no effect on asthma. [*Ind J Med Res* 1979;69:981–9]

Boswellia: Best known for its actions against rheumatoid arthritis, boswellia has also been shown to have a beneficial effect on asthma. A double-blind study of 80 people with mild asthma found that the frequency of attacks and their breathing capacity both improved when taking a dose of 300 mg of boswellia three times a day. [*Eur J Med Res.* 1998;3:511-514]

Notable Herbs

Tylophora

Boswellia

Other Nutraceuticals That May Work:

Vitamin C

Magnesium

Benign Prostate Hyperplasia

This condition is a non-cancerous growth of the prostate that causes obstruction of the bladder and urine flow. It is predominantly seen in men over 50 years of age, as it is relatively common for the prostate gland to become enlarged as men age. It can be painful and serious, and it is characterized by the inability to start or stop a urine stream, painful urination, incontinence, urinary retention, and a frequent and/or urgent need to urinate. This is because an enlarged prostate causes the gland to press against the urethra, and the bladder wall becomes more irritable. It begins to contract more often (even though there may be small amounts of urine) and may eventually weaken to the point where it loses the ability to empty itself. It isn't known exactly what causes this condition, but several theories have it that testosterone may play a role. Most herbal treatments act as anti-inflammatories. BPH is one of the few conditions where herbal medicine has been firmly linked as an appropriate treatment.

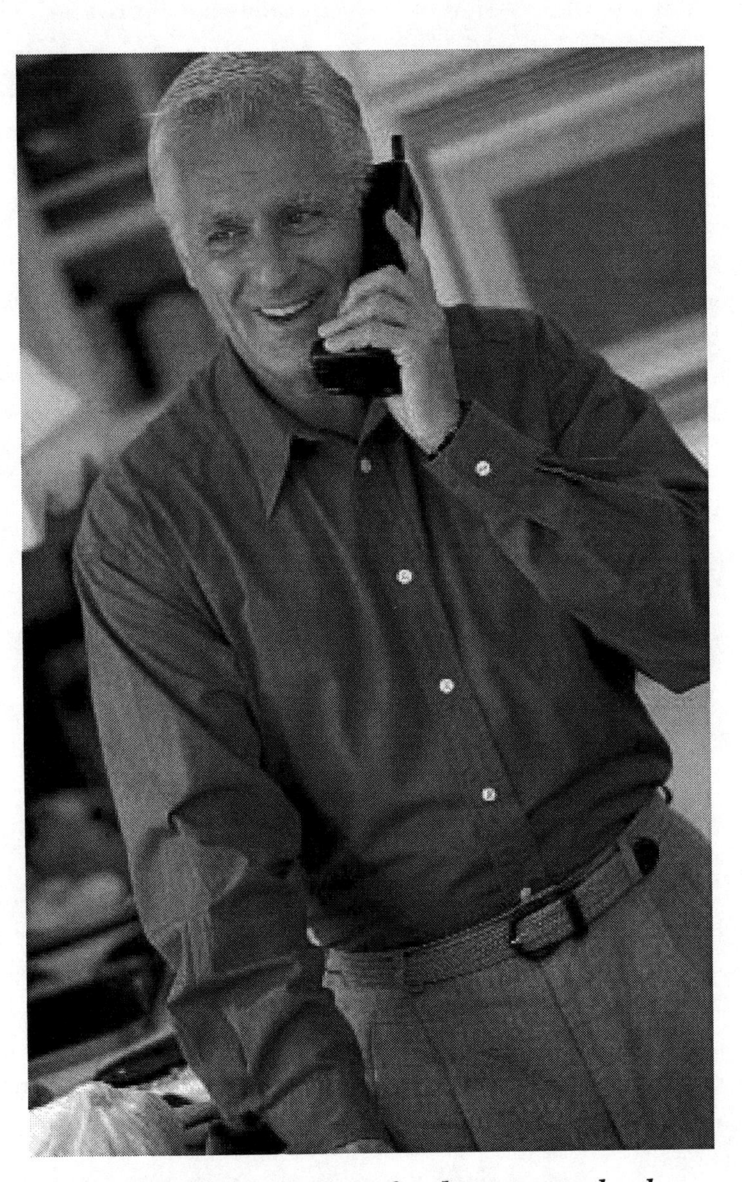

It is relatively common for the prostate gland to become enlarged as men age.

HERBS TO TRY:

Saw Palmetto: Many doctors, in the east and west, prescribe this herb to relieve BPH because it can be so beneficial. It is a bushy plant that typically grows in sandy soil in the Southeastern U.S., the Caribbean, and in the Mediterranean. Its partially dried black berries are the source of the plant's medicinal properties. It may stop testosterone from converting to DHT in the prostate and helps improve all symptoms of BPH. A Russian study found that five-year therapy with saw palmetto extract proved highly effective and safe in 26 patients with symptoms of BPH. [*Urologiia* 2002;(1):23-5] In 85 men taking either saw palmetto or placebo, there was statistically significant improvements in urinary symptoms for men taking the herb without any adverse affects. [*Urology* 2001;58(6):960-4] Many other studies have proven the herb's effectiveness as well.

Pygeum: Traditional African medicine dictates that sipping tea made from this tall evergreen tree will control urinary disorders in men. That's where it comes from. Since the 1970s, it's been approved for treating mild to moderate BPH in Europe. Pygeum has been found to be safe and effective for BPH treatment, and studies have typically used 50 to 100 mg of extract twice a day. [*Curr Ther Res* 1995;56:796–817] The herb contains compounds that have a diuretic action, anti-inflammatory activity, and a unique ability to dispose of any built-up cholesterol deposits.

Nettle: Nettle root contains compounds that inhibit the action of sex hormones thought to stimulate prostate tissue growth. It helps with urine flow as well by assisting the bladder's ability to empty itself in men with early-stage BPH. [*Urologe* 1994;334:90–5] It's also been successfully combined with both herbs mentioned above to treat BPH in double-blind studies. [*Urologe*1996;36:292–300]

Notable Herbs

Saw Palmetto

Pygeum

Nettle

Other Nutraceuticals That May Work:

Grass Pollen

Beta-Sitosterol

Vitamin E

Selenium

Zinc

Burns and Scalds

Simply put, a burn is an injury to the tissue caused by heat or flame. There are three degrees of burns. First degree burns are characterized by redness, swelling, and pain, and they involve only the top layer of skin, the epidermis. Second degree burns cause redness and blisters and involve both the epidermis and the dermis. Third degree burns affect the entire thickness of the skin, including underlying muscle tissue, subcutaneous fat, and bone. Even after the surface wounds heal, pain and scarring can be ongoing afflictions. It is important to see a doctor if you've been burned, no matter how serious it appears. In the beginning, run cool water over the burn, and don't let clothes touch it. Cover the burn with a clean and dry bandage and don't put creams or any topical ointments on it. Herbal treatments often include anti-inflammatories and pain relievers, as well as immune system boosters.

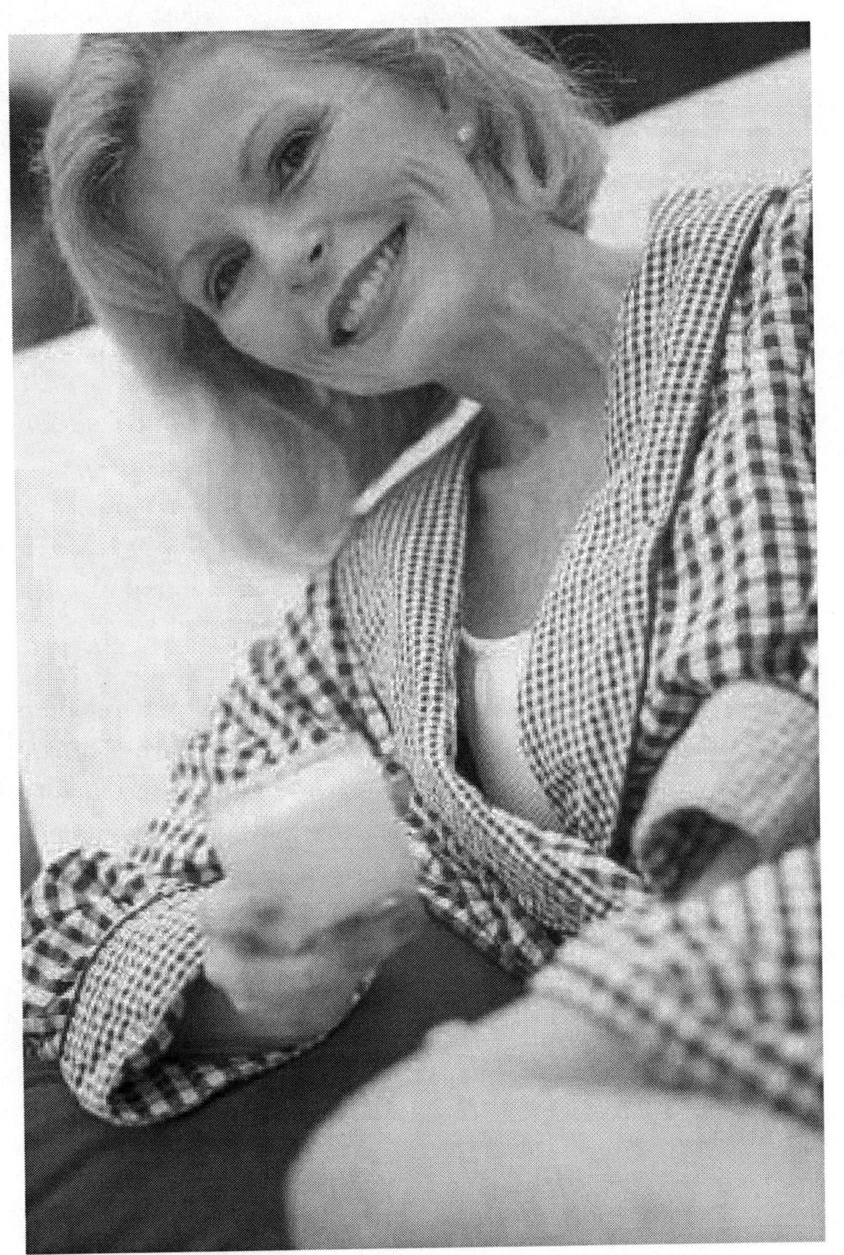

Even after the surface wounds heal, pain and scarring can be ongoing afflictions.

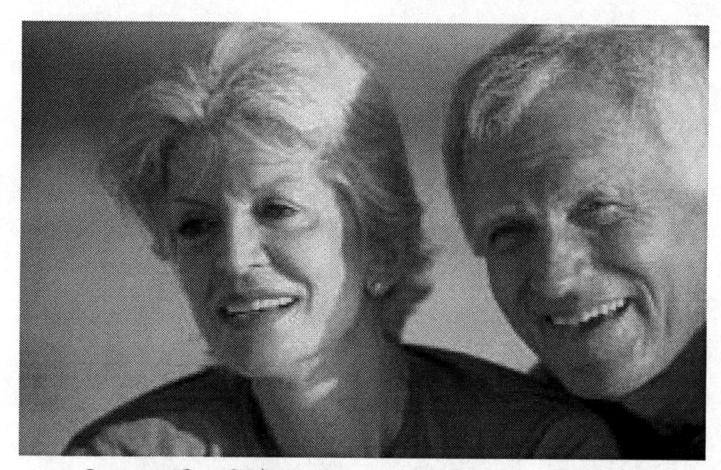

One study of 27 patients with burns compared aloe to Vaseline gauze and found the herb to have a healing time of about 11 days compared to the latter's 18 days.

HERBS TO TRY:

Gotu Kola: This herb is widely thought to help heal skin and other connective tissues. It contains many glycosides that help with wound healing and promote the development of healthy skin. It has been used in the treatment of second and third degree burns because of its ability to heal and reduce the formation of scar tissue. It has been clinically found to promote rapid wound healing. [*Perfusion* 1998; 11:508-20]

Aloe Vera: This fleshy plant is not fully understood by researchers, but it is often applied to the skin to promote the healing of minor burns, scalds, and cuts. One study of 27 patients with burns compared aloe to Vaseline gauze and found the herb to have a healing time of about 11 days compared to the latter's 18 days. This study showed aloe to be effective in a partial thickness burn wound. *[J Med Assoc Thai.* 1995 Aug;78(8):403-9] In a review of the effectiveness of using plants to heal skin problems, aloe vera was mentioned as specifically having the ability to heal burns. [*Adverse Drug React Toxicol Rev* 2001;20(2):89-103]

Note on Tea Tree Oil: Many sources indicate that tea tree oil is marginally effective in treating minor burns, as it may have the ability to soothe a burned area. It should be noted, however, that several major studies have found this herb to be ineffective for treating burns. Two studies from the journal *Burns* conclude that tea tree oil is not recommended. [*Burns, 1997;23(4): pp.349-351... Burns* 1998 Feb;24(1):80-2]

Notable Herbs

Aloe Vera

Gotu Kola

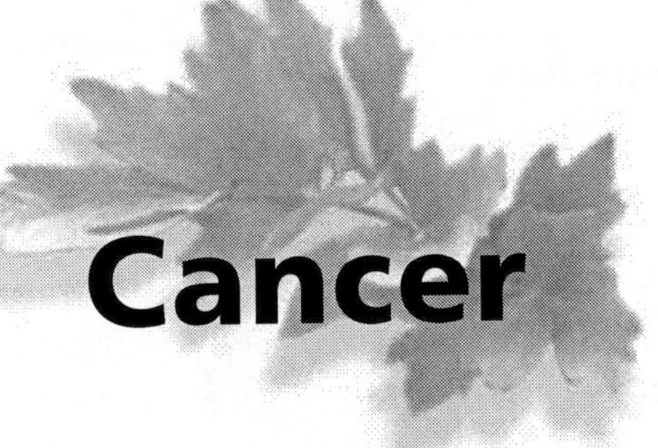

Cancer

Cancer is not just a single disease, but rather a group of over 100 diseases, characterized by uncontrolled, abnormal growth of cells. Of course, we all know there isn't yet a cure. These cells can spread locally or through the bloodstream and lymphatic system. The earlier cancer is diagnosed, the greater your chance of survival. That said, cancer is still the second leading cause of death in the United States. Herbal therapies for cancer strengthen the immune system and help battle the negative side effects of radiation or chemotherapy treatments. Because of the money put into the ongoing research battle against cancer, many herbs have come under the microscope in a whole host of countries. Some listed below are generally beneficial against cancer's effects, and some are specifically tailored to a specific cancer of which lung, breast, colon, and prostate are the most widespread.

The earlier cancer is diagnosed, the greater your chance of survival.

HERBS TO TRY:

Korean Ginseng: The type of ginseng found in Korea – "Panax" – is singled out because it is one of the most heavily tested herbs in cancer research. One study in 2003 found results that "strongly suggested" Korean ginseng had specific cancer preventive effects on any organ in the body. It succeeded in identifying the ingredient as well that had the biggest effect: ginsenoside. This herb is perhaps best used to combat gastric and lung cancers, as the relative risk for any side effects is lowest. [Mutat Res. 2003 Feb-Mar;523-524:63-74] This study came on the heels of *a Lancet* article that described Korean ginseng's protective effects and all the preliminary studies that had looked into its ability to ward off major cancers. [*Lancet Oncol.* 2001;2(1):49-55] The year before that, a study found that ginseng inhibited prostate cancer and at the same time prompted the body to incite cell death in those tumor cells. [*Life Sci.* 2000;67(11):1297-306]

Boswellia: The acid from this herb may be able to induce cell death in leukemia patients. One study found boswellic acid to strongly stop cancerous cells from growing. Researchers called it a "powerful agent" in the treatment of leukemia. [*Leuk Res.* 1999;23(1):43-50]

Omega-3 Fatty Acids: For a long time now, people who eat a lot of fish in their diets have been shown to have lower risks of getting mouth, throat, stomach, colon, rectum, pancreatic, lung, breast, and prostate cancers. Fish is high in omega-3 fatty acids, as are fish oil supplements. These acids are thought by many researchers to be the mysterious ingredient in fish that protects against cancer. [*Pharmacol Ther* 1999;83:217–44]

Sun Spurge: This is a rare weed that studies have suggested could play a role in stopping tumor cells from advancing and growing. In mice, it showed an "anti-tumor" effect and actually prolonged the life-span of mice that had cancer. What else? It boosted the immune function within these mice, further protecting them against foreign invaders like cancer-causing viruses. Sun spurge, untested so far on humans, may be considered a potent anti-cancer herb. [*Zhong Yao Cai.* 1999;22(11):579-81]

Hemsleya amabilis: This is a medicinal herb that has been used for a long time in Asia to treat cancer and other conditions. How it does so remains rather mysterious. In a 2002 study, an extract from this herb significantly inhibited tumor cell growth at a bunch of different doses. When cancerous cells were seeded near this herbal extract (even at a very low dose) those cells had an extremely tough time spreading. Hemsleya amabilis also promoted tumor cell death. [*Life Sci.* 2002;71(18):2161-70]

Garlic & Onion: These herbs, as well as leeks and chives, are members of a group of plants called "Allium." In preliminary studies, eating Allium herbs may have a link to cancer. Garlic and onion have shown effects on the gastrointestinal tract, and preliminary studies have found that the more Allium vegetables you eat, the less risk you have of getting colon cancer – one of the world's greatest killers of men. [*Br J Cancer* 1999;79:1283–7] Eating these herbs also may reduce the risk of getting precancerous growths in the colon. [*Am J Epidemiol* 1996;144:1015–25].

Echinacea: In mice, it's been shown to boost the number of "natural-killer cells" – the ones that instinctively destroy problematic cells, like ones with tumors. A study in 2001 tried to see what would happen if echinacea was part of the diet of mice with leukemia (a tumor that these killer cells love to target). They found mice fed echinacea had "highly significant" protection against leukemia. Thus, this herb has a lot of potential in cancer therapy. [*J Altern Complement Med.* 2001;7(3):241-51]

Turmeric: Turmeric and its central ingredient, curcumin, are the substance that turns curry yellow. Turmeric is known throughout medicine as having healing qualities. Not tested on humans, it has been shown in lab and animal studies to throw a wrench into the growth of cancerous cells associated with the breast, skin, and colon. Daily doses of turmeric have been shown to decrease the level of "mutagens" in the body – it is these increased mutations that can cause cancer. In the late 1990s, an animal study showed that curcumin almost entirely prevented skin cancer from spreading – possibly in relation to its antioxidant activity. [*Cancer Lett* 1999;141:159–65]

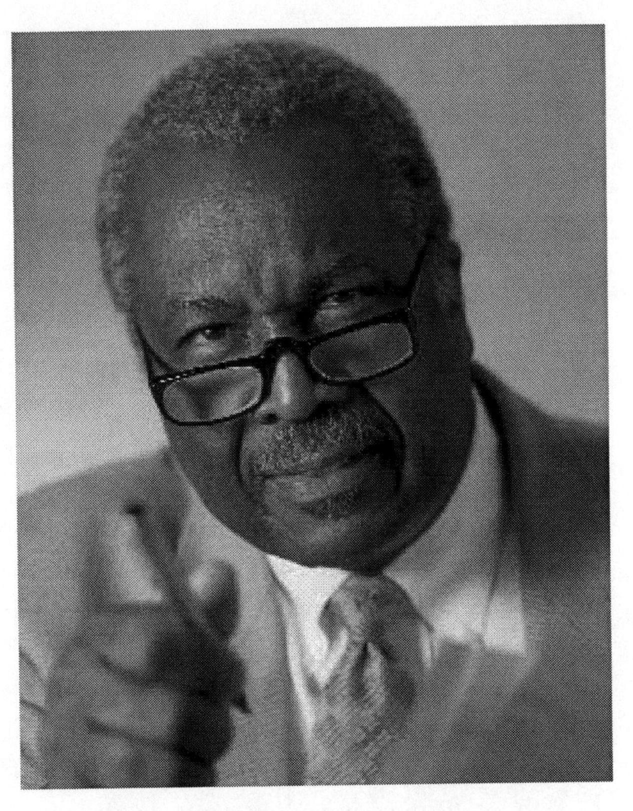

Injecting lentinan in prostate cancer patients has helped increase survival rates by five years in Japan.

Astragalus: According to *The Journal of Urology*, scientists discovered the potential of astragalus in treating cancer as early as the 1950s. This herb is an excellent source of the mineral "selenium," and it is interesting to note that places in the world where selenium content in food was *high*, the rate of many different cancers was *low*. It could be that selenium protects cells from toxic damage. Its antioxidant effect is thought to be about 500 times that of vitamin E. The dried root of this herb has been found to inhibit gastric cancers cells, but it doesn't seem to actively kill those cells. [*World J Gastroenterol.* 2003 Apr;9(4):670-]

Motherwort: This herb had to be mentioned, because a study has come back with some exciting results – as exciting as they get in the realm of cancer. It seems an extract from the Chinese herb motherwort wound up inducing cell death in every type of tumor (seven) on which it was tested. The study was extremely technical, but the mitochondrion was singled out as being involved in this cancer cell-killing activity. [*J Altern Complement Med.* 2003 Aug;9(4):511-8]

Green Tea: One Japanese study found that drinking green tea led to prolonged life and a reduced spread of cancer in women that had early stages of breast cancer. It didn't have such beneficial effects, however, in women who had more advanced stages. [*Jpn J Cancer Res* 1998;89:254–61] Women who drank at least five cups of green tea a day had the lowest chance of cancer recurring in their breast. What isn't known is if green tea holds an ability to help patients with breast cancer or prevent healthy women from getting it.

Shiitake Mushrooms: A carbohydrate found in these grocery store mushrooms, "lentinan," may have an anti-cancer effect. But, it is only seen when lentinan is *injected* into cancer patients. Two studies found that these injections allowed people with serious, advanced cancers to live much longer. [*Anticancer Res* 1997;17:2751–6] Injecting lentinan in prostate cancer patients has helped increase survival rates by five years in Japan. Still unknown: Can eating shiitake mushrooms, or even taking oral lentinan supplements, have the same effects?

Milk thistle (*Silybum marianum*) is a botanical that may be useful in the prevention or treatment of liver dysfunction in patients undergoing chemotherapy. It might stimulate appetite and reduce nausea.

Huanglian: This widely used Chinese herb is often used to treat gastroenteritis. It has also been found to inhibit the growth of tumors in colon, gastric, and breast cancer lines. Huanglian is a good indication that traditional Chinese herbs may hold the key to specific cellular processes involved in cancer therapy.

Notable Herbs

Korean Ginseng

Boswellia

Sun Spurge

Hemsleya amabilis

Garlic/Onion

Echinacea

Turmeric

Astragalus

Motherwort

Green Tea

Shiitake Mushrooms

Milk Thistle

Huanglian

Other Nutraceuticals That May Work:

Omega-3 Fatty Acids

Selenium

Candidiasis

Candidiasis is a fungal/yeast infection that can affect any moist area of the body, including the mouth, sinuses, underarms, inner thighs, between fingers, and the vagina. It often affects people with weakened immune systems, such as those with HIVAIDS or those who have been treated with antibiotics. It is generally not very serious and almost completely curable. As for chronic candidiasis, women are eight times more likely than men to get it. For them, the common vaginal symptoms include itchiness, burning urination, redness, and odor. Herbal treatments act as anti-fungals and immune boosters.

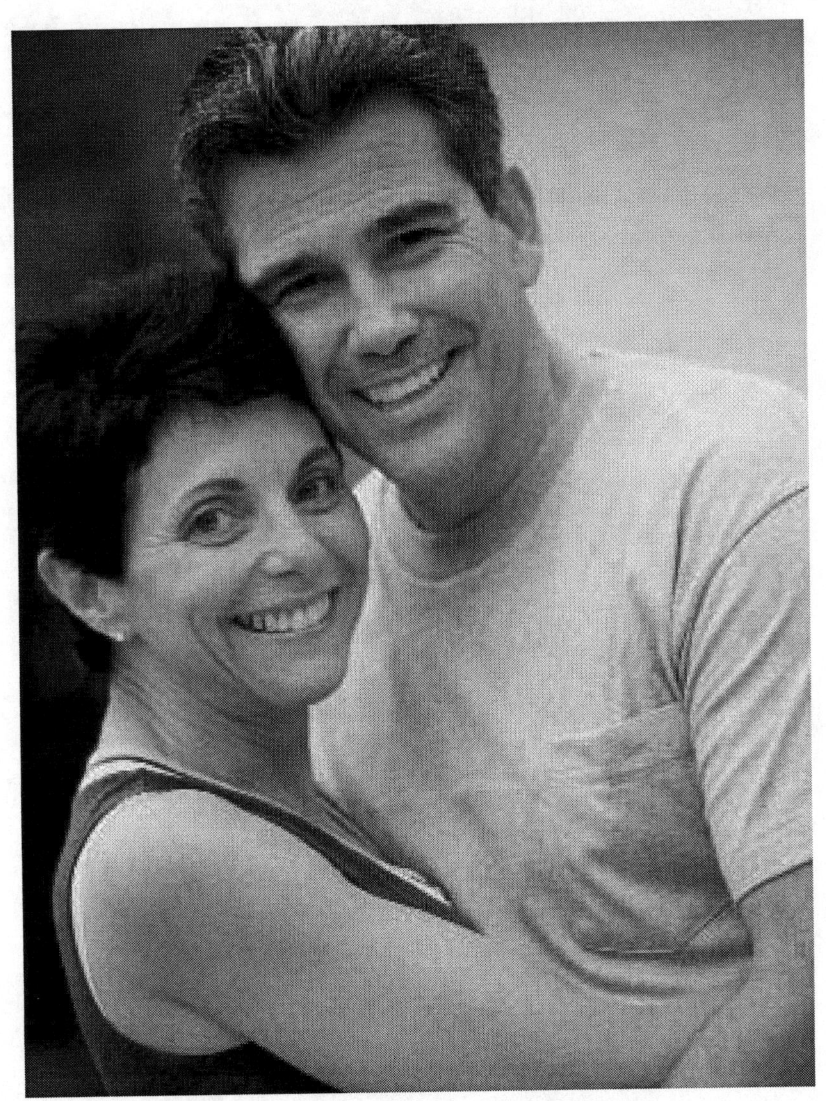

Women are eight times more likely to get chronic candidiasis than men.

HERBS TO TRY:

Garlic: Despite there being no studies on humans yet, garlic is one of the first botanical remedies that is mentioned in relation to candidiasis. Eating the pungent cloves may stop yeast organisms from growing and may help the body resist vaginal yeast infections. It has antibacterial, antiviral, and antifungal traits to it. The

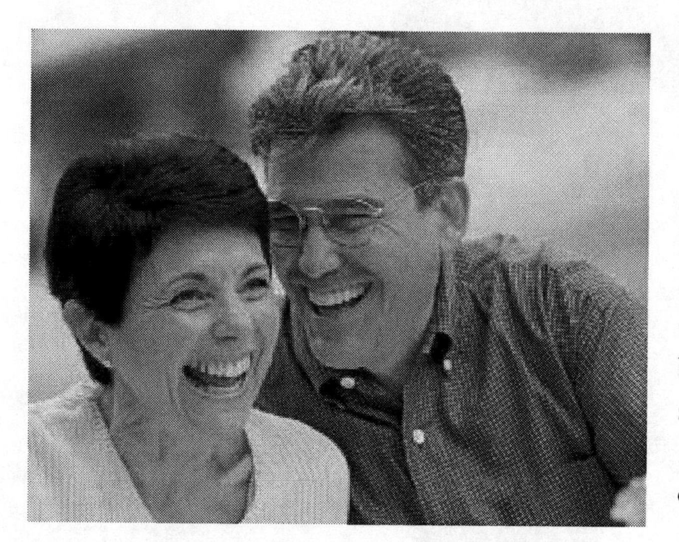

Volatile oils culled from these herbs are thought to play a role in relieving candidiasis: tea tree, thyme, peppermint, rosemary, and oregano.

Garlic's antifungal activity has been demonstrated in test tube studies. [*Mycologia* 1977;69:341–8… *Mykosen* 1980;23:691–8]

Certain oils: Volatile oils culled from these herbs are thought to play a role in relieving candidiasis: tea tree, thyme, peppermint, rosemary, and oregano. All of them have been found relatively effective in test tube studies. [*J Antimicrobial Chemother* 1998;42:591–5] In a separate study, oregano turned out to be 100 times more effective than a regularly used acid against candidiasis. [*J Applied Nutr* 1995;47:96–102]

Echinacea: The juice of the echinacea plant, when taken orally, has been proven to help prevent the recurrence of vaginal yeast infections. A double-blind trial found that adding this to treatment with a typical nitrate-based cream reduced the recurrence significantly more than the cream alone. [*Therapiewoche* 1986;36:3352–8] Similar benefits may be yielded for Yeast Syndrome.

Notable Herbs

Garlic

Tea tree oil

Thyme oil

Peppermint oil

Rosemary oil

Oregano oil

Echinacea

Other Nutraceuticals That May Work:

Probiotics

Cataracts

Cataracts are a type of visual impairment, often seen in elderly patients. It is characterized by a clouding of the lens in the eye, affecting vision, and can lead to blindness. Other symptoms include faded colors, glare, lamps and sunlight seem overly bright, night vision is poor, double vision in one eye, and frequent changes in your prescription. Cataracts are caused by protein clumping up in the lens, reducing the amount of light that reaches the retina, or a clear lens simply colors with age, and with it there seems to be a brownish tint to everything one sees. More than half of people over the age of 80 have a cataract or have had surgery to correct one. Cataracts can occur in one or both eyes, but can't spread from one eye to another. Supplemental remedies are often preventative, and they deal with general eye health.

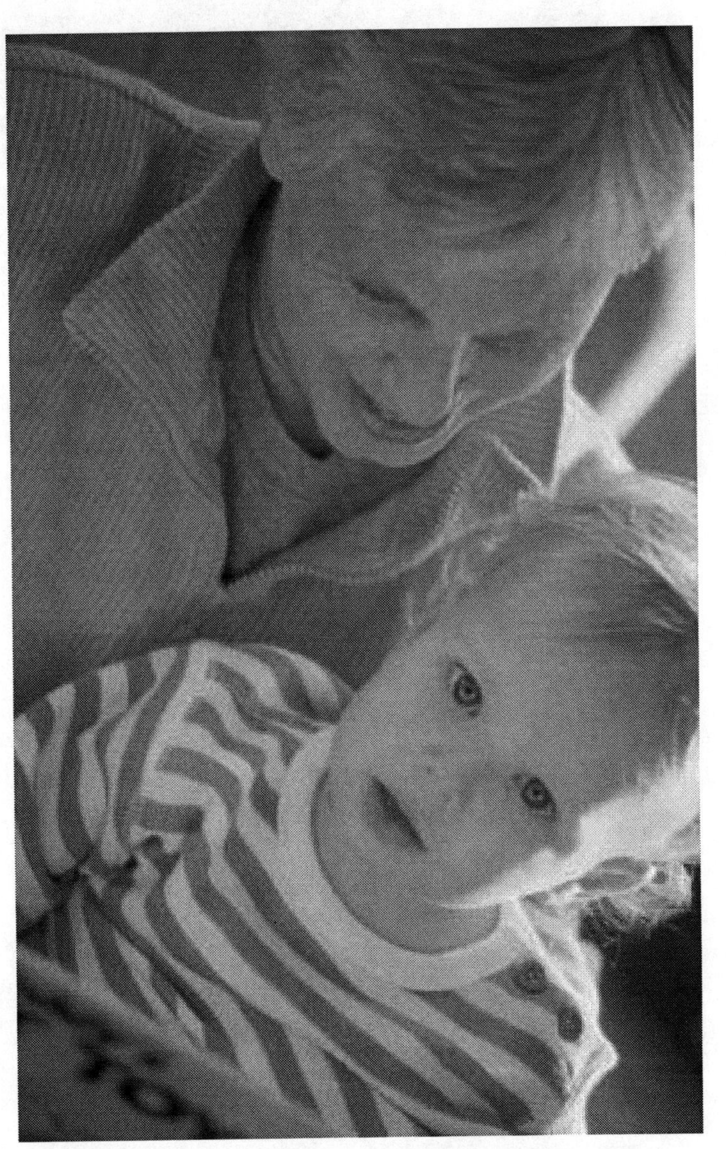

More than half of people over the age of 80 have a cataract or have had surgery to correct one.

HERBS TO TRY:

Bilberry: Within this berry (a member of the blueberry, huckleberry, and cranberry family) are flavonoids that may protect the lens from cataracts. Bilberry is one of the most commonly used supplements for vision. It's thought to be very useful in a variety of ways for the eye, and its popularity persists although there is not much

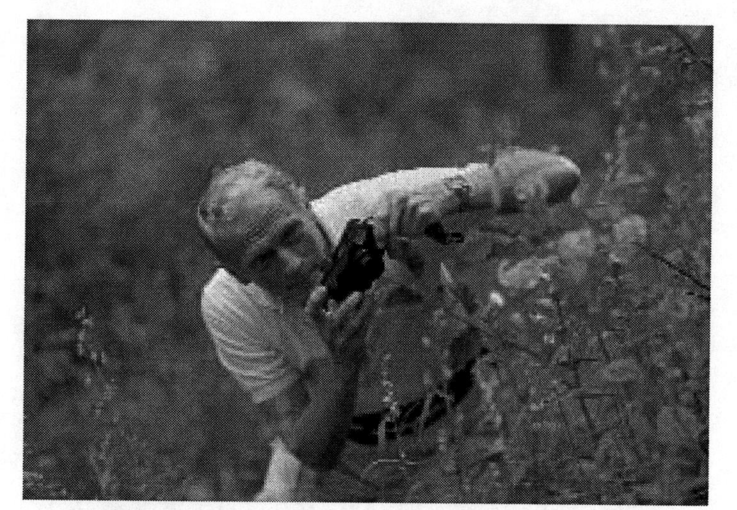

A combination of bilberry extract and vitamin E supplements halted the progression of cataracts in nearly all of the 50 patients studied.

evidence backing it up. One Italian study, though, did find that a combination of bilberry extract and vitamin E supplements halted the progression of cataracts in nearly all of the 50 patients. It's unclear, though, which of the treatment's ingredients was primarily responsible.

Carotenoids: Is it folklore? Perhaps not – carrots may be good for your eyes. A few studies have hinted that carotenoids may be effective at preventing cataracts. In a lengthy study of 500 women aged 53 to 73, it was found generally that those with higher levels of carotonoids and vitamin C were less likely to have cataracts. [*Am J Clin Nutr*. 2002;75:540-9] Two carotenoids, lutein and zeaxanthin, are thought to be specifically involved in protecting vision. They are found in many fruits and vegetables, not only carrots (they provide the pigmentation). These two carotenoids were found in a study of U.S. men to achieve a modestly lower risk of cataracts severe enough to require extraction. [*Am J Clin Nutr* 1999:70:517-24]

Vitamin C: Although not a herb, this one needs to be mentioned because of its connection to cataract prevention. In a Tufts University study, vitamin C, age, and risk for the common "cortical" cataracts were all linked together. Women under 60 who had more than 362 mg of the vitamin a day had a 57% reduced risk of getting cataracts than those taking 140 mg a day. Those taking C supplements for more than a decade had 60% lower chances of cataracts than those who took no supplements. [*Am J Clin Nutr*. 2002;75:540-9]

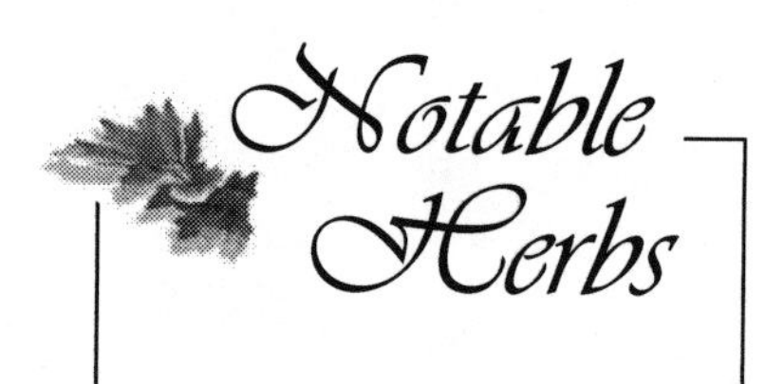

Bilberry

Other Nutraceuticals That May Work:

Carotenoids (especially lutein & zeaxanthin)

Vitamin A

Vitamin C

Selenium

Chicken Pox & Shingles

Contrary to popular belief, chicken pox does not just affect school-aged children. It ranges in severity from very mild to quite serious. The disease itself is a very common, highly infectious and contagious viral infection. It is also known as "varicella" – named after the virus that spreads through the air and by physical contact. You are more likely to get chickenpox in early spring and in late winter; in other words, during moderate temperatures when viruses tend to thrive. The classic symptom is a blistery red rash that is very itchy. In healthy children, the virus lasts two weeks at most, but in adults who have never had it, chickenpox can pose a more serious problem. Complications can be fatal, and about 100 people die a year in the U.S. from the virus. Shingles are caused by the same virus, herpes zoster, and about 90% of those who've had chicken pox are at risk of developing shingles later in life, a disease the springs to life after the varicella virus, lying dormant in the body, is awakened by a weakened immune system. The symptoms include: tingling, shooting pain, itchiness, rash, and blisters. There is not a wealth of evidence into herbal treatments, but some topical herbal remedies will help relieve the itching and pain caused by varicella and promote quick skin healing. Caution: herbal medicines are not always appropriate for children, so speak to a health care practitioner before administering any herbal medicine to a child.

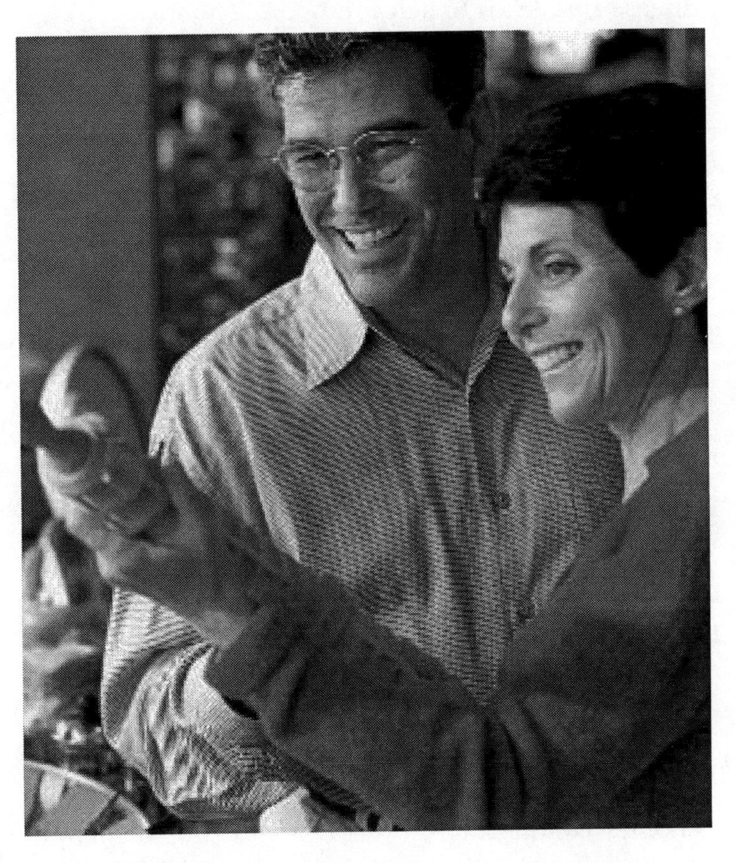

In healthy children, the virus lasts two weeks at most, but in adults who have never had it, chickenpox can pose a more serious problem.

HERBS TO TRY:

Capsaicin: Also known as cayenne, this cream made from the spicy pepper is a proven powerful pain reliever when it's rubbed onto the skin around sore joints and muscles. It may help relieve "post-herpetic neuralgia", which is a potential complication of shingles. Not studied too much for chickenpox, capsaicin cream has been looked at in treating psoriasis, another dermatologic disease that leads to itchy, red skin. The idea is that itching follows the same pathway as pain – thus if the cayenne pepper helps relieve pain, it will do so for itching too. It was proven in a study of 200 patients with psoriasis – even a 0.025% capsaicin cream significantly reduced itching, scaling, thickness, and redness compared to the effects of a plain cream.[*Journal of the American Academy of Dermatology*, Sept. 1993;29:438-42]

Chamomile: German chamomile, in particular, is a traditional remedy for skin conditions such as chickenpox. Research again is lacking, so we must turn to chamomile's effects and why it could be useful in treating these conditions. One part of chamomile, "chamazulene", has been found to have anti-inflammatory and antiseptic activities, which can help reduce infection. [*Aust J Med Herbalism* 1993;5:33-9] A double-blind study found that chamomile is effective in superficial wound healing. [*Z Hautkr* 1987;62:1262-71] The essential oil of chamomile is found in many skin creams and it is a good choice for preventing skin infections. It is nontoxic.

Peppermint Oil: A recent study suggested this may be effective in treating post-herpetic neuralgia, the shingles complication that not everyone contracts, but those who do suffer from it for years. A case study on a 76-year-old woman found that after painkillers, acupuncture, and medicine failed to relieve the shingles complication, two to three drops of peppermint oil three times a day led to almost complete pain relief for about six hours. When pain returned, more oil brought it down again. [*The Clinical Journal of Pain* 2002;18:200–2].

Goldenseal: This herb, taken internally, usually dissolved in water or tea, or applied to the skin, is a powerful antibiotic and is known to help clear infection. Without much evidence to back it up, goldenseal may be of value in fighting viral skin ailments such as chickenpox and shingles.

Notable Herbs

Capsaicin

Chamomile

Peppermint Oil

Goldenseal

Other Nutraceuticals That May Work:

Lysine

Vitamin C

Zinc

B Vitamins

Bromelain (enzyme)

Papain (enzyme)

Chlamydia

Chlamydia is the most common sexually transmitted disease in both men and women, with an estimated four million people in the U.S. infected every year. Rapidly spreading and reproducing bacteria cause it, and it can be passed on during any sexual contact. Symptoms include mucus or pus within the urine, but often are so mild they go unnoticed, thus the condition goes untreated. This is dangerous, as the infection could move inside the body and cause pelvic inflammatory disease in women and epidydimitis in men. Herbal treatments work to soothe the symptoms and act as an antifungal to fight the bacteria that cause the infection.

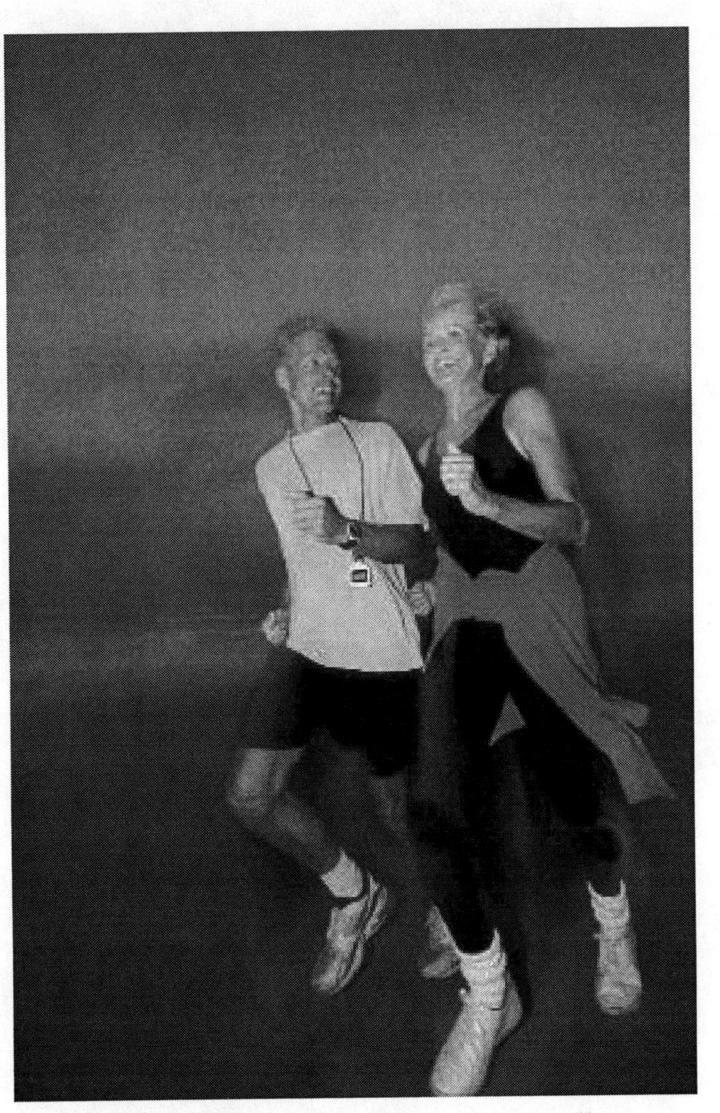

Chlamydia is the most common sexually transmitted disease in both men and women.

HERBS TO TRY:

Goldenseal: One of this plant's active ingredients, "berberine" is responsible for goldenseal's ability to help relieve the effects of chlamydia. Berberine is known to stimulate the immune system, help kill the chlamydia bacterium, and help the urinary tract (disturbed by chlamydia). It has been shown to be helpful in preventing bacteria from building on the bladder wall and resolving bladder infections. [*Antimicr Agents Chemother* 1988; 32:1274–7] And in a study of 51

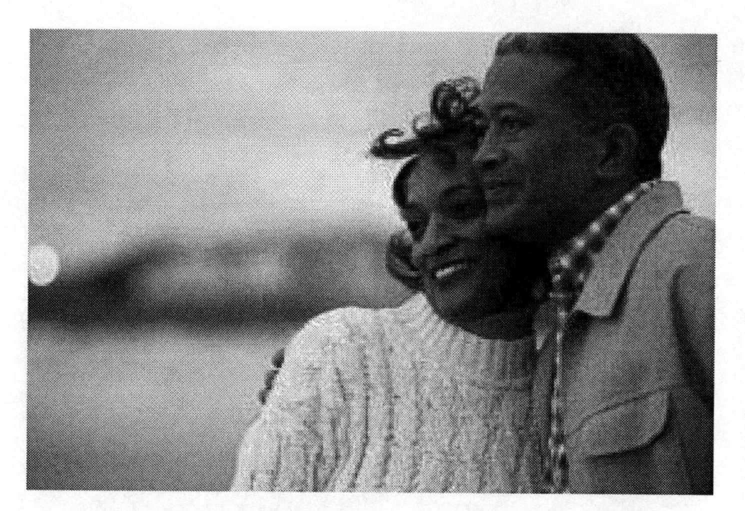

The infection could move inside the body and cause pelvic inflammatory disease in women and epididydimitis in men.

people with a chlamydia infection, berberine helped kill the organism – perhaps by stimulating the body's own protective mechanism. [*Rev Int Trach Pathol Ocul Trop Subtrop Sante Publique* 1992;69:147-165]

Cranberries: Long used to treat urinary tract infections (caused by chlamydia), these small red berries may be useful in alleviating symptoms of this sexually transmitted disease. In one study, 16 ounces of cranberry juice a day led to beneficial effects in 73% of people with urinary tract infections. [*The Healing Power of Herbs*, 1992]. Of those who stopped drinking the juice, 61% had a recurrence of the infection. Cranberries appear to prevent bacteria from "adhering" to the lining of the bladder and urethra.

Saw Palmetto: It won't target chlamydia per se, but it is known for its urinary antiseptic abilities, and is used for a variety of urinary tract ailments. The mechanism by which this herb helps with urinary problems remains unknown. In one double-blind study, the herb led to a statistically significant improvement in urinary symptoms in men over the age of 45 who had lower urinary tract symptoms. [*Urology* 2001;58(6):960-4]

Notable Herbs

Goldenseal

Cranberries

Saw Palmetto

Chronic Fatigue Syndrome

While researchers are still debating the exact cause, and indeed the question of whether or not chronic fatigue syndrome really does exist, people suffering from the illness understand just how debilitating it can actually be. Officially, CFS occurs when fatigue lasts for at least half a year, and is accompanied by other symptoms such as sore throat, chronic cough, sleep disturbances, an intolerance to alcohol, mysterious aches and pains, headaches, and tender lymph nodes. It's a difficult condition to treat, both nutritionally and medically. This is because it has no clear cause and there is nothing to measure – this means it's a virtual guessing game trying to figure out which treatments, which herbs, to use in an effort to stimulate such a fatigued body. Women get CFS two to four times as often as men, and overall about half a million people in the U.S. have a condition that at least resembles CFS. No herbal remedies have been tested for CFS in particular, but many can help with symptoms of this mysterious illness.

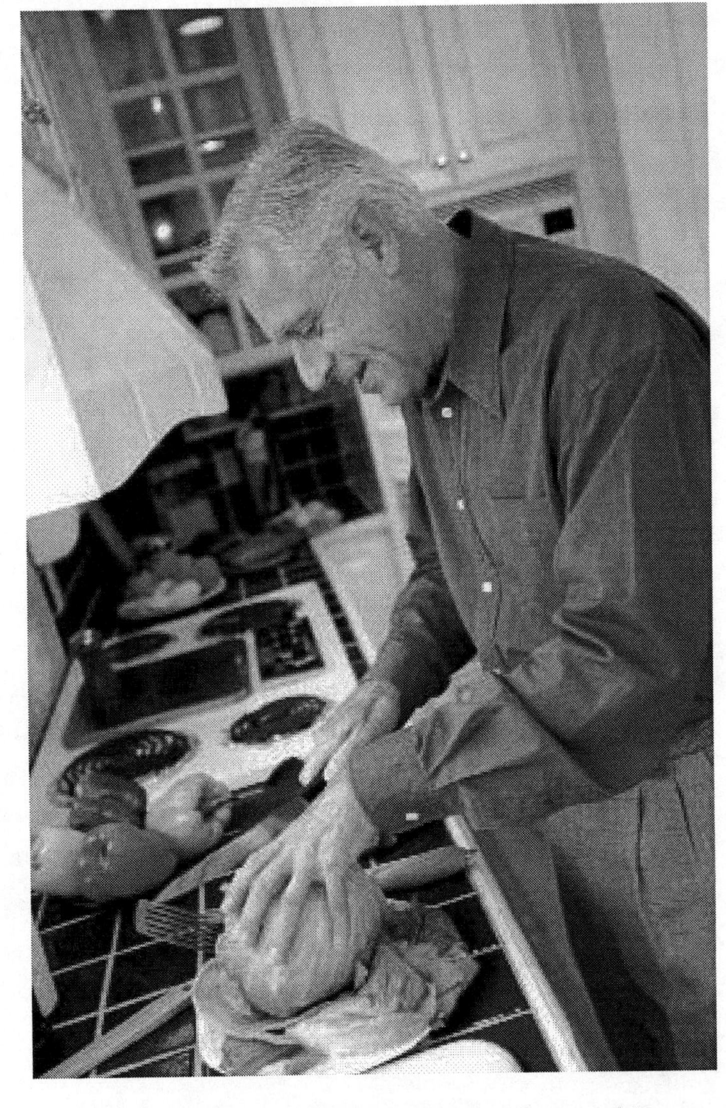

People suffering from the illness understand just how debilitating it can actually be.

HERBS TO TRY:

Evening primrose oil: This supplement has in it gamma-linolenic acid (GLA), which is proven to reduce inflammation. Primrose oil is documented to reduce pain associated with a number of conditions, such as rheumatoid arthritis and diabetes-related nerve pain, and its proven ability to help pain may reduce the mysterious aches and pains associated with chronic fatigue syndrome. Other sources of GLA, such as fish oil, could be useful as well.

Valerian: This tall perennial plant is known best as a sedative and thus can help with any sleep disturbances caused by CFS – quite a frustrating symptom considering one is too tired to be active, yet cannot sleep. A big double-blind study found that valerian root help patients get a higher quality sleep and allowed them to fall asleep faster with no lethargy in the morning. [*Psychopharmacology* 1992; 108:248-55] For this reason, it seems valerian could be a keeper for CFS patients.

Astragalus: Those with CFS are known to have weakened immune systems, and astragalus can help with that. It's a known immune booster, commonly used in Chinese traditional medicine as a tonic for the immune system. It is so powerful that it's being studied for use against AIDS. One clinical example is in more than 1,100 chronic bronchitis patients, there was a significant immune enhancement when astragalus was used with interferon, than with interferon alone. [*Chin. Med. J.* 1981;94(1):35-40] Several Chinese studies have shown astragalus to benefit immune function and actually influenced survival of cancer patients. [*Alt Med Alert* 1999;Nov:125-8]

Echinacea: This herb (whose real name is "purple coneflower") is also known as an immune booster and in this way may benefit CFS patients. It is easily one of the most widely used herbs for the immune system in the world. Many studies have documented its ability to do so, although it's still unclear what conditions it is best used for, and what doses may be most effective. One report said its immune-stimulating properties were complex and attributable to several of its ingredients. It has been found to directly stimulate white blood cell production as well. [Alt. Med. Review 2001;6 (4):411–414]

Notable Herbs

Evening Primrose Oil

Valerian

Astragalus

Echinacea

Other Nutraceuticals That May Work:

Coenzyme Q_{10}

Beta-carotene

DHEA

Chronic Obstructive Pulmonary Disease

COPD is an umbrella term for several diseases that cause lung damage including bronchitis and emphysema. The first has to do with inflammation and scarring of the airway tubes (bronchi) and the latter is due to an enlarged and damaged alveoli (air sacs) within the lungs. About 16 million Americans have COPD. These are characterized by a difficulty in expiring air from the lungs, with shortness of breath generally the first sign that something is wrong in the air pipes. Other symptoms include a chronic cough, feelings of fatigue, wheezing, respiratory infection, weight loss, and a lack of appetite. It is most often caused by smoking and the lung damage caused is most of the time irreversible – however, quitting smoking and some treatments can help stop the progression of diseases such as emphysema. Herbal therapies work as an anti-inflammatory, easing the breathing process.

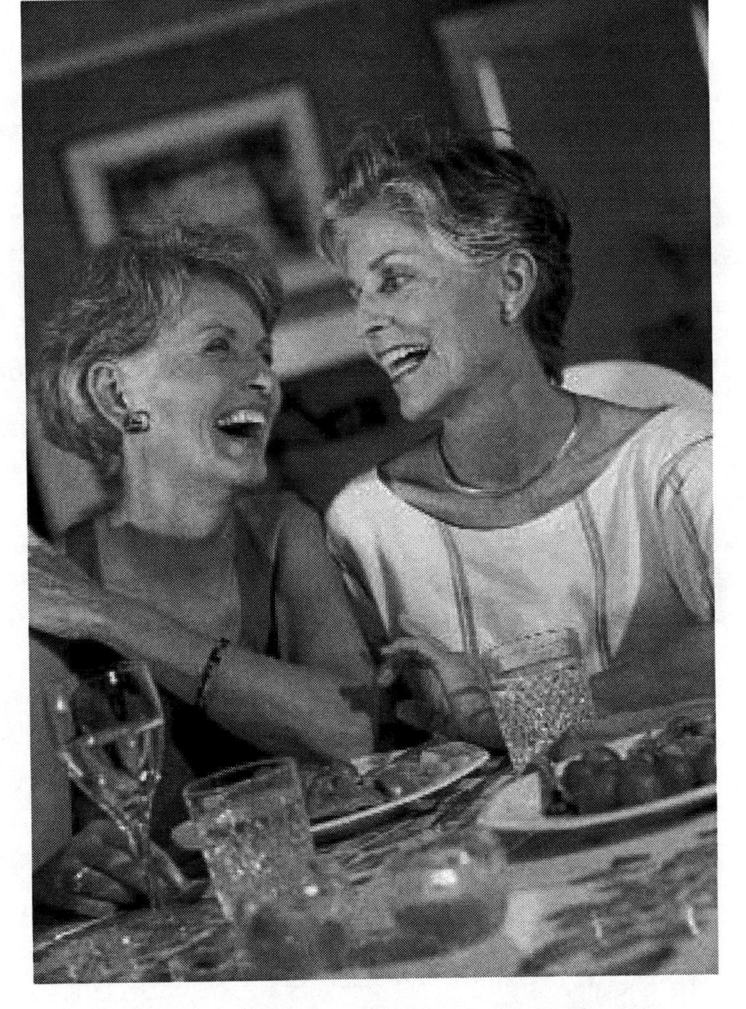

About 16 million Americans have COPD.

HERBS TO TRY:

Licorice: Battling infections, lowering fevers, licorice root is figured to have antiviral properties that helps shorten respiratory conditions such as bronchitis. It can exert a soothing effect on the linings of the throat and respiratory tract, helping eliminate cough. Its primary ingredient, glycyrrhizin, acts almost like a steroid in its anti-inflammatory and anti-allergic properties. It is an expectorant as well, useful for relieving respiratory problems. Expectorants are used in strong cough and sore throat medicines.

Echinacea: Researchers generally agree that this well-known and well-used herbal remedy boosts the immune system and shortens the duration of an upper respiratory tract infection. It is helpful in preventing viral bronchitis and similar COPDs from progressing into a more severe state because of its ability to enhance macrophage function and increase T-cell response. [*Immunopharmacol* 1997;35:229–35] Data from a German study suggests also that echinacea reduces the risk of getting an infection by 12% and decreases the length of a COPD by about two days. [*Am J Med* 1999;106:138-43]

Plantain: Not to be confused with the banana-like vegetable of the same name, this plant acts as an expectorant and a demulcent, approved in Germany for use in relieving coughs and irritation association with respiratory infections. Two Bulgarian studies have found it useful in helping people who have chronic bronchitis. [*Probl Vatr Med* 1983;11:61–9...*Vutr Boles* 1982;21:133–7]

Garlic: This pungent herb is known to help with such COPDs as bronchitis. It may relax the smooth muscle cells in the lungs, thus loosening up the bronchi to allow more air to pass. Garlic extracts have been found to kill off bacteria in the lungs, which helps relieve and prevent COPD. [*Appl Microbiol Biotechnol* 2001;57:282-6] Garlic is a traditional treatment for bronchitis, possibly related to the fact that its active ingredients are secreted straight to the lungs when you eat it.

Ginseng: A recent study found that Korean ginseng was more effective in treating bronchitis than antibiotics alone. With all 75 patients treated with antibiotics, but only half with the addition of ginseng, researchers found those on ginseng experienced far smaller bacteria counts in their lungs. Ginseng seemed to clear up the bacteria that caused bronchitis more quickly than just antibiotics. [*Clin Drug Invest.* 2001;21:41-45] In another study, 1,500 workers in Russia who took ginseng daily had significantly fewer bouts of cold, flu, bronchitis, and sinus infections than those not taking the herb. [*The Healing Herbs*, 1991]

Notable Herbs

Licorice Root

Echinacea

Plantain

Garlic

Ginseng

Other Nutraceuticals That May Work:

Vitamin C

Zinc

Coenzyme Q_{10}

Vitamin E

Magnesium

Circulation (impaired)

Circulation problems are often a symptom of other diseases, like heart disease, peripheral arterial disease, or diabetes, but they can also appear on their own. Symptoms often include cold extremities (hands and feet), dizziness, and fatigue. The movement of blood through the vascular system can be hampered by clogged arteries, inflammation, dilated blood vessels, or a weakened heart, among other factors. This is a very serious condition, likely to be an indicator of an underlying disease, and you should consult your doctor before initiating any alternative treatment yourself. There are herbal remedies you can try that may decrease inflammation, regulate the heart, and increase blood flow.

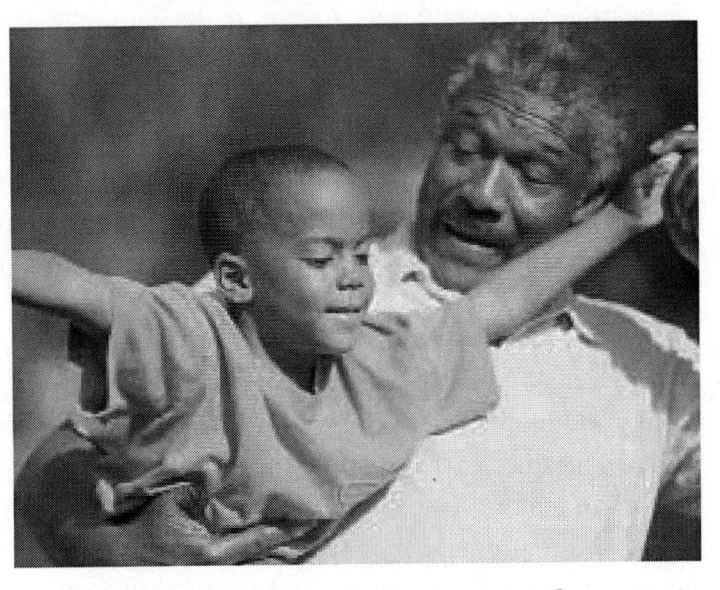

There are herbal remedies you can try that may decrease inflammation, regulate the heart, and increase blood flow.

HERBS TO TRY:

Hawthorn: The berries, flowers, and dried leaves of this herb all show benefits to the heart and circulation. High in flavonoids, hawthorn may work by widening the arteries and thus improving the flow of blood – an action otherwise known as "dilation." That theory was backed up by the results of one study out of Germany [*Arzneirninelforschung* 1995;45:842-845]. Because of its cardiovascular health benefits, hawthorn is one of the most prescribed natural remedies in Europe. The Germans are really on top of this herb, as another study showed that hawthorn tended to mildly lower blood pressure in those who took it [*Fortschr Med* 1993;111:352-354]. Hawthorn acts as a "vasodilator" by opening blood vessels and increasing blood flow. It both relaxes the smooth muscles in artery walls and inhibits an enzyme that tends to constrict blood vessels.

Garlic: This herb is well known for its cardiovascular and circulation-improving traits. A major journal by the American Heart Association reported that garlic can maintain the elasticity of aging blood vessels, which tend to lose their ability to stretch with time. [*Circulation* 1997;96(8):2649-2655] Garlic helps widen blood vessels as a result of relaxing the muscles that surround the walls, which is why it's a major herb for hypertension. Garlic has gone through a tremendous number of tests, including one for "intermittent claudication", which is restricted blood flow in the leg. In the double-blind trial, those who received garlic powder were able to walk significantly farther than others, the herb allowed greater blood flow to the leg and reduced pain. [*Clin Investig 1993;71: pp.383-6*]

Ginger: Researchers have found that ginger root may inhibit prostaglandins and leukotrienes, which are involved in inflammation and pain. Thus, the spice is an anti-inflammatory. In terms of arthritis, a condition where impeded blood flow is a problem, patients receiving ginger extract had fewer gastrointestinal side effects and needed far fewer pain killers. [*Arthritis Rheum* 2001;44(11):2531-8] Ginger may work by slicing substance P levels. Herbalists in North America consider it an excellent circulatory stimulant, helping blood flow throughout the body.

Turmeric: What makes curry yellow may also treat inflammation. Turmeric is part of the ginger family and has been proven in animal studies to reduce inflammation, a belief held for centuries in India. The spice, taken internally, may work by inhibiting the production of prostaglandins, which are inflammatory chemicals. It reduces inflammation by lowering histamine levels and perhaps by boosting the production of cortisone by the adrenal glands. [*Ind J Med Res* 1971;59:1289–95] Its main ingredient is curcumin, which is primarily responsible for this histamine-lowering ability. The herb has been found to prevent platelets from clumping up, which guards against atherosclerosis and improves blood circulation. [*Thromb Res* 1985;40:413–7]

Cayenne: Also known as capsaicin, the spicy cayenne is well known for its benefits to the circulatory system. It's traditionally used as a central ingredient in circulatory tonic. It has the ability to open up capillaries that allow blood to reach areas previously restricted because of poor circulation.

Boswellia: This Ayurvedic herb can defend against inflammation and restore blood vessels in connective tissue. It can improve circulation to parts of the body, especially joints that are inflamed due to arthritis. It's the boswellic acid, in particular, that is thought to reduce inflammation. A review of unpublished studies into this herb found double-blind trials deduced that is was effective in relieving rheumatoid arthritis symptoms. [*Phytomed* 3(1): 67–70, 1996]. A number of scientific studies have confirmed the effectiveness of boswellia. In a study of 175 people with arthritis, four weeks of boswellia treatment helped 122 of them reduce pain and stiffness.

Notable Herbs

Hawthorn

Garlic

Ginger

Turmeric

Cayenne

Boswellia

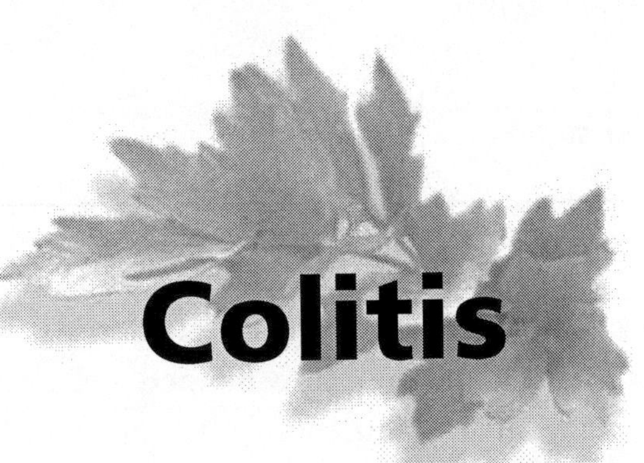

Colitis

Under its full name, "ulcerative colitis," this means a chronic disease of the colon, characterized by inflammation or tiny open sores that form on the surface of the colon's lining. Immediate symptoms include bloody diarrhea, cramping, urgency to move bowels, and abdominal pain. Causes are not known precisely, but it may be hereditary or due to environmental antigens or a person's immune system. Other symptoms may include loss of appetite, weight loss, fatigue, joint pain, anemia, malnutrition, nausea, and fever. It could affect other bodily systems leading to joint pain, mouth sores, skin sores, and inflammation. The unpredictable nature of the disease makes it tricky for doctors to figure out if a treatment has been effective or not.

HERBS TO TRY:

Specific Herbal Concoction: A Bulgarian study looked at the effects of some well-known natural herbs on patients with non-specific colitis. The concoction included dandelion, lemon balm, marigold, and fennel. In half a month, focused pain in the large intestine disappeared in 95% of the patients. As well, regular bowel movements were regained. [*Vutr Boles.* 1981;20(6):51-4]

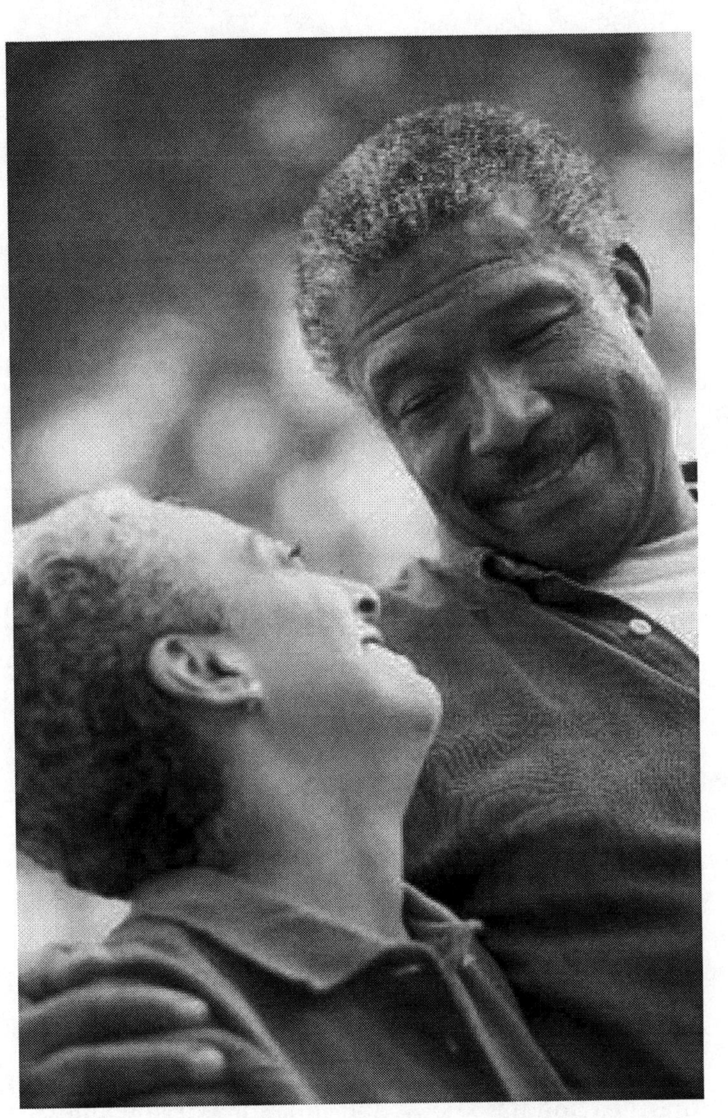

Causes are not known precisely, but colitis may be hereditary or due to environmental antigens or a person's immune system.

Aloe Vera: The aloe plant helps clean mucus from colon walls and acts as a laxative to help improve bowel function and quell the diarrhea effects of colitis. It was proven in a study of 35 men and women randomized to a treatment that combined aloe vera with psyllium – otherwise known as fiber, the well known laxative. Those on the aloe vera combination had more frequent bowel movements with softer stool. It showed aloe vera was an effective laxative. [*Digestion* 1991;49(2):65-71] However, aloe vera does not appear to reduce abdominal pain.

Fish Oil: Although not necessarily a herb, it's been studied as a treatment for ulcerative colitis. In one notable study, patients experienced a decrease in inflammation and wound up less dependent on drugs. Researchers concluded that fish oil was an effective colitis therapy. [*Am J Gastroenterol* 1992 Apr;87(4):432-7]

Boswellia: This herb may help lower inflammation in the colon, which is part of the colitis problem. In one study, 82% of patients taking 350 mg of boswellia three times a day found that inflammation completely disappeared. [*Eur J Med Res.* 1997 Jan;2(1):37-43] Could it be the mystery of the disease, or the herb's effects? It may be worth a shot.

Peppermint Oil: This is a known antispasmodic that can relax intestinal muscles. Study results are not always consistent, but several have pointed to its ability to soothe colitis-type problems. One report found it eased cramping and irritation in the intestines. [*Lancet* 1982;ii:989] In two controlled trials, peppermint oil relieves symptoms of irritable bowel syndrome, closely tied to colitis. [*Gastroenterol* 1998;93:1131–5… *Aliment Pharmacol Ther* 1994;8:499–510] Peppermint is usually best taken in enteric-coated pills that supply between 0.2 and 0.4 ml of oil.

Ginger: Ginger is reputed to help relieve abdominal pain and soothe the digestive tract. Stimulating digestive enzymes, it is an aid in moving food through the body. It also helps relieve diarrhea and has known anti-inflammatory qualities.

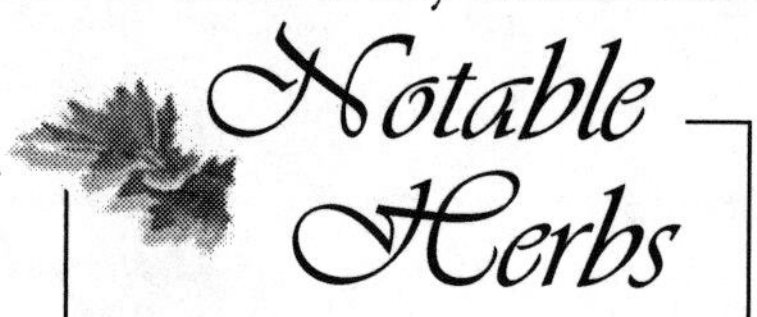

Dandelion

Lemon Balm

Marigold

Fennel

Aloe Vera

Fish Oil

Boswellia

Peppermint Oil

Other Nutraceuticals That May Work:

Probiotics

Blue-Green Algae

Glucosamine

Bromelain

Common Cold & Flu

A cold is a viral upper respiratory infection that is caused by the inflammation of the mucous membranes of the nasal cavity. It's obviously quite common and mostly harmless, with symptoms that include coughing, sneezing, runny nose, sinus congestion, fatigue, muscle aches and pains, and headaches. What separates it from other viral infections is that a cold won't lead to a high fever. Cold treatments work to battle the infection, strengthen the immune system, prevent further infection, and reduce symptoms. Adults get about two to four colds a year, while children may have between five and 10. Symptoms generally improve within a week, and if it last longer than two weeks you should see your doctor. A flu, on the other hand, can become serious for the elderly and people with chronic illnesses such as diabetes or AIDS. Most people recover from the flu in under two weeks. Flu shots can help, but they need to be done each year because the virus constantly mutates.

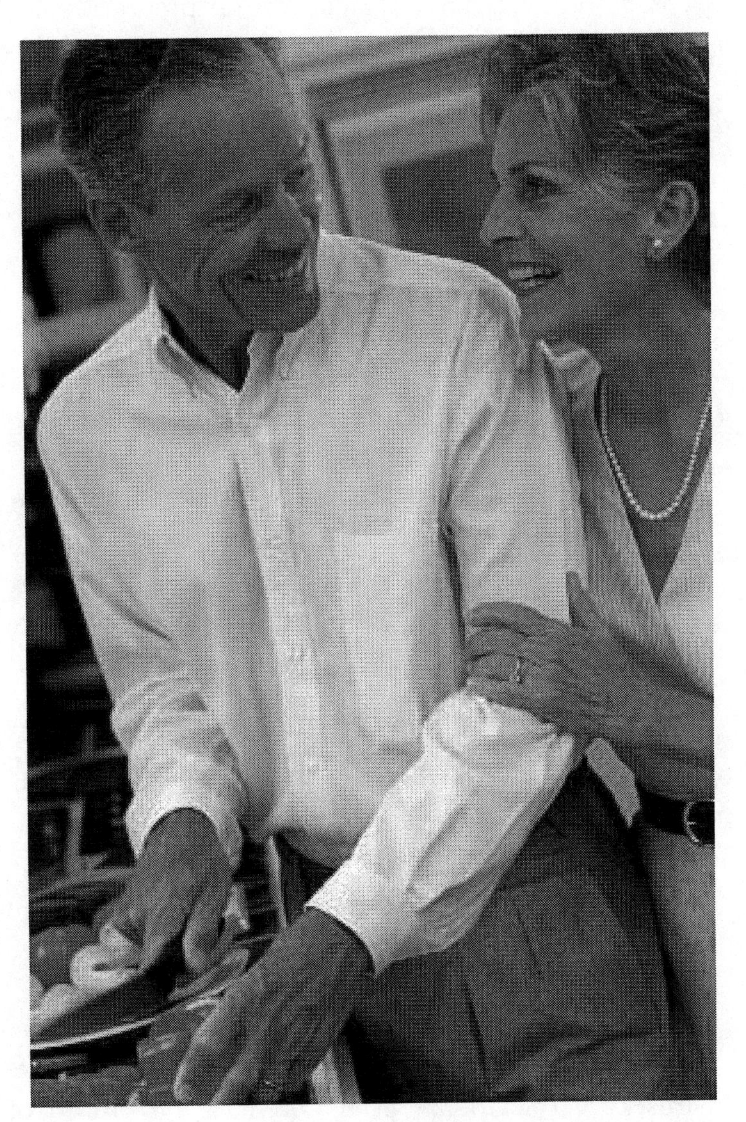

Most people recover from the flu in under two weeks.

HERBS TO TRY:

The Echinacea Debate: This herb helps bolster the immune system to protect against colds and flu. It's been shown to shorten the duration of each when taken at first sign of symptoms. Some studies have proven its effectiveness. One study found that people who regularly get colds reduced their annual number by 35% when taking echinacea. Another study, double-blind, found that echinacea shortened colds by about three days when it was taken at the onset. All is not so magical, though, as one recent major study observed no difference in healthy subjects who took echinacea. In fact, the cold lasted longer in the herbal group than in those taking placebo. [*Annals of Int. Med.* 2002; 137: 939-946] Four years earlier, a study found echinacea ineffective in preventing colds. [*Arch. of Fam. Med.* 1998:7(6);541-5]. Whenever this herb is studied, it makes big news because of its reputed benefits. It won't hurt to take it and see if it works for you.

Garlic: Garlic has long been used as a traditional way to prevent and fight colds and their symptoms. The claims of garlic boosting antibodies to defend against viruses weren't backed up clinically until 2001. A study found that those taking a garlic supplement every day – one that contained its principle health ingredient, allicin – reduced the risk of them catching a cold by more than 50%. According to the Garlic Center in the U.K., over a three-month period during the winter, when most colds strike, only 24 colds were recorded in those taking garlic compared to 65 taking placebo. Although more research is needed, numbers don't lie!

Goldenseal: The root of this plant is a traditional cold-fighter, which appears to reduce inflamed mucous membranes and fight viruses and bacteria by active white blood cells. It is also high in berberine, an alkaloid thought to bolster the immune system (similar to echinacea). It does lack in scientific studies, unfortunately.

Ginseng: Forms of this herb are though to help strengthen the body, allowing it to better contend with viruses such as the common cold. A double-blind study found that those taking 100 mg of Asian ginseng extract, along with flu vaccine, had a lower number of colds and flu compared to people taking only the vaccine. [*Drugs Exptl Clin Res* 1996;22:65–72]

Astragalus: The Chinese have long used this root to boost the immune system, strengthening the body against bacteria and viruses. Astragalus has been linked to the growth of active immune cells as well as increasing the number of stem cells in bone marrow. It also might boost interferon in the body, which can prevent or shorten a bout of cold or flu. No controlled studies on humans have confirmed its effects, but basic science and animal studies suggest its effectiveness.

Notable Herbs

Echinacea

Garlic

Goldenseal

Sinseng

Astragalus

Other Nutraceuticals That May Work:

Vitamin C

Zinc

Vitamin A

Andrographis (Indian shrub)

Constipation

Constipation is most easily described as infrequent or difficult bowel movements. In most cases, constipation arises from insufficient fiber and fluids in the diet. Fiber is best found in fruits, vegetables, and whole grains. Experts usually recommend about 20 to 35 grams of fiber a day. Inadequate liquid makes stool more difficult to pass. Constipation can also be a side effect of some drugs such as iron tablets, pain killers, and antidepressants. Some symptoms include bloated sensations, a sudden decrease in bowel movements, difficulty in passing stool, and less than three bowel movements a week. Herbal treatments work in their own laxative-like way to stimulate the intestines and provide relief from symptoms.

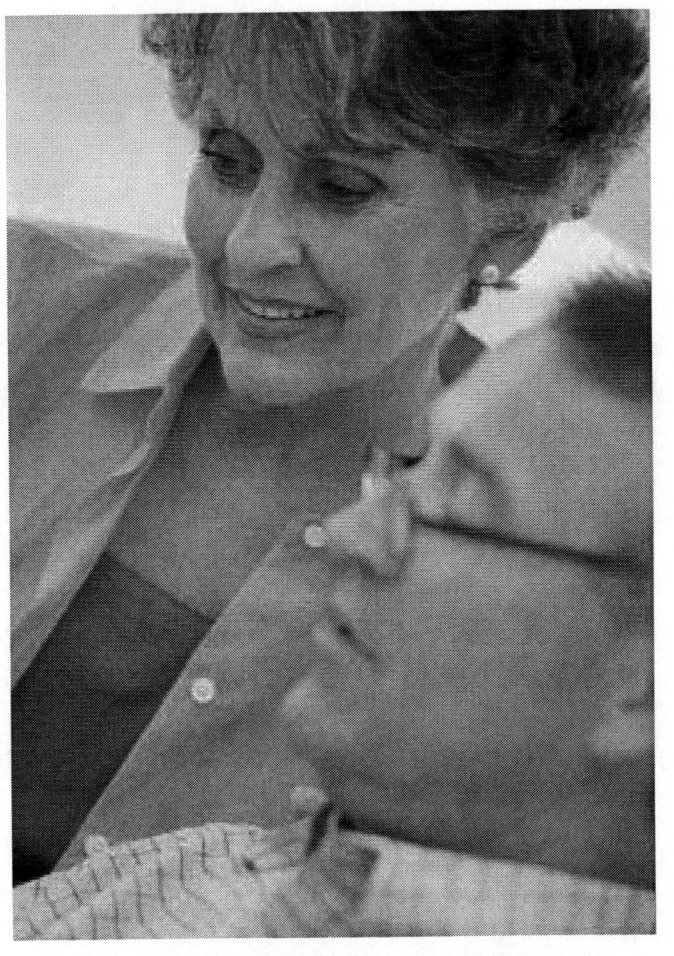

Fiber is best found in fruits, vegetables, and whole grains. Experts usually recommend about 20 to 35 grams of fiber a day.

HERBS TO TRY:

Aloe Vera: The aloe plant helps clean mucus from colon walls and acts as a laxative to help improve bowel function and quell the diarrhea effects of colitis. It was proven in a study of 35 men and women randomized to a treatment that combined aloe vera with psyllium – otherwise known as fiber, the well known laxative. Those on the aloe vera combination had more frequent bowel movements with softer stool. It showed that aloe vera is an effective laxative. [*Digestion* 1991;49(2):65-71] However, aloe vera does not appear to reduce abdominal pain.

Psyllium: This seed is extremely high in soluble fiber and is the main ingredient in such laxatives as Metamucil. Inside the seed is a gel that bulks up the intestinal tract because it is not digested. Combined with water, it swells up and provides lubrication. In a study of more than 170 patients with chronic constipation, psyllium was a superior treatment to a regular over-the-counter laxative called docusate sodium. [*Aliment Pharmacol Ther*. 1998;12(5):491-7] Another study found that psyllium – also known as ispaghula husk – was highly effective in relieving simple constipation. Its use also results in less diarrhea and abdominal pain than the laxative it was tested against. [*Curr Med Res Opin*.1998;14(4):227-33] About four million Americans take psyllium.

Senna: In a study of people in nursing homes, treatment with senna and psyllium worked effectively in relieving chronic constipation. [*BMJ* 1993; 307:769–71] Also an ingredient in many over-the-counter laxatives, this herb alone has been used in ancient Chinese and Indian medicine. Within its chemical structure, it contains glycosides, which are strong laxatives that soften stool, provide a cathartic action and make the intestinal muscles contract. Therefore, you get increased bowel movements. In 1980, a study proved senna effective in about 95% of women who had postpartum constipation. [*South African Med. J.* 1980;57(3): 78-80] The *South African Medical Journal* shows that treatment with senna was successful in 93%-96% of women suffering from postpartum constipation. The year before, senna prevented or treated constipation with patients who underwent proctologic surgery. [*Diseases of the Colon and Rectum* 1979;22(3):149-51]

Flaxseed: Not unlike psyllium, it swells and bulks up in the intestines, creating a laxative effect. When taking this herbal remedy, water is needed throughout the day. Flaxseed helps the passage of stool and clears constipation. It is very high in fiber and is considered safe.

Basil: The seed from this well-known member of the spice rack may actually work as a laxative. One preliminary study found it relieved constipation by bulking up stool in the intestinal tract. [*Maharaj Nakornratchasima Hosp Med Bull* 1985;9:120–36] That was backed up by basil seeds showing similar usefulness when taken by elderly patients post-surgery who had constipation. [*Ramathibodi Med J* 1985;8:154–8]

Notable Herbs

Aloe Vera

Psyllium

Senna

Flaxseed

Basil

Other Nutraceuticals That May Work:

Dandelion

MSM

Cascara sagrada

Congestive Heart Failure

Related to heart disease, congestive heart failure (CHF) is a disease characterized by a decline in heart function, specifically in how it transports blood to other tissues. The heart is unable to empty (pump) blood properly into the vascular system, and there is also trouble accepting blood back into the heart. Underlying conditions include coronary artery disease or hypertension. Common symptoms include fatigue, exercise intolerance, cough upon waking, excessive nighttime urination, shortness of breath, and leg swelling. CHF is the number one cause of death in people over the age of 65. In the U.S. about five million people have heart failure, and roughly 250,000 die every year because of it. The first step is to make lifestyle changes that include a better diet with less salt, exercise, and weight loss. Herbal treatments help blood pressure, circulation, and heart rate.

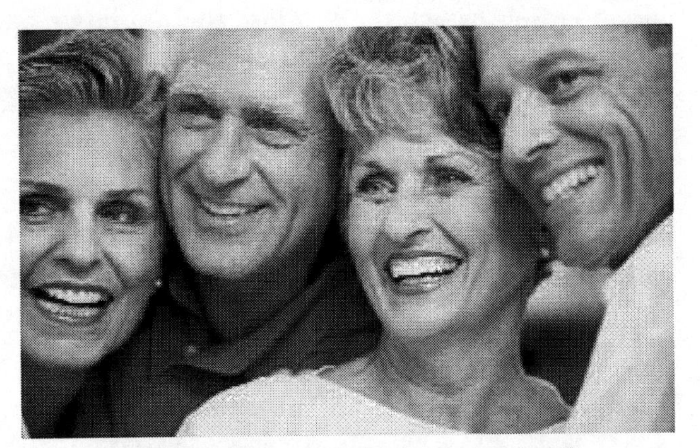

The first step in preventing congestive heart failure is to make lifestyle changes that include a better diet with less salt, more exercise, and weight loss.

HERBS TO TRY:

Hawthorn: *American Family Physician* says this is a "highly promising" herb. Flavonoids, a major ingredient in hawthorn, are widely used in Europe to improve circulation. A study in 1994 found the herb effective in treating patients with CHF. [*Phytomedicine* 1994; 1: 17-24] In a 1996 review of literature, German researchers concluded that clinical trials have shown hawthorn to be beneficial in symptoms of stage II CHF. [*Fortschr Med* 1996;114:27-9] Hawthorn has been linked to better blood pressure and a higher quality of life and mental well-being.

Coenzyme Q_{10}: Of course not a herb, this coenzyme (that occurs naturally in the body) is nonetheless a supplement with much promise against congestive heart failure. Evidence is not all agreeable though, with some studies refuting others. Some of the beneficial results include a 1999 study that showed 22 patients with an increased stroke index at rest and at work and a decreased pulmonary capillary wedge at rest when taking coenzyme Q_{10}. It concluded that those with congestive heart failure may benefit from supplementation of Q_{10}. {*Biofactors* 1999;9:285-9] This and several other studies have prompted *American Family Physician* to believe Q_{10} may have a beneficial role in CHF, but so far its role appears "modest."

Garlic: This herb is well known for its cardiovascular and circulation-improving traits. A major study by the American Heart Association reported that garlic can maintain the elasticity of aging blood vessels, which tend to lose their ability to stretch with time. [*Circulation* 1997;96(8):2649-2655] Garlic helps widen blood vessels as a result of relaxing the muscles that surround the walls, which is why it's a major herb for hypertension. Its effect on blood vessels signals why it may be appropriate for patients with CHF.

Turmeric: What makes curry yellow may also treat inflammation. Turmeric is part of the ginger family and has proven in animal studies to reduce inflammation, a belief held for centuries in India. The spice, taken internally, may work by inhibiting the production of prostaglandins, which are inflammatory chemicals. It reduces inflammation by lowering histamine levels and perhaps by boosting the production of cortisone by the adrenal glands. [*Ind J Med Res* 1971;59:1289–95] Its main ingredient curcumin is primarily responsible for its histamine-lowering ability. The herb has been found to prevent platelets from clumping up, which guards against atherosclerosis and improves blood circulation. [*Thromb Res* 1985;40:413–7]

Cayenne: Also known as capsaicin, is well known for its benefits to the circulatory system. It's traditionally used as a central ingredient in circulatory tonic. It has the ability to open up capillaries that allow blood to reach areas previously restricted because of poor circulation.

Boswellia: This Ayurvedic herb can defend against inflammation and restore blood vessels in connective tissue. It can improve circulation to parts of the body, especially joints that are inflamed due to arthritis. It's the boswellic acid, in particular, that is thought to reduce inflammation. A number of scientific studies have confirmed the effectiveness of Boswellin, although not specifically for CHF.

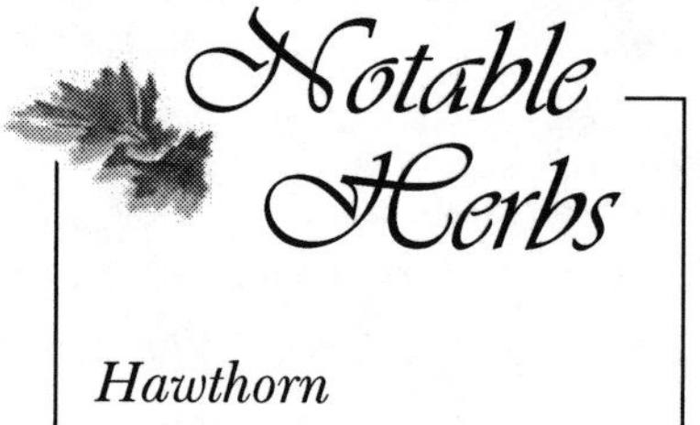

Hawthorn

Garlic

Turmeric

Cayenne

Boswellia

Other Nutraceuticals That May Work:

Coenzyme Q_{10}

Vitamin B-1

Vitamin C

Vitamin E

Carnitine

Taurine

Arginine

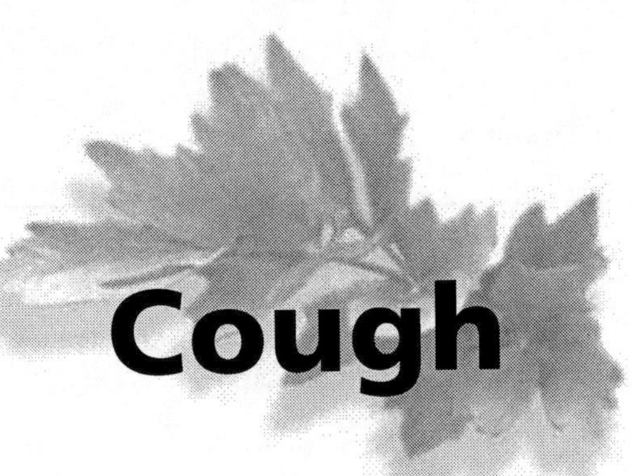

Cough

A cough is a symptom, not a disease, but it can be painful and aggravating nonetheless. A person coughs either to expel mucus, fluid, or other materials from the lungs or due to a physical irritation or allergy. Herbal remedies can soothe irritated airways, help expel fluids, and effectively stop the cough.

HERBS TO TRY:

Echinacea: This herb helps bolster the immune system to protect against colds and flu. It's been seen to shorten the duration of each when taken at the first sign of symptoms. Some studies have proven its effectiveness. One study found that people who regularly get colds reduced their annual number by 35% when taking echinacea. Another study, double-blind, found that echinacea shortened colds by about three days when taken at the onset. All is not so magical, though, as one recent major study observed no difference in healthy subjects who took echinacea. In fact, the cold lasted longer in the herbal group than in those on placebo. [*Annals of Int. Med.* 2002; 137: 939-946] Four years earlier, a study found echinacea ineffective in preventing colds. [*Arch. of Fam. Med.* 1998:7(6);541-5].

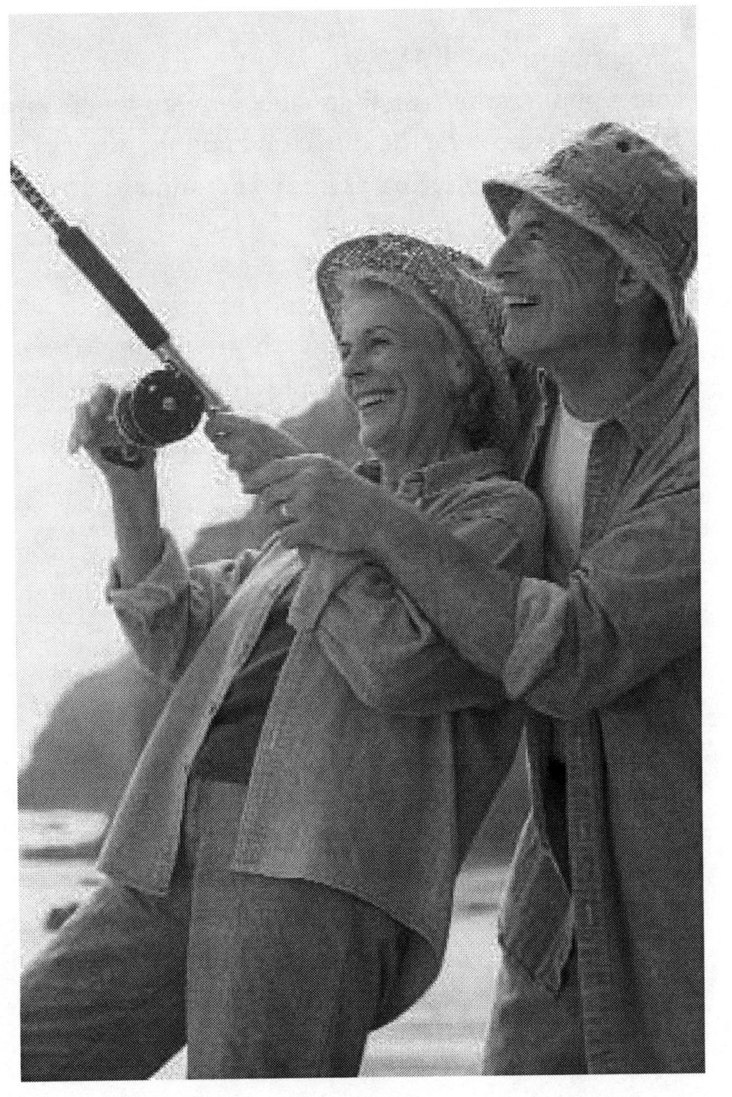

People who regularly get colds reduced their annual number by 35% when taking echinacea.

Slippery Elm: Growing just east of the Rocky Mountains, from Canada down to Mexico, slippery elm grew in popularity in the 1700s and 1800s as a remedy for coughs and colds. The FDA has recognized this herb as safe and effective for sore throats and coughs. Slippery elm, of which the reddish bark is used medically, is thought to alleviate the respiratory dryness that comes with coughing. Although there is a lack of clinical studies, with what is already known, there isn't much use in studying slippery elm. It has soothing properties and is a safe substance to use.

Peppermint: The FDA recognizes this supplement as well in the ability to relieve symptoms of cold – peppermint is an ingredient in many cough and throat lozenges and nasal decongestants. It is meant to soothe the throat and add moisture to the respiratory tract. The soothing effect of peppermint is no secret, as it is common in toothpaste, mouthwash, lotions, aromatherapy, and cosmetics.

Mullein: Not studied scientifically, it is known to act as a demulcent to soothe irritated throat tissues, which in turn brings down the cough. Most evidence of its effectiveness is anecdotal or based on observations. It is approved in Germany for use in colds and coughs. It is best taken in tea form.

Licorice: Battling infections, lowering fevers, licorice root is thought to have antiviral properties that helps shorten respiratory conditions such as bronchitis. It can exert a soothing effect on the linings of the throat and respiratory tract, helping eliminate cough. Its primary ingredient, glycyrrhizin, acts almost like a steroid in its anti-inflammatory and anti-allergic properties. It is an expectorant as well, useful for relieving respiratory problems. Expectorants are used in strong cough and sore throat medicines.

Plantain: Not to be confused with the banana-like vegetable of the same name, this plant acts as an expectorant and a demulcent, approved in Germany for use in relieving coughs and irritation association with respiratory infections. Two Bulgarian studies have found it useful in helping people who have chronic bronchitis. [*Probl Vatr Med* 1983;11:61–9...*Vutr Boles* 1982;21:133–7]

Notable Herbs

Echinacea

Slippery Elm

Peppermint

Mullein

Licorice

Plantain

Cystic Fibrosis

About 30,000 Americans are living with cystic fibrosis, a genetic disease that causes the body to produce an abnormally thick, sticky mucus that clogs the lungs. These thick secretions obstruct the pancreas, preventing digestive enzymes from reaching the intestines to help break down and absorb food, and can cause serious, and even fatal, lung infections. Thus it is a life-threatening disorder leading to nutritional deficiencies and lung damage – respiratory failure is its most extreme consequence. It is a condition that infants are born with, and it can drastically reduce quality of life and lifespan. There have been research leaps recently though, with patients living into their 30s, 40s and beyond as a result of more information on the genetic basis of cystic fibrosis. There is very little evidence about herbal treatments, but below are possibilities.

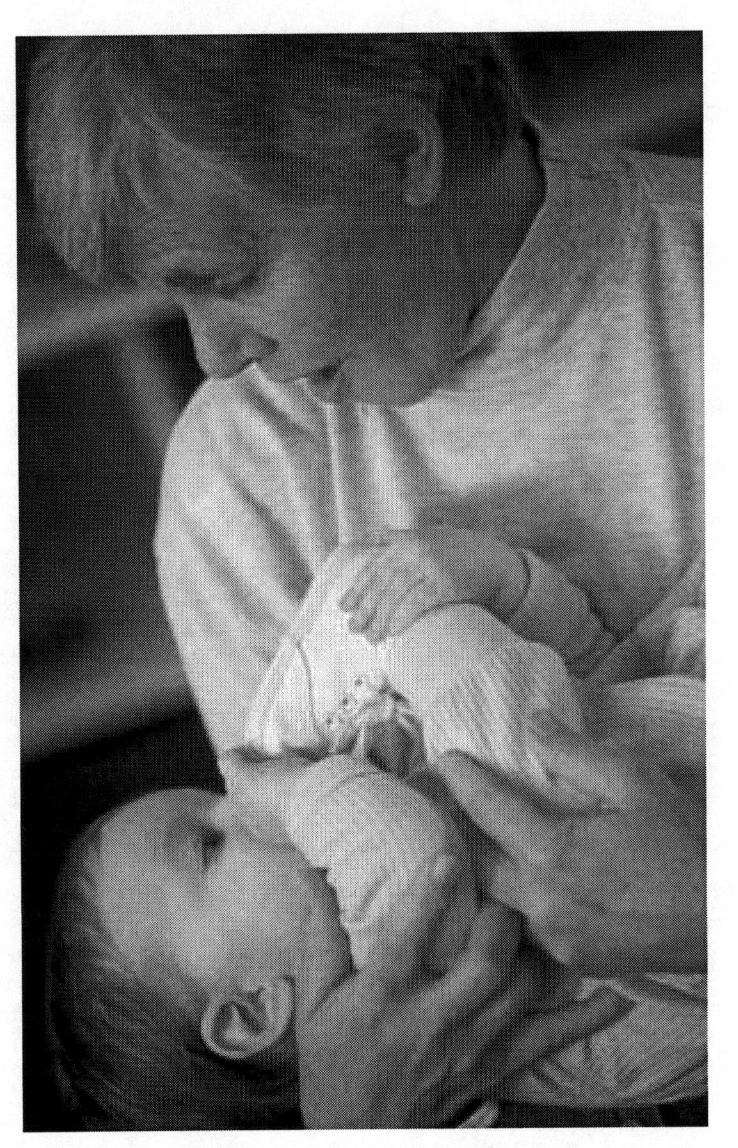

About 30,000 Americans are living with cystic fibrosis.

HERBS TO TRY:

Fish Oil: These supplements contain "eicosapentaenoic acid" (which comes with a far less burdensome acronym, "EPA"), which was found in a double-blind trial to reduce sputum and improve lung function in children who were experiencing respiratory infection because of cystic fibrosis. [*Lancet* 1993;342:465–9]

Vitamins: The malabsorption difficulties associated with cystic fibrosis often leaves patients with a deficiency in fat-soluble vitamins. One study, whose conclusion is supported by most experts, suggested that orally supplementing these nutrients is critical in maintaining good nutrition. [*Clin Gastroenterol* 1998;12:805–22 [review] It's thought that patients with cystic fibrosis need from 5,000 to 10,000 IU/day of vitamin A. For vitamin D, they need 1,000 to 2,000 IU/day. For vitamin E, it's 100 to 300 IU/day. For vitamin K, about 5 mg every three days.

There appears to be particular herb that has any notable affect on cystic fibrosis, but you may find interesting the following natural concoctions suggested by the University of Maryland Medical School:

To help liquefy mucus, they recommend mixing four of these six herbs together:

1. Thyme
2. Indian tobacco
3. Anise
4. Hyssop
5. Licorice root
6. Rosemary

To stimulate the pancreas, they recommend mixing these three herbs in warm water:

1. Dandelion
2. Blue flag
3. Fringe tree

For acute infections, they recommend these six herbs in a mixture:

1. Echinacea
2. Goldenseal
3. Thyme
4. Wild Indigo
5. Elecampane
6. Cayenne

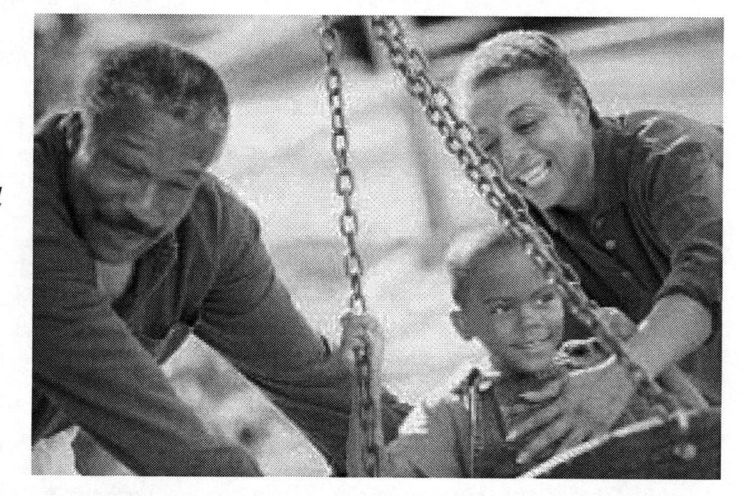

There have been research leaps recently with cysticfibrosis patients living into their 30s, 40s and beyond as a result of more information on the genetic basis of cystic fibrosis.

In cystic fibrosis, it's important to consult you doctor. If you decide to take the herbal path of treatment, have your doctor or a health care provider recommend dosages.

Depression

Depression is a serious psychological disease, characterized by frustration, anger, sadness, hopelessness, lack of sleep, poor concentration, hyperactivity or inactivity, low self worth, suicidal thoughts, fatigue, poor appetite, weight loss or weight gain, or a combination of any of the aforementioned symptoms. There are many types of depression, the most frequent being major depression, dysthymia and bipolar disorder. Life events, illnesses, and a genetic predisposition can cause depression, not the least of which are life-threatening diseases that offer scant hope for the future. This is how much depression can vary. Up to 20% of the population can be affected by depression at some time or another. It can be a temporary affliction or a lifelong battle. Important risk factors include: family history of depression, alcohol abuse, substance abuse, postpartum, and stressful life events. It is believed to be caused by low levels of certain neurotransmitters or the brain's inefficient use of these neurotransmitters. It is much more than just feeling "sad." Herbal treatments target the mind, assisting with brain functioning and acting as sedatives to relax, quiet, and help focus the mind. Treatment of depression is a distinct area, and has potential for side effects – it's best if anyone wishes to begin a herbal treatment, they should first consult a doctor.

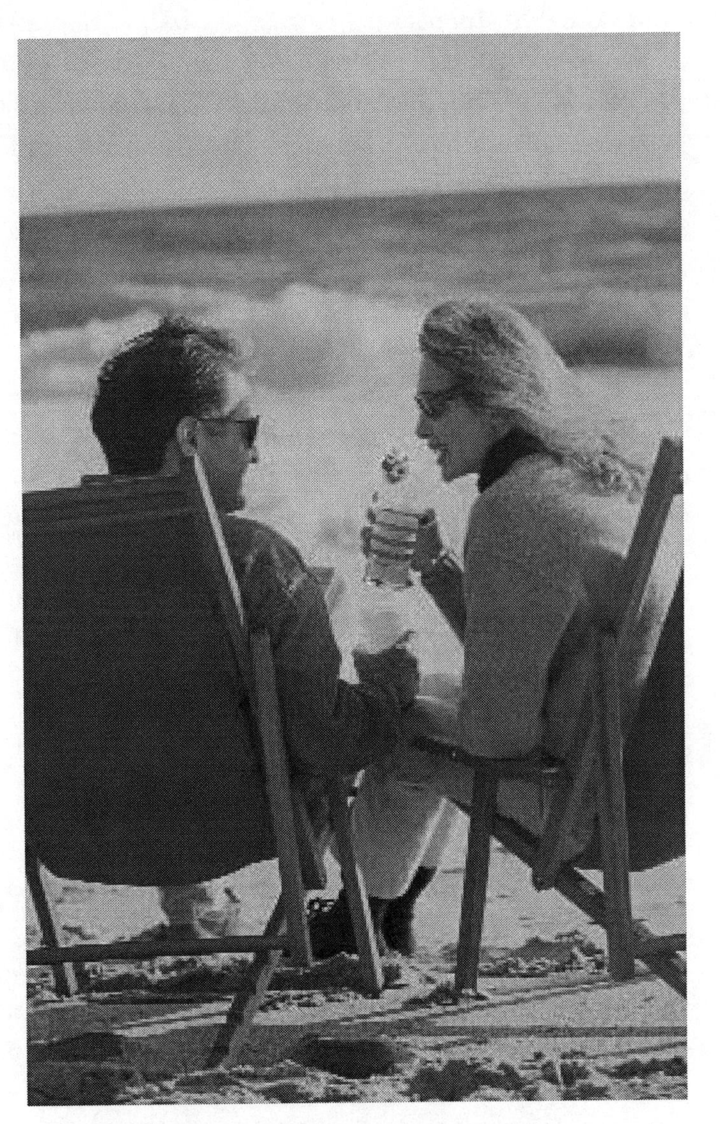

One study showed that St. John's wort extract did relieve depression symptoms, allowing an improvement in mood and a decrease in feelings of sadness, hopelessness, and poor sleep.

HERBS TO TRY:

St. John's Wort: Here's the lowdown: Two studies in the past few years, appearing in the *Journal of the American Medical Association (JAMA)*, declared St. John's wort to be an ineffective treatment for depression. They got a lot of publicity, and definitely should be considered – but they aren't the sole and final word on this herbal remedy. A few previous studies can't be ignored. One showed that St. John's wort extract did relieve depression symptoms, allowing an improvement in mood and a decrease in feelings of sadness, hopelessness, and poor sleep. [*Phytomedicine* 1995;2:67–71] And, in a double-blind trial comparing the herb to Prozac, researchers found the prescribed drug to be only half as effective as St. John's wort in treating people aged 60 to 80. [*Arzneimittelforschung* 1999;49:289–96] Still another study found St. John's wort to be as effective as Prozac – with far fewer side effects. The final note is that this herb should only be used under medical guidance if you have mild to moderate depression. It has been shown to be effective, and in Germany it is regularly used as a medical treatment.

Ginkgo Biloba: It's unclear how this herb works to clear depression, although it may have something to do with increasing the circulation of blood to the brain. The major study backing this herb was conducted on 40 patients, aged 51 to 78, who received either 240 mg of ginkgo or placebo for two months. There were significant improvements in the ginkgo patients' depression as well as an improvement in their overall mental state. There were no side effects. [*Geriatr Forsch* 1993;3:45–53] Ginkgo is sometimes used for "resistent depression" – the kind that is unresponsive to drugs or St. John's wort.

SAMe: This molecule (not a herb) is an amino acid that impacts the brain chemicals serotonin and dopamine, which are thought to elevate mood and lift it above depression. SAMe may be faster in overcoming depression than mainstream drugs such as SSRIs and Prozac. Major clinical trials, including one in the *British Journal of Psychiatry*, demonstrated that SAMe had significant antidepressant effects on patients. [*Br J Psychiatry* 1987;150:724–5.] Unfortunately, mania is a side effect that occurs in some patients taking SAMe, so this should also be taken under the guidance of a doctor.

Notable Herbs

St. John's Wort

Ginkgo Biloba

Other Nutraceuticals That May Work:

5-hydroxytryptophan (5 HTP)

S-adenosylmethionine (SAMe)

Phenylalanine

DHEA

Fish oil

Diabetes

This is certainly a condition that is escalating in the population. It is actually a group of diseases that affect insulin production and use and the processing of sugars within the body. Sugar is your body's central source of fuel and insulin, produced by the pancreas, is a hormone that lets blood sugar enter cells. There are of course two types of diabetes. Type I diabetes is an insulin dependence that usually occurs before the age of 30 and accounts for 10% of all cases. Far more prevalent is Type II diabetes – this occurs in those over 40 or in those who are overweight. These patients have normal insulin supplies, but their bodies fail to use it because of insulin sensitivity. Common symptoms include: frequent urination, increased risk of infection, fatigue, blurred vision, weakness, and leg cramps. ***It's important to note that no one herb has been proven effective in treating diabetes. Many, such as the ones listed below, have shown preliminary signs that they may help regulate blood sugar levels.***

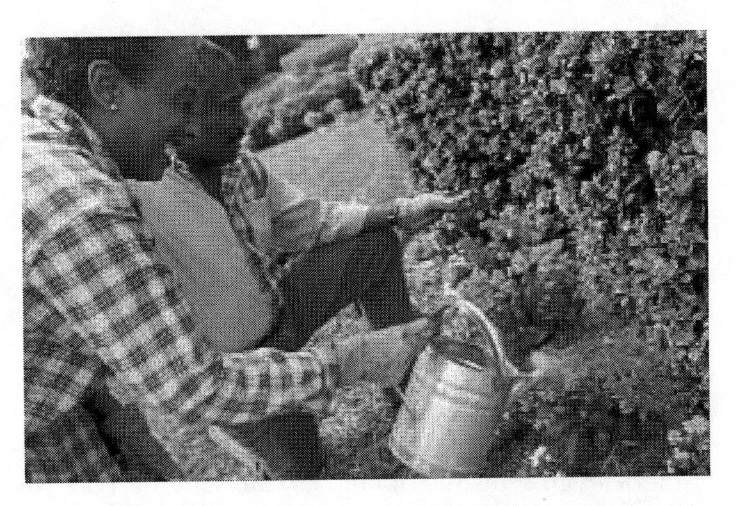

Type II diabetes occurs in those over 40 or in those who are overweight.

HERBS TO TRY:

Cinnamon: One study has shown that cinnamon, taken at one, three, or six grams a day, helps reduce glucose, triglycerides, LDL cholesterol, and total cholesterol in type Type II diabetic patients. The data suggests that including cinnamon in a diet will lower the risk factors associated with both diabetes and cardiovascular diseases. [*Diabetes Care* 2003;26:3215-3218]

Aloe Vera: Taken internally, aloe vera juice may help lower blood sugar and triglyceride levels in patients with diabetes. Two studies were conducted out of the University of Bangkok in the mid-1990s. In the first, with 72 patients aged 35 to 60, researchers noted significantly reduced blood glucose levels in those taking aloe vera, a reduction that continued throughout the trial. [*Phytomedicine* 1996; 3,3:241-243] In the second, with 72 patients aged 35 to 70, blood glucose levels were again significantly reduced in those taking the herb's juice. [*Phytomedicine* 1996; 3,3:245-248]

Chromium: Not a herb, but rather a mineral, this one should be noted as it is backed by some of the strongest evidence to date. One study suggested chromium can help those with both hypoglycemia and Type II diabetes. [*Int. J. of Bio. Med. Res.* 1989;11(2):163-180] Two years earlier, chromium was tested in 180 people in China with Type II diabetes. They found that high doses of the mineral normalized glucose and insulin levels in participants, results that the lead investigator called "spectacular." *[Metabolism: Clin. and Exp.* 1987;36(4):351-355]

Ivy Gourd: A study in India reported that there were major changes in glycemic control after six weeks of using the dried leaves of this herb against Type II diabetes. [*Bangladesh Med Res Counc Bull* 1979;5:60-66] Another study found that 12 weeks of using dried ivy gourd led to changes in glycemic control similar to conventional drugs. [*J Res Ayurveda Siddha*. 1996;XVII:77-84]

Ginseng: There have been a number of small trials looking into American ginseng as a potential treatment for Type II diabetes. There are two longer trials that administered the herb for eight weeks, and both reported there to a decrease in "fasting blood glucose." [*Diabetes Care* 1995;18:1373-1375... *J Am Coil Nutr* 2001;20:370S-380S] There have been others that pointed to ginseng-related glucose reductions as well.

Gymnema Sylvestre: This herb comes from Ayurveda medicine in India. After early animal studies hinted at a possibility in regulating blood sugar levels, two clinical trials indeed did show improved glycemic control when using a gymnema extract than those who used conventional treatment. The data is limited, but it is promising.

Note: Most of these come from a major clinical review published by *Diabetes Care* in 2003. Researchers looked at more than 100 trials investigating 36 herbs and nine vitamin/mineral supplements and their possible affects on Type II diabetes. Although there is insufficient evidence for all herbs, they do appear to be safe. The ones listed above had the most positive results.

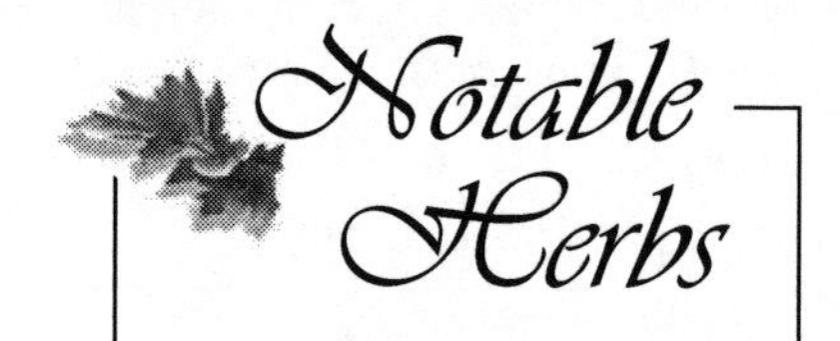

Cinnamon

Aloe Vera

Ivy Gourd

Ginseng

Gymnema Sylvestre

Other Nutraceuticals That May Work:

Chromium

Niacinamide

O. Strepta-cantha

For Diabetic Neuropathy:

Lipoic Acid

Evening Primrose Oil

Vitamin E

Diarrhea

Diarrhea is characterized by urgent, loose and/or fluid bowel movements. Cramping often accompanies it. Diarrhea can be caused by an allergy, virus, mild food poisoning, or improper digestion. It can also be a side effect of a medication or drug, or a symptom of a more serious condition. Herbal treatments help soothe the stomach and intestines and firm stool.

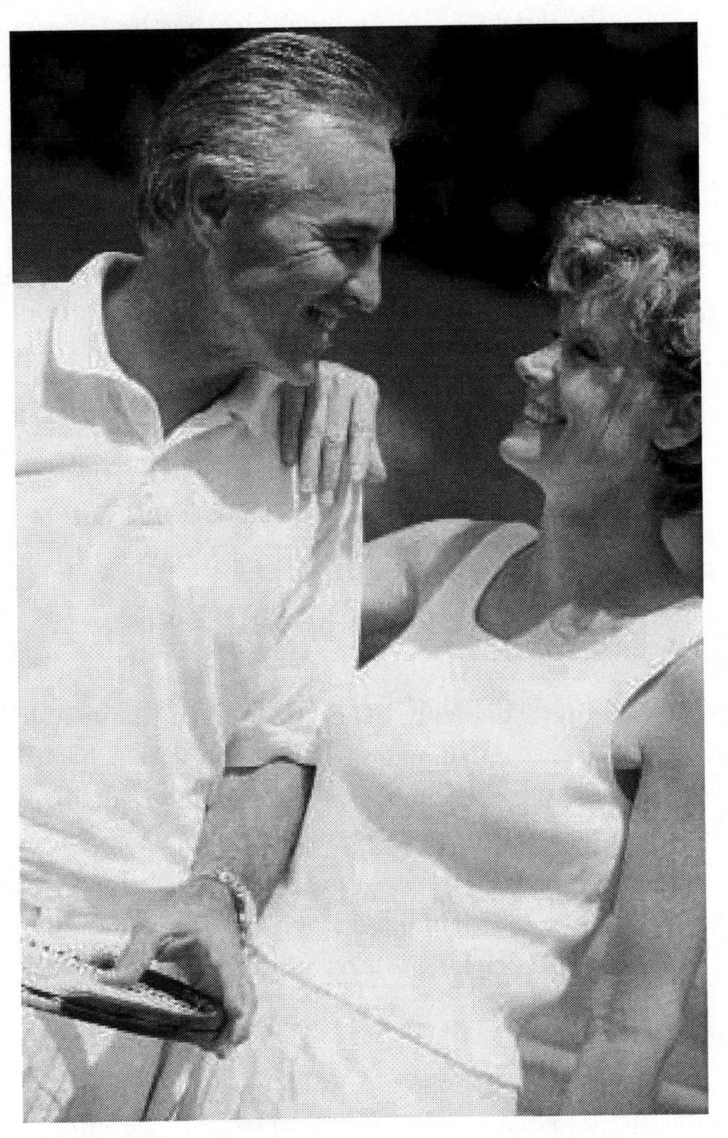

About four million Americans take psyllium.

HERBS TO TRY:

Psyllium: This seed is extremely high in soluble fiber and is the main ingredient in such laxatives as Metamucil. It has been found to reduce symptoms of non-infectious diarrhea. [*Gastroenterol* 1993;104: 1007–12] Inside the seed is a gel that bulks up the intestinal tract because it is not digested. Combined with water, it swells up and provides lubrication. Another study found that psyllium – also known as ispaghula husk – was highly effective in relieving simple constipation. It also resulted in less diarrhea and abdominal pain than the laxative it was tested against. [*Curr Med Res Opin.* 1998;14(4):227-33] About four million Americans take psyllium.

Bilberry: High in "tannins" this relative of the blueberry may have astringent actions that cause proteins to be deposited on membranes lining the intestinal tract. This theory holds that the proteins ward off irritation and restore normal bowel movement. In addition, a fiber within bilberry firms up the stool. It's used traditionally in Germany for diarrhea, and only dried berries or juice should be used.

Aloe Vera: The aloe plant helps clean mucus from colon walls and acts as a laxative to help improve bowel function and quell the diarrhea effects of colitis. It was proven in a study of 35 men and women randomized to a treatment that combined aloe vera with psyllium – otherwise known as fiber, the well known laxative. Those on the aloe vera combination had more frequent bowel movements with softer stool. It showed that aloe vera was an effective laxative. [*Digestion* 1991;49(2):65-71]

Flaxseed: Not unlike psyllium, it swells and bulks up in the intestines, creating a laxative effect. When taking this herbal remedy, water is needed throughout the day. Flaxseed helps the passage of stool and clears constipation. It is very high in fiber and is considered safe.

Green Tea: Contains "tannins", which are thought to help normalize bowel function. It also packs some "theophylline", which is a muscle relaxant that may calm diarrhea by limiting the movement of the intestines. Not tested specifically for diarrhea, green tea appears to be effective in relieving the condition, when studied for an illness that causes diarrhea.

Chamomile: This herb, generally used in tea, may help ease irritation and inflammation in the intestines that can cause diarrhea. It has, though, only been backed up in test tube studies. [*Planta Med* 1980;39:38–50] Many doctors recommend dissolving two to three grams of powdered chamomile or adding three to five milliliters of a chamomile liquid extract to hot water and drinking it three or more times per day, between meals.

Basil: The seeds from this well-known member of the spice rack may actually work as a laxative. One preliminary study found it relieved constipation by bulking up stool in the intestinal tract. [*Maharaj Nakornratchasima Hosp Med Bull* 1985;9:120–36] That was backed up by basil seeds showing similar usefulness when taken by elderly patients who had constipation post-surgery. [*Ramathibodi Med J* 1985;8:154–8]

Notable Herbs

Psyllium

Bilberry

Aloe Vera

Flaxseed

Green Tea

Chamomile

Basil

Other Nutraceuticals That May Work:

Quercetin

Marshmallow root

Licorice Root

Goldenseal

Digestion

Like many other health concerns, digestion problems are usually a symptom of another disease or disorder. However, even those people with a clean bill of health can suffer from the occasional bout of indigestion, flatulence, or stomach cramping. If you have ongoing problems with digestion, it is wise to see your health care practitioner for a professional opinion. Some herbs work wonders for soothing the stomach and aiding digestion, no matter what the cause of your discomfort or concern.

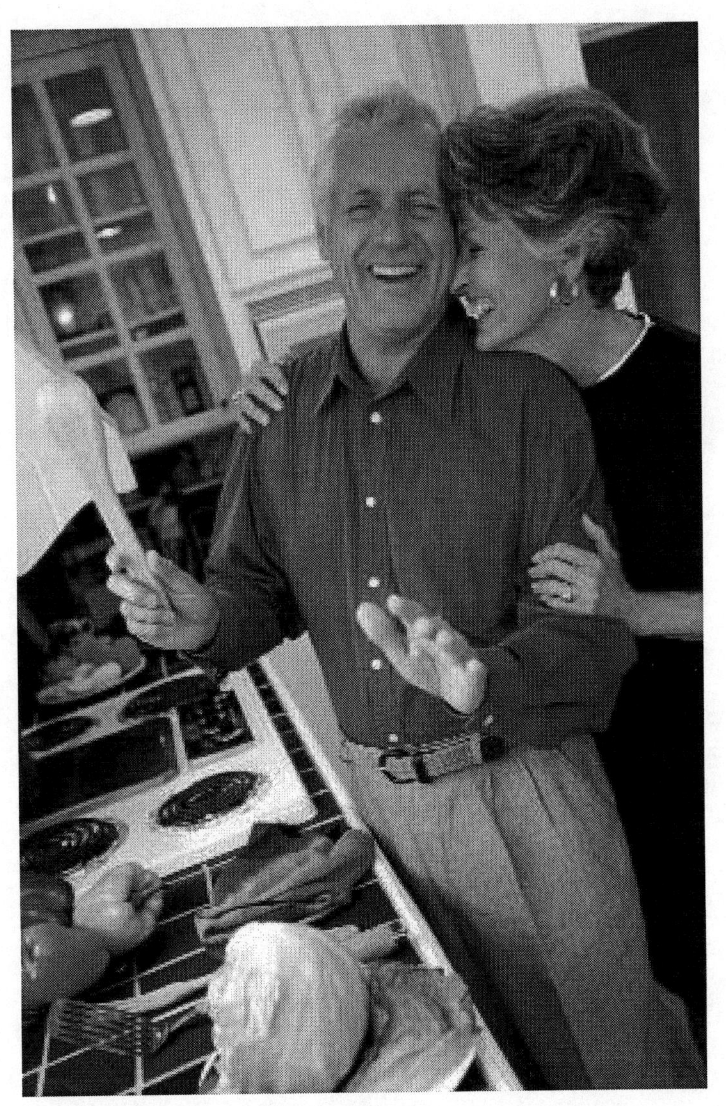

Some herbs work wonders for soothing the stomach and aiding digestion, no matter what the cause of your discomfort or concern.

HERBS TO TRY:

Greater Celandine: This herb has been found to relieve – significantly more than placebo – abdominal cramping, nausea, and that feeling of being full as a result of indigestion. [*Comp Ther Med* 1993;1:189–93] *Caution: This herb has been associated with increased risk of hepatitis.*

Artichoke: This vegetable is mildly bitter, and its extracts have shown time and again to be useful for indigestion. Double-blind trials [*Phytomedicine* 1997;4:370–8] and other evidence shows that artichoke may be especially good when there is liver malfunction and not enough bile is being produced.

[*Phytomedicine* 1994;1:107–15.] The active ingredient for this purpose is "cynarin". So ensure supplements are chalked full of this.

Peppermint, Caraway, Fennel: A combination of these three "carminatives" (which means they relieve gas) has been shown in a double-blind trial to reduce gas and cramping associated with indigestion. [*Phytomedicine* 1996;2:285–91] Two German studies have backed up this conclusion in the late 1990s. Mix three to five drops of essential oils from these herbs, taken with water a few times a day works well. Or, try grinding the seeds of fennel, caraway, and peppermint leaves into a tea. The tea is best taken before meals.

Turmeric: This yellow taint of curry may also play a role in aiding digestion. At least one major study has concluded that turmeric, at 500 mg of powder four times a day (in pills), relieved indigestion. [*J Med Assoc Thai* 1989;72:613–20]

Ginger: This well-known spice has long been suggested for gastrointestinal complications, but it also may be able to help digestion. Specifically, ginger's ability to ward off nausea and inflammation means it can enhance the normal movements of the intestines, which make digestion easier. [*Int J Clin Pharmacol Ther* 1999;37:341–6]

Licorice: In particular, "deglycyrrhizinated licorice" (or DGL) can be useful in stomach ulcers and acid reflux. Its effect on the stomach is proven, and in this case may protect the membranes that line your digestive tract by helping the body produce more "mucin" that shields the negative effects of stomach acid and other harmful substances. [*Biochem Physiol* 1996;113C:17–21] Generally, a few chewable pills of DGL before meals and bedtime are recommended. Unfortunately so far, evidence into licorice's particular effect on digestion remains largely anecdotal.

Notable Herbs

Greater Celandine

Artichoke

Peppermint

Fennel

Caraway

Ginger

Turmeric

Licorice

Other Nutraceuticals That May Work:

Lipase

Eczema

Eczema is an inflammatory disease of the skin. It can affect any part of the body, and its severity ranges from very mild to rather serious. Many infants are afflicted with eczema. Symptoms include dry, red, itchy skin, thickened skin, oozing, lesions, scales, flaking, and peeling. Risk factors include: physical or psychological disorders, vitamin or mineral deficiencies, drugs, and allergies (food, plants, chemicals). It is not contagious, although unfortunately its appearance belies that fact to other people. The condition can be reduced by treatment, although it will always be prone to future flare-ups. There are many types of eczema, and what is also known as dermatitis. Causes also vary, from allergens to heredity to a problem with blood circulation in the legs. Herbal treatments are typically anti-inflammatories, and many make soothing external applications as well.

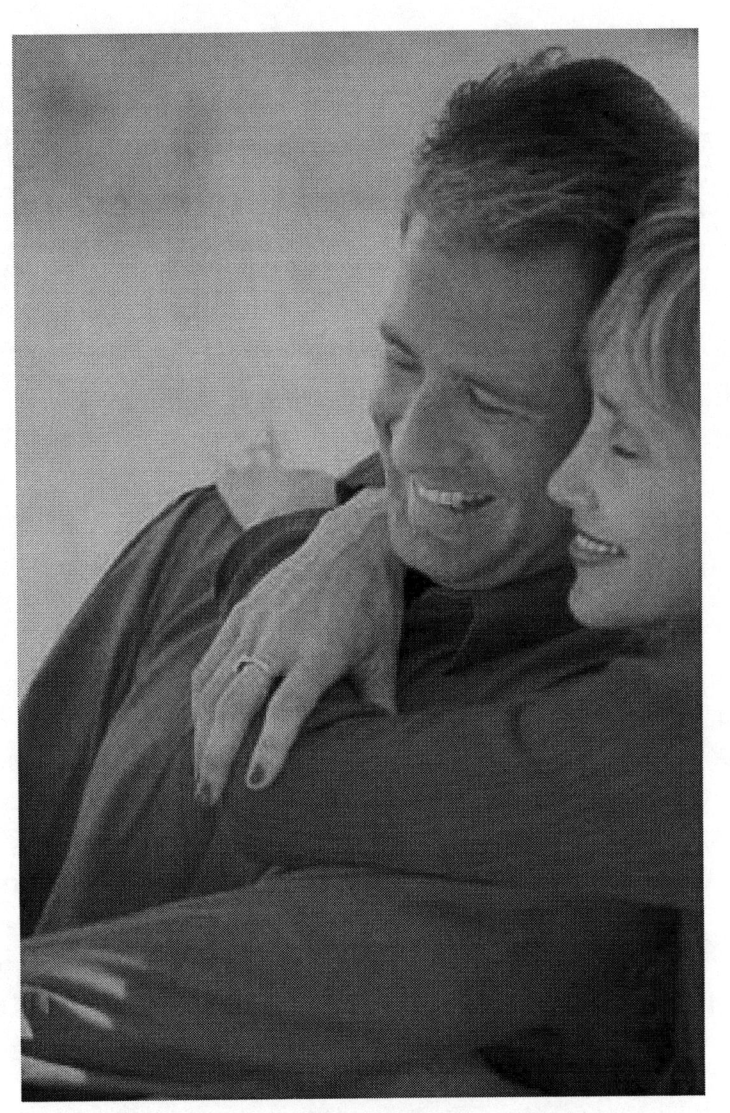

When applied to the skin, the soothing herb chamomile has proven moderately effective in treating eczema.

HERBS TO TRY:

The Evening Primrose Question: The key ingredient here is "gamma-linolenic acid" (or GLA, also found in borage seed oil) which produces a less inflammatory environment. Taking this oil means you are trying to alter the level of prostaglandins in your body, the substances that contribute to many inflammatory diseases, such as dermatitis. Sometimes the skin condition occurs when the body can't properly convert fats into GLA. Thus, supplemental GLA from this oil may be helpful in averting eczema. The *British Journal of Dermatology* reported that patients with eczema had significant improvements when treated with evening primrose oil and were less dependent on steroids. [*Br J Derm* 1984;110:643] Another report in that publication looked at a review of nine trials – all of which reported less itching when changes were made to GLA and fatty acid levels. [*Br J Dermatol* 1989;121:75–90]

Other studies, though, have had less definitive results. Several major ones, that are more recent than those above, have found no benefit of GLA from evening primrose. This would seem to lessen the positive results of previous studies. With no research consensus, see what your doctor thinks about this herb.

Ginkgo Biloba: It may be certain molecules in this herb that act against chemical components of eczema. Applied twice a day, an ointment that contained mostly ginkgo showed that 70% of participants had significantly less skin reactivity compared to placebo. [*Contact Dermatitis* 1998;38(3):123-6] Other evidence has suggested significant anti-allergy affects on the part of Ginkgo.

Omega-3 Fatty Acids: Certain omega-3 fatty acids play a role in the process by which skin cells convert acids into an anti-inflammatory hormone that is used to treat eczema. The fatty acids have proven to have an effect on patients with one type of eczema, atopic dermatitis. [*J. Intern. Med. Suppl.* 1989;69(4):359-62] When fish oil that provided 1.89 grams of EPA (one of the omega-3s) was given to eczema patients for three months, it led to significant improvements. [*Br J Dermatol* 1987;117:463–9] All is not so definite, however, as two major double-blind studies failed to confirm this effectiveness

Chamomile: When applied to the skin, the soothing herb chamomile has proven moderately effective in treating eczema. [*Z Hautkr* 1988;63:184–90] Compared to a typical cream whose central ingredient was cortisone, chamomile proved 60% as effective. [*Meth Find Exp Clin Pharmacol* 1983;5:75]

Notable Herbs

Evening Primrose Oil

Borage Seed Oil

Ginkgo Biloba

Omega-3 Fatty Acids

Chamomile

Other Nutraceuticals That May Work:

Vitamin E

Vitamin C

Erectile Dysfunction

At one time or another, the majority of men have to deal with erectile dysfunction. The problem can be intermittent or chronic. For most men, it is normal and eventually passes. For others, feelings of desire, an erection, arousal, and an orgasm seem like impossibilities. It can be caused by a vascular disorder, an endocrine or hormone imbalance, or is can be psychological (depression, anxiety), physical, structural, or neurological. In most cases, the dysfunction can be treated. Herbal medicines stimulate circulation and work as a nerve tonic to help with blood flow and to lessen the stress and anxiety that some men experience when they feel a pressure to "perform." There is very little clinical evidence to support any herbal remedy specifically for ED, because major journals have not yet attempted to back up what smaller, more focused clinical research journals have conculded. But there are a few options to help increase blood flow. Herbs for this condition should generally be used with the advice of a physician.

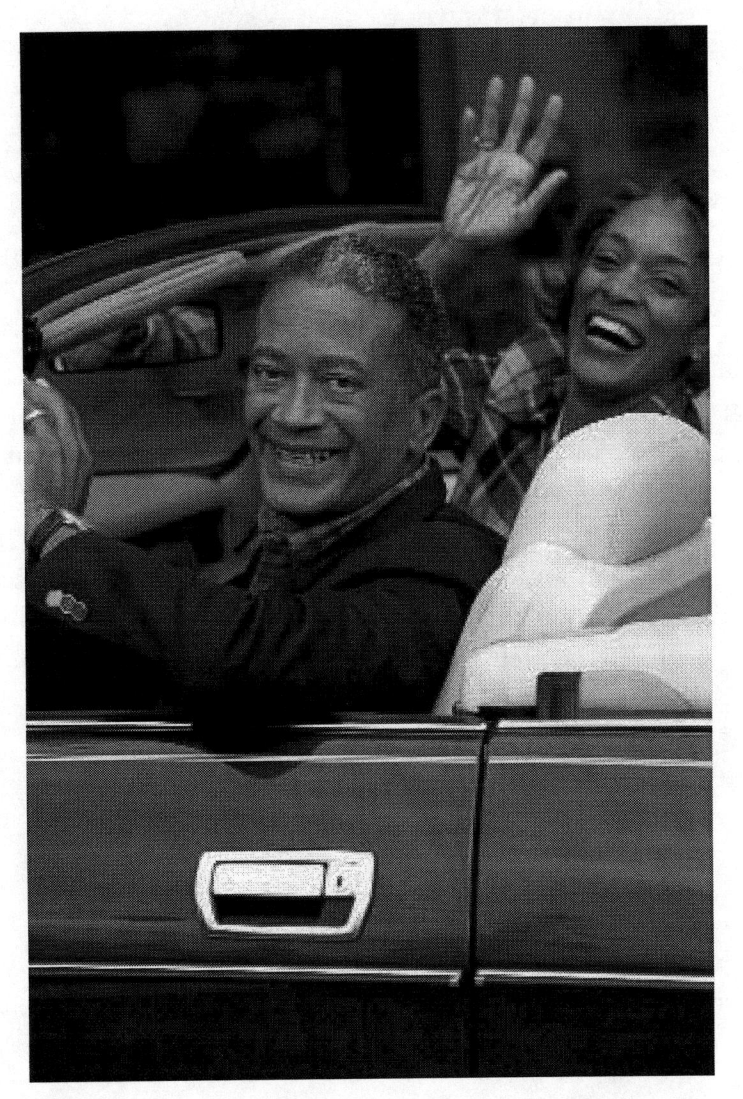

Herbal medicines stimulate circulation and work as a nerve tonics to help with blood flow and to lessen the stress and anxiety that some men experience when they feel a pressure to "perform."

HERBS TO TRY:

Yohimbe: Otherwise known as the bark of an African tree, this supplement contains an alkaloid that increases blood flow – thus is could help stimulate an erection. The ingredient, "yohimbe", has been shown to help treat men with ED in a double-blind trial in the mid 1990s. [*Arch Sex Behav* 1996;25:341] Some people claim it is a sexual stimulate, although scientific study hasn't backed this claim up. It should also be noted that some trials have not come to the same conclusion as that double-blind study. Nonetheless, yohimbe does dilate blood vessels and may help to do so in the pelvic region, regardless of why a man has ED.

Ginkgo Biloba: This herb may be useful, but its effect has been suggested only by preliminary trials. Ginkgo does have an ability to promote blood flow, which could be useful in gaining an erection. Men taking a ginkgo extract (240 mg a day) for nine months experienced improvement in their erections, according to one double-blind (but still preliminary) study. [*J Sec Educ Ther* 1991;17:53–61] A small study of 30 men with ED that was a side effect of medication concluded that about 200 mg a day of extract led to beneficial results in erection in just over three-quarters of the patients. [*J Sex Marital Ther* 1998;24:139–43] Ginkgo is thought by some to be the best herbal remedy for ED caused by pharmaceutical use, especially antidepressants.

Asian Ginseng: Widely believed to help increase libido, ginseng goes back centuries in the Asian culture as part of a tonic that treats sexual problems. There are many kinds of ginseng – American, Siberian, Asian, and more – and some doctors who believe in its effects may suggest rotating between some of the different species. Here, the Asian species has been singled out, because it appears it's been the only one studied clinically (albeit, again, preliminary). A daily dose of 1,800 mg of Asian ginseng extract, taken for three months, helped improve libido in men with ED, as well as showing an ability to promote and keep an erection. [*Int J Impotence Res* 1995;7:181–6]

Notable Herbs

Yohimbe

Ginkgo Biloba

Asian Ginseng

Other Nutraceuticals That May Work:

Arginine (amino acid)

DHEA

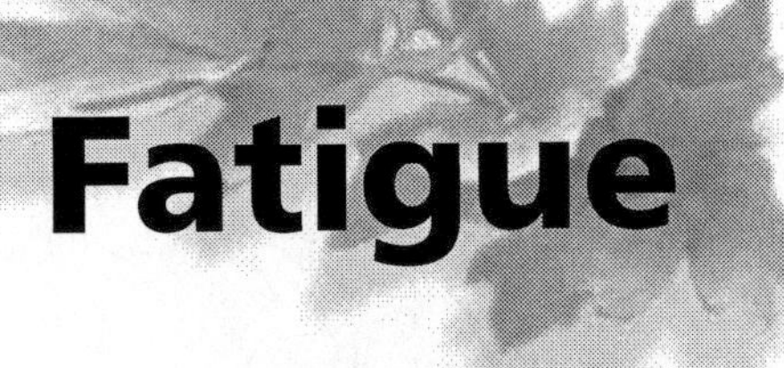

Fatigue

Everybody knows this feeling. Fatigue can be caused by illness, stress, depression, and inadequate sleep. Ongoing fatigue can affect quality of life, relationships, productivity, and general health. For a typical adult, six to eight hours of uninterrupted sleep is critical to health and well-being. It is said that every hour of sleep deprivation causes a 25% decline in overall productivity the next day. Herbal treatments can help "wake you up," but proper rest and relaxation are the real answer to your fatigue questions. For chronic fatigue problems, see the chapter on "Chronic Fatigue Syndrome."

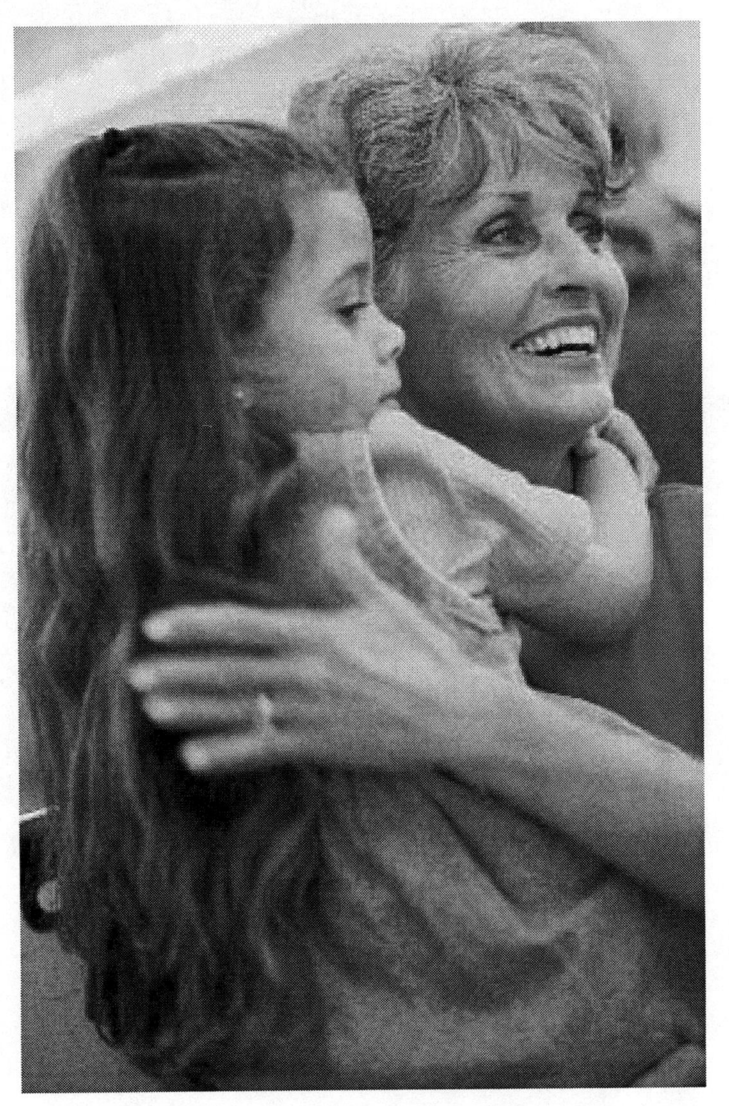

Ongoing fatigue can affect quality of life, relationships, productivity, and general health.

HERBS TO TRY:

St. John's Wort: Widely recommended for treatment of depression, this herb found in the fields near the capital of Newfoundland was tested in patients who had fatigue that had been going on for at least two weeks, but who did not consider themselves depressed. So, could this herb play a role in fatigue only? In 17 women and three men, St. John's wort extract was seen to significantly reduce fatigue after two weeks of treatment, then significantly more than that after six weeks. This herb needs more research to back up this finding. One patient had dizziness

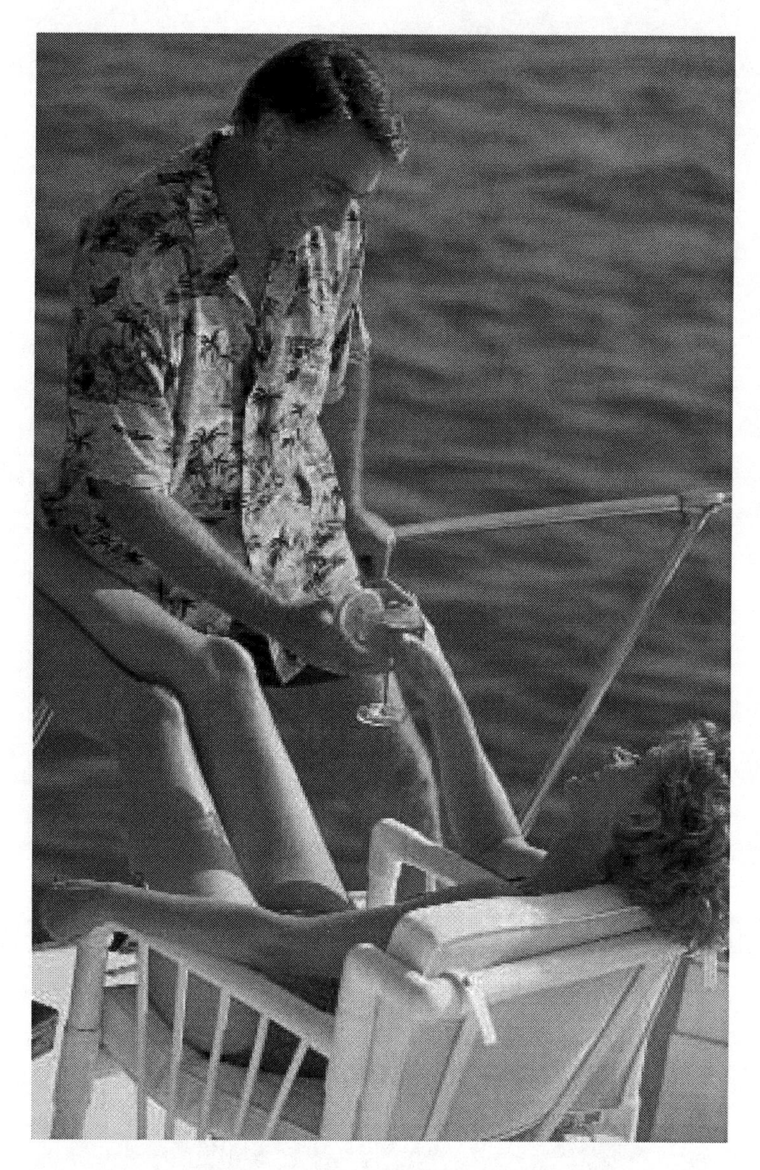

Rhodiola has an anti-fatigue effect with no side effects.

and needed to stop treatment, but other than that no side effects occurred. [*Phytomedicine* 1998; 5(6): 443-447]

Rhodiola: There may be just one study that has looked into the herb Rhodiola and its anti-fatigue capability. It looked at the herb's ability over time to reduce fatigue in a work-like setting – it was a double-blind study on 56 physicians who were performing night duty. Using a special fatigue index, the herb successfully reduced symptoms of fatigue with results measuring memory, calculation, concentration, senses, and total mental performance. Though it was only a two-week trial, researchers believe that Rhodiola has an anti-fatigue effect with no side effects. [*Phytomedicine* 2000;7(5):365-371]

Notable Herbs

St. John's Wort

Rhodiola

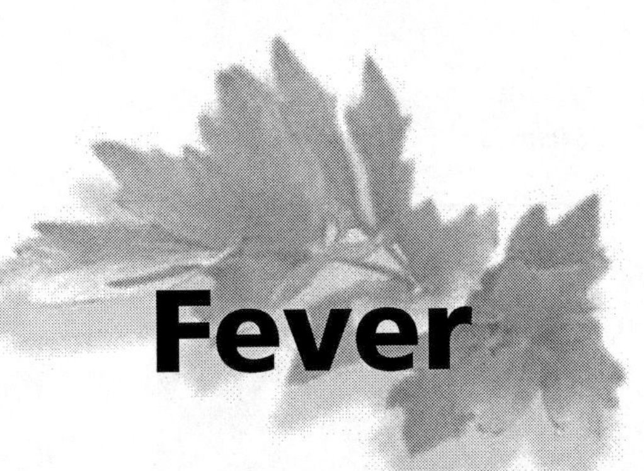

Fever

This is, of course, when your body temperature rises above what's considered the average – 98 degrees F. Normal for you, though, may be slightly higher or lower than this figure, so it's not a definitive benchmark. Fevers become significant if they reach 102 degrees F., measured via the mouth or ear. For children, it's a bit different, as even mildly high temperatures could signal a serious infection. Fever is not a condition, but a symptom and if it's combined with other symptoms – such as nausea, vomiting, phlegm – it may signal an illness. If you have fever plus several other symptoms of sickness, see a doctor.

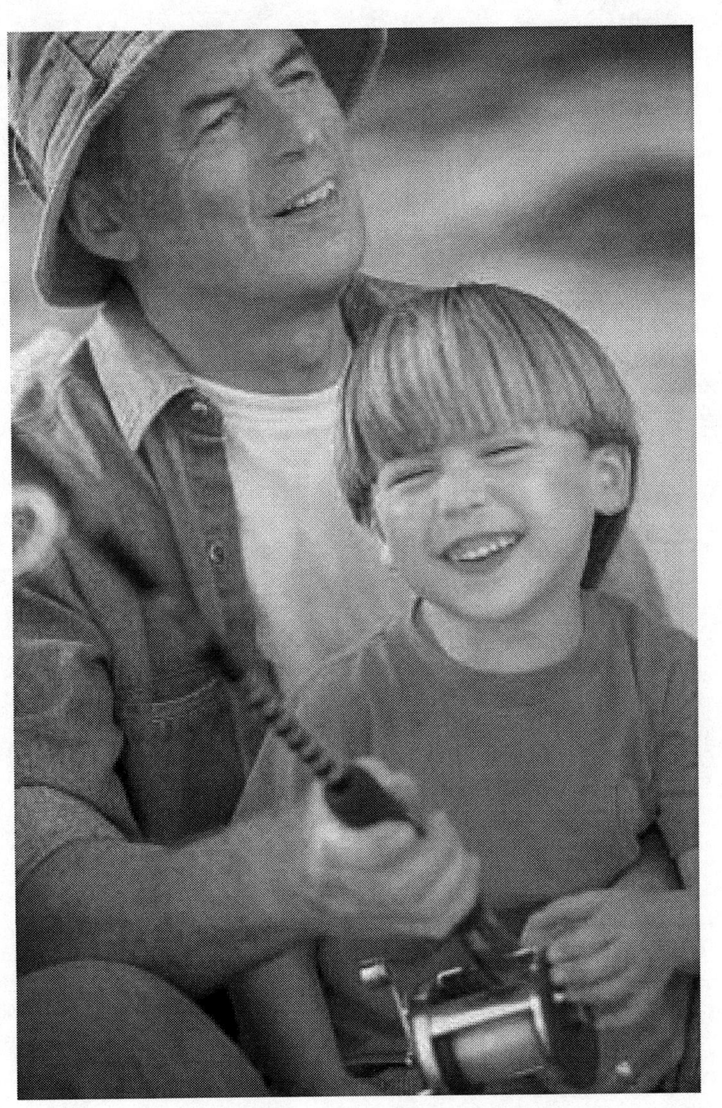

For children even mildly high temperatures could signal a serious infection.

WHY HERBAL REMEDIES AREN'T A GOOD IDEA:

Although certain herbs, such catnip, echinacea, elderberry, and ginger are sometimes used to help reduce fever, it's not generally the best way to go about things. Here's why. When there is a virus in your body, it often thrives in cooler temperatures – your body may be raising the heat to fight it off. Thus, cooling your body temperature is not always the way to go, and this is what herbal remedies are said to do. Fevers typically diminish after a day or two.

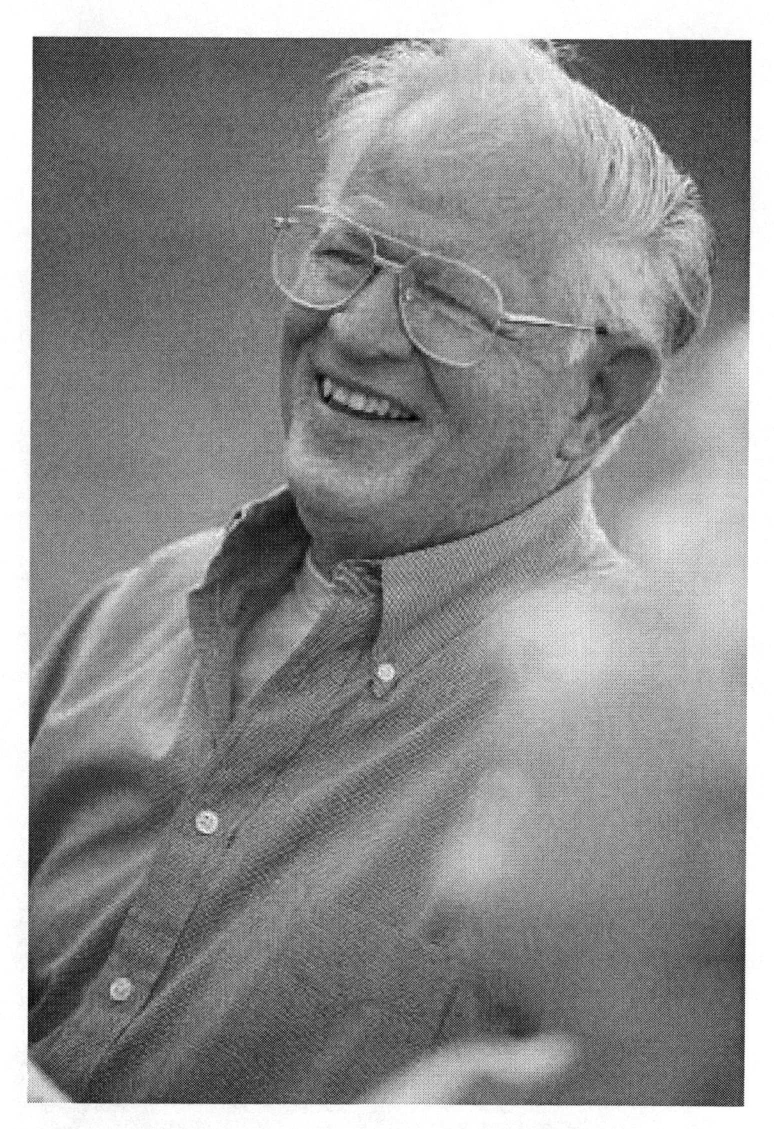

High temperatures are a sign that something is wrong and the body is having trouble fighting if off.

There is no clinical evidence supporting any herbal treatments specifically for fever. High temperatures as indicated above are a sign that something is wrong and the body is having trouble fighting if off. In cases of high fever (especially infants and children!) you should see your health care provider immediately. Herbs shouldn't be taken to lower temperature without first getting medical advice.

Fibromyalgia

This mysterious disease continues to baffle doctors. Affecting between three and eight million Americans and the second biggest cause of join pain, its cause is still unknown. Hereditary factors, physical trauma, and depression may all play a role in fibromyalgia. It's a bit of a mystery as to how many people actually have the condition as it can easily go undiagnosed. Eight out of 10 people with fibromyalgia are women, but it can strike either gender at any age. The complex condition is characterized by chronic, widespread pain in the muscles and soft tissues in the joints, most often centering on the neck, shoulders, spine, and hips. Pain and discomfort continue to reoccur through the body, you wake up in the morning with stiffness, and symptoms are almost always worse in extreme weather – cold or humid. It often induces chronic fatigue, a loss of energy and often severe depression. The symptoms also can include headaches, bloating, irritable bladder, difficulty concentrating, and alternating diarrhea and constipation. Herbal cures, and other supplements target the inflammation and alleviate the depressive symptoms associated with a degenerative, chronic disease. None have been specifically tested against fibromyalgia.

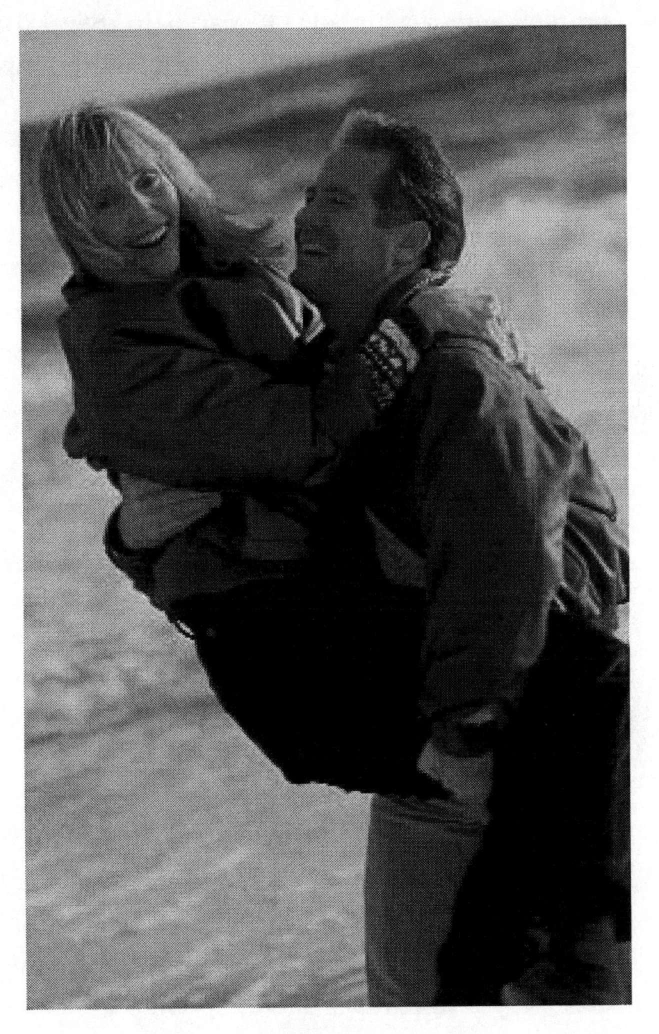

Eight out of 10 people with fibromyalgia are women, but it can strike either gender at any age.

HERBS & OTHERS TO TRY:

SAMe: Study found that S-adenosyl-methionine (SAMe) – not a herb but an activated form of an amino acid – reduced the number of trigger points and painful sites in fibromyalgia sufferers, and placebo did not. Depression was also limited. They concluded it was a safe, effective therapy for fibromyalgia, although the study is now 17 years old. [*Am. J. of Medicine* 1987:83(5A):39-49] But since then, two other studies have backed up SAMe's ability to decrease symptoms and lower depression with 200 mg injected and 200 to 400 mg orally twice daily.

5-HTP: Because fibromyalgia sufferers often show low levels of serotonin in their blood, supplementing with 5-HTP may help. Several trials, including a double-blind trial in 1990, found that 300 mg of 5-HTP a day relieved symptoms of the painful joint disease. [*J Int Med Res* 1990;18:201–9]

Amino Acids: These are the essential building blocks of protein and can be linked to hormonal imbalances, mood swings, lack of sleep, and pain. Low levels are associated with the possibility of fibromyalgia. One in particular, tryptophan, is thought to help relieve pain in these patients, as patients with low levels were in more distress. Tryptophan is critical in the production of serotonin also – and serotonin deficiency may be a reason that pain transmitters are far higher in fibromyalgia patients.

Ginkgo Biloba & Coenzyme Q_{10}: A controlled study into this supplemental combination is now in the works after a preliminary study found 200 mg of each led to positive results in fibromyalgia patients. Ginkgo is thought to improve mental clarity, cognitive function, and help reduce depression in fibromyalgia patients. In the study, patients reported improved quality of life – 64% claimed to be better and only nine percent did not. This matched a clinical "quality of life score" that improved for most patients. [J Int Med Res 2002 Mar-Apr;30(2):195-9]

Cayenne: Also known as capsaicin, this cream (sold over the counter) is meant to provide short-term relief of arthritis and fibromyalgia. One of its primary ingredients is found in chili peppers—it's what makes them hot—and can lessen pain when put on the skin. Capsaicin works by decreasing the level of substance P, which is a neuropeptide that communicates pain sensations. With fewer impulses sent via substance P, you feel less pain. It needs to be applied three or four times a day. In one study, 100 arthritic patients received capsaicin cream or placebo – those taking the chili pepper ingredient had significantly more relief from pain, 80% of them experiencing pain reduction after two weeks. [*Clin Ther.* 1991;13(3):383-95]

Notable Herbs

Ginkgo Biloba

Cayenne

Other Nutraceuticals That May Work:

Coenzyme Q_{10}

SAMe

5-HTP

Various Amino Acids

Vitamin E

Blue-Green Algae

Gallstones

Although women are most often affected by gallstones, they also occur in men. Gallstones are hard formations of calcium, cholesterol, and bile salts that form in the gallbladder. Gallstones can block the bile duct, causing infection and even death. Fever, jaundice, nausea, vomiting, loss of appetite, and constant pain following meals are common symptoms. First course of action should include dietary changes: more water, less fat, and low cholesterol (this means as close to vegetarian as possible). Herbal remedies, which have not received a vast amount of attention from medical literature, may help to break up the stones, as well as alleviate the pain associated with the condition.

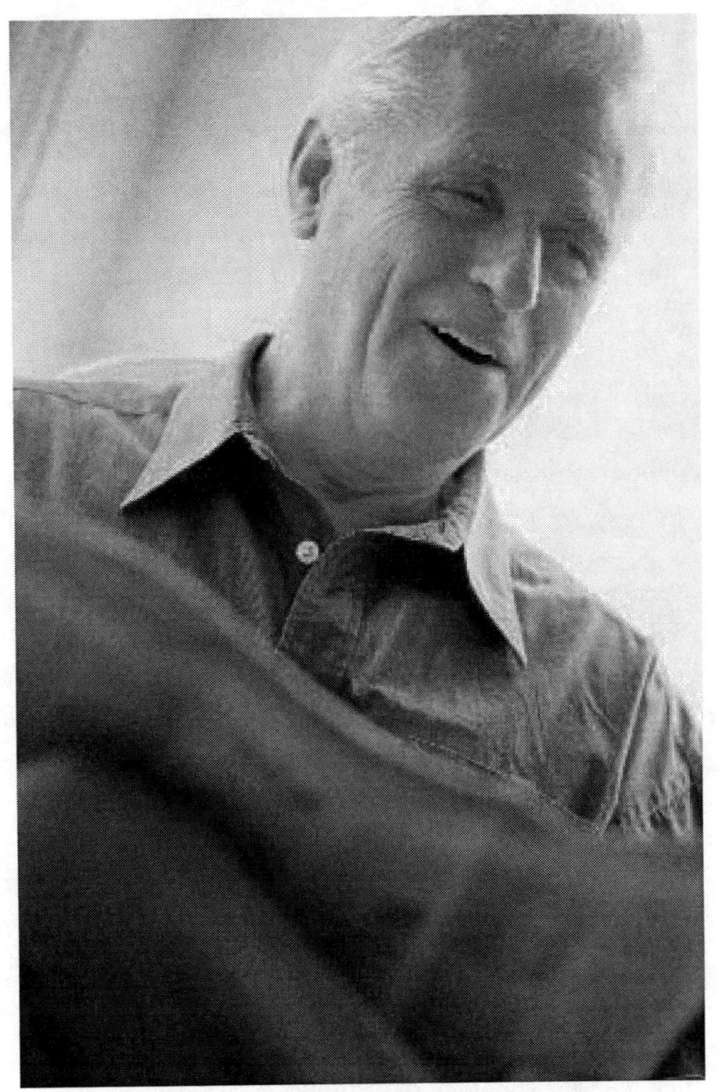

Although women are most often affected by gallstones, they also occur in men.

HERBS TO TRY:

Milk Thistle: This prickly herb grows worldwide, and its seeds are used medicinally. It is known to treat diseases of the liver and gallbladder. It stimulates the production of bile and increases its solubility. Herein lies its potential effect on gallstones. One study that looked into "silymarin" (the active ingredient in milk thistle) concluded that 420 mg a day helped lower the level of cholesterol in bile. [*J Hepatol* 1991;12:290-5] This is an effective way to reduce the formation of

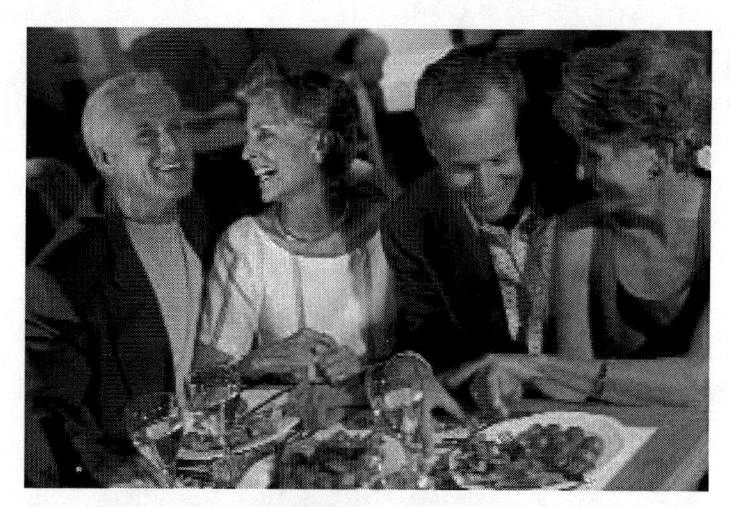

Patients taking 420mg a day of Silymarin for 30 days effectively reduced the formation of gallstones.

gallstones. Patients took that dosage for 30 days.

Peppermint: Another substance that has tested positive for preventing cholesterol crystals from forming in bile are "terpenes" – namely, the compounds found in menthol. What's menthol got to do with it? It happens to be a major component of peppermint. So, as we break it down to the terpenes level, we find that it reduces the risk of gallstones within bile. [*Klin Wochenschr* 1987;65:458-62] What else? One study showed that a mix of essential oils were effective in actually dissolving gallstones that did form! [*Postgrad Med J* 1985;61:313-6] As it turns out, peppermint is the closest available herbal oil to the mixture that was used. *Caution: consult your doctor before using this to treat gallstones.*

Turmeric: The spice that contains "curcumin" and turns curry dishes yellow has been tested on treating gallstones. In Germany, whose approach to herbal cures is more progressive than any other country, turmeric has been endorsed for use on gallstones. It has reduced the size of gallstones significantly in animal studies. Turmeric has shown an ability to protect the liver from toxic compounds.

Celandine: This herb is widely touted for its ability to treat gallstones and help the liver function properly. There are compounds within the herb that may soothe the muscles along the biliary tract, which will help with the flow of bile and relieve stress on the abdomen. Its principle ingredient, chelidonine, has been linked to significantly helping with symptoms of gallstones.

Notable Herbs

Milk Thistle

Peppermint

Turmeric

Celandine

Other Nutraceuticals That May Work:

Vitamin C

Lecithin

Taurine
(an amino acid)

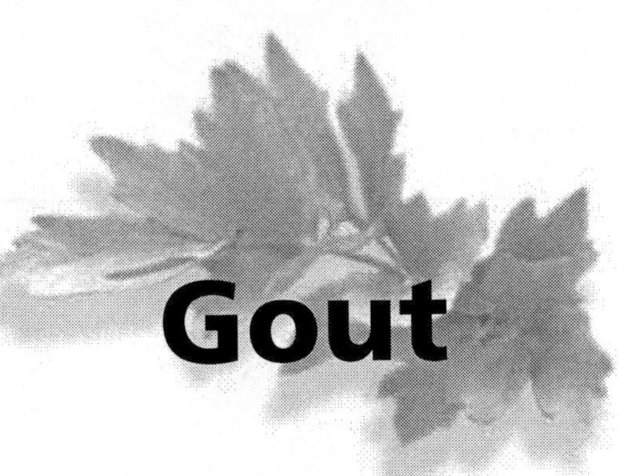

Gout

Often afflicting the big toe, gout is a type of arthritis. It can affect anyone, but is most common in men over 40. Women occasionally suffer gout following menopause. The best news about gout is that it affects less than one percent of the population. A report in the British Medical Journal *(1995) said if a doctor has 2,000 patients, 15 men and three women will have a tendency to gout. It also said the condition has long periods of absence, then will suddenly spring to life: when it comes, it does so quickly and violently, without any warning at all. Within a day one or two of your joints will appear swollen, and will be very painful. In fact, gouty arthritis can be excruciating and has been described as feeling like a part of you is on fire. Visibly, the main signs of gouty arthritis are a swollen joint and red, scaly skin. If there is pain, gout is a strong possibility. It is caused by a build-up of uric acid in the blood stream due to over-production – this is most often linked to too many "purines" in the diet. Risk factors include: family history, leukemia, or the use of certain drugs. What happens is that uric acid deposits form crystals in joints in the feet and hands – this is what the pain and inflammation is. The principle course of action is to alter your diet – eat less items that are chalked full of purines. Ask your doctor what diet he recommends. Very few herbs have been linked to helping with the pain of gout and inflammation, and minimal clinical evidence, yet there are several supplements that might help relieve you from the agony of gout.*

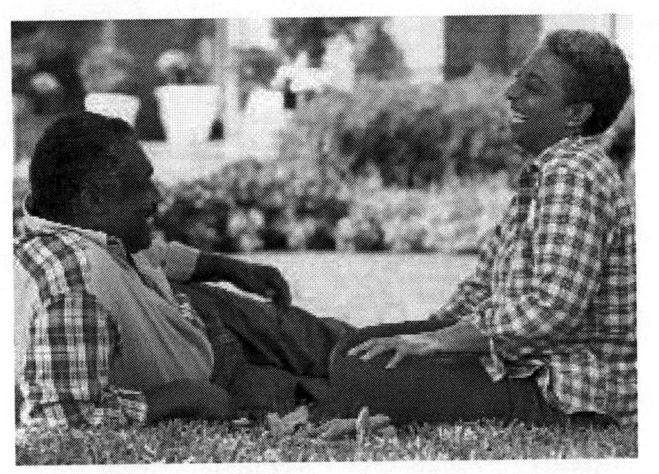

If a doctor has 2,000 patients, 15 men and three women will have a tendency to gout.

SUPPLEMENTS TO TRY:

Bromelain: This enzyme found in pineapples is available as a supplement. Because of what's known about its action, some experts recommend bromelain for someone with gout, at about 200 to 400 mg daily, to be used between meals as many as three times a day. (If you take it while eating it will not act as anti-inflammatory, and instead aid digestion.) Bromelain inhibits the proteins that promote inflammation. It may help relieve the swelling and the pain of a gout attack. Regular use of bromelain could prevent gout as well.

Flaxseed oil: Also known as linseeds, flaxseeds have therapeutic value in the oil derived from them. It comes from the flax plant, historically a healing herb first found in Europe. This oil is high in omega-3 fatty acids, one of which – eicosapentaenoic acid (or "EPA") – helps stop inflammation. In regards to gout, flaxseed oil may lessen the pain and reduce swelling.

Cod liver oil: Taking these pills has long been thought to help reduce the level of enzymes that cause arthritic damage. As reported by the BBC, a study in early 2004 out of Cardiff University (U.K.) found that cod liver oil may help prevent arthritis – 86% of arthritic patients taking this oil showed significantly reduced enzyme levels that cause cartilage damage compared to just 26% on placebo. Since gout is a form of arthritis and both are linked to inflammation, cod liver oil's anti-inflammatory action may be useful in gout.

Cayenne: Also known as capsaicin, this cream (sold over the counter) is meant to provide short-term relief of arthritis. One of its primary ingredients is found in chili peppers—it's what makes them hot—and can lessen pain when put on the skin. Capsaicin works by decreasing the level of substance P, which is a neuropeptide that communicates pain sensations. With fewer impulses sent via substance P, you feel less pain. It needs to be applied three or four times a day. One study found that just a 0.025% capsaicin cream worked significantly better than normal cream for osteoarthritis of the knee. [Seminars in Arthritis and Rheumatism 994;23:Suppl 3:25-33]. In another study, 100 arthritic patients received capsaicin cream or placebo – those taking the chili pepper ingredient had significantly more relief from pain, 80% of them experiencing pain reduction after two weeks. [*Clin Ther*. 1991;13(3):383-95]

Quercetin: A bioflavanoid and a natural antihistamine, quercetin may have some anti-inflammatory properties, and is thought to inhibit a particular enzyme that creates uric acid. It hasn't been tested in humans, but studies in test tubes are fairly positive. It succeeded in inhibiting an enzyme that plays a big role in gout [J *Allergy Clin Immunol* 1984;73:801–9] More research needs to be done into this supplement.

Autumn Crocus: It's possible this herb may help with a case of gout. The drug colchine, which is a conventional treatment for gout, originally came from this plant. Colchine helps limit the amount of white blood cells that swarm to the gouty area, because once they arrive they make inflammation and pain much worse. It has high toxicity though, and should only be used under medical guidance.

Notable Herbs

Cayenne

Autumn Crocus

Other Nutraceuticals That May Work:

Bromelain

Flaxseed Oil

Cod Liver Oil

Quercetin

Vitamin E

Vitamin C

Grave's Disease

An autoimmune disease, Grave's is characterized by the overfunctioning of the thyroid gland – it is the most common form of "hyperthyroidism." In this disease, your immune system mistakenly attacks the thyroid gland, forcing it to produce too much "thyroxine" (a thyroid hormone). Too much thyroxine can cause the body's metabolism to increase dramatically, and that can bring on any number of significant health problems. Grave's is fairly rare, and not usually life-threatening. Symptoms can include insomnia, weight loss, fever, heat intolerance, fast heart rate, nervousness, shakiness, menstrual changes, and anxiety. There unfortunately is no real way to prevent the immune system from attacking the thyroid, but herbal cures will help boost the immune system function. For herbal remedies on insomnia, fever, and anxiety, see the chapters on each in this book.

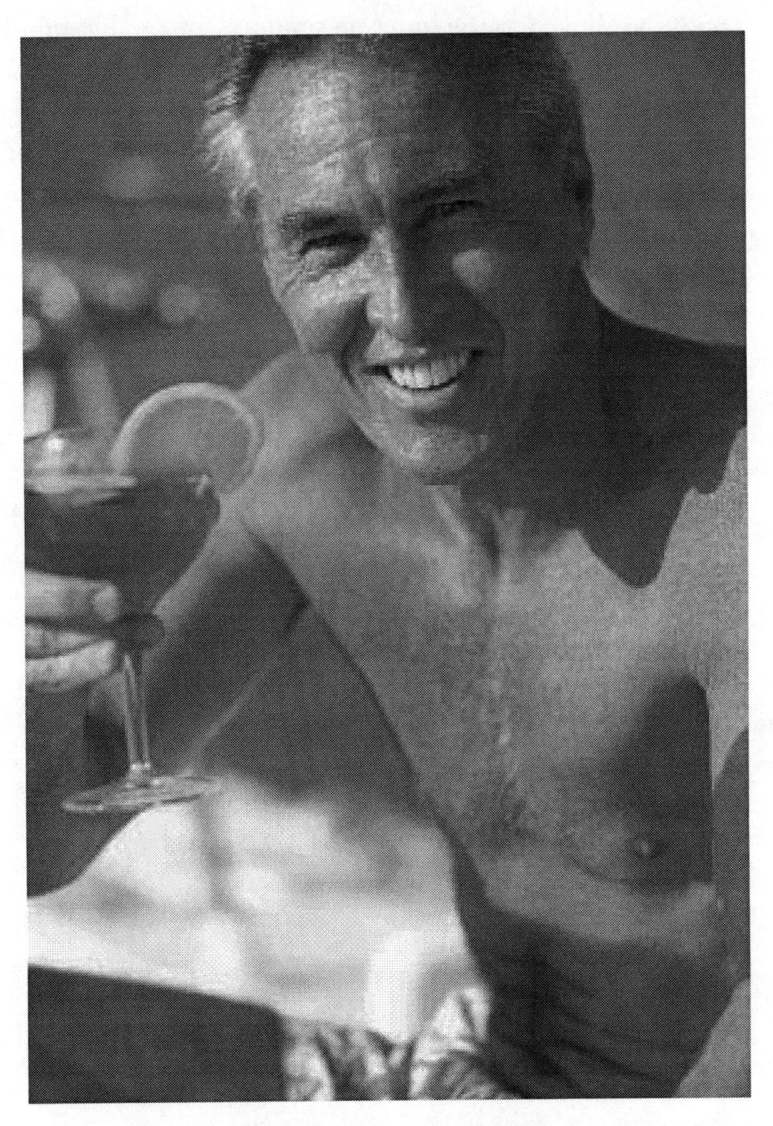

Grave's is fairly rare, and not usually life-threatening.

HERBS TO TRY:

Lemon Balm: It should be noted that clinical trials have not looked into lemon balm's effectiveness in treating Grave's, however studies in test tubes found that lemon balm helps stop antibodies from attaching to thyroid cells – the process by which Grave's disease begins. [*Endocrinol* 1985;116:1687–93] It may also block signals from the brain to the thyroid, which will avoid further stimulation of the thyroid gland.

Ginseng: Trials in the Far East on healthy volunteers indicate that ginseng may make certain immune cells more active in people. The herb has a long history of preventing and treating conditions linked to the immune system. One double-blind study found that 100 mg twice a day boosted immune function in 60 healthy people. [*Drugs Exptl Clin Res* 1990;16:537–42] Six years later, a study of 227 healthy people backed that result up, finding those on ginseng had higher antibody counts and lower incidence of immune-related disorders. [*Drugs Exp Clin Res* 1996;22:65-72] Five years after that, a study of 75 patients with chronic bronchitis found that ginseng removed bacteria faster than antibiotics. [*Clin Drug Invest* 2001;21:41-5]

Cat's Claw: This vine, native of South America, derives its name from the claw-like hook that it forms. It is commonly used to boost the immune system in fighting diseases. Certain alkaloids are primarily thought to produce its medicinal benefits. There is little clinical evidence to support this herb, but some reports say that HIV patients have increased levels of helper T cells, reduced viral loads, and increased vitality when taking cat's claw. What is known is the cat's claw is high in oxyindole alkaloids that have been proven to stimulate the immune system. [US Patent no. 5,302,611, April 12, 1994] It isn't known whether this is enough to have an effect on disease.

Astragalus: This is a known immune booster, commonly used in Chinese traditional medicine as a tonic for the immune system. It is considered useful as a *complementary* treatment for cancer therapy and immune deficiency syndromes. [*J Biol Respon Modif* 1983;2(3):227-37] Astragalus has been found to result in a significant immune enhancement when combined with interferon, than with interferon alone. [*Chin. Med. J.* 1981;94(1):35-40] Because of its powerful immune effects, this herb is being studied for use against AIDS.

Notable Herbs

Lemon Balm

Ginseng

Cat's Claw

Astragalus

Headaches

Also See Migraines

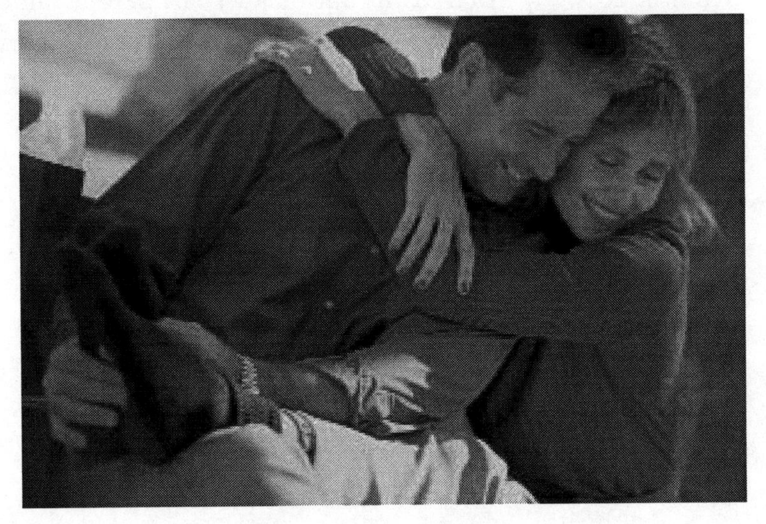

About 90% of headache sufferers can be treated successfully.

"Headache" is a term that is used by almost everyone from time to time to describe pain that originates in the nerve pathways located in the face, head, and neck. The pain isn't in the skull or tissue, but rather it is located in the nervous system. Such pain can be temporary and mild, or chronic and completely debilitating. If you don't suffer from headaches, you may think that headaches are more of a minor inconvenience than a category of disease. However, if you are headache prone, you know the reality behind this painful affliction. Headaches can be caused by injury to the head, dilated blood vessels, inflammation, or any number of other factors. Headaches are sometimes difficult to treat because the symptoms, triggers, and level of pain varies so much from person to person. Fortunately, about 90% of headache sufferers can be treated successfully. Herbal remedies help minimize inflammation, relieve pain, and take away other common symptoms like nausea and dizziness.

Sinus vs. Tension Headaches

Sinus Headache

Symptoms: pain in the front of your head; yellow discharge from nose, fever, not feeling well.

Causes: A virus or bacteria that has planted in your sinuses.

Tension Headache

Symptoms: Pain at back of the head – feels like a dull pressure or squeezing sensation in the back of head – and it tends to spread elsewhere.

Causes: Bad posture, low blood sugar, stress, depression, anxiety, PMS, food allergies.

HERBS TO TRY:

Feverfew: This popular medicine for headaches acts as an antithrombotic and anti-inflammatory. Feverfew's effectiveness might lie in its ability to stop serotonin from secreting and also reduce the size of inflamed blood vessels in the brain (they cause the throbbing pain). In 2000, researchers reviewed clinical studies into the herb's ability to relieve headaches or migraines. [*Cochrane Database Syst Rev*. 2000;(3):CD002286] Four major trials were included in the review, and all were found to suggest feverfew was more beneficial than placebo in treating headaches. Feverfew led to less frequent, less severe, and shorter migraines. The only problem was that the largest and most focused trial found no significant difference between the herb and placebo. Still, there is much to suggest feverfew could work for you.

Peppermint Oil: Smoothing this oil across your temples might just help to relieve a tension-related headache. So said one preliminary study, as well as a double-blind one that found that a 10% peppermint oil lotion rubbed over the temples three times every half-hour was more effective than Tylenol in relieving headache pain. [*Nervenarzt* 1996;67:672–81] Yet another study found that peppermint oils – including its central ingredient, menthol – were just as effective as over-the-counter pain medication, and also better than placebo. [*Aust Fam Physician* 1996;25(2):216-220]

Cayenne: This one should only be used with the guidance of a doctor, because it is inhaled through the nose. Meant to help relieve "cluster headaches" (recurring in bunches), this spice rack regular inhibits the work of substance P – the nerve chemical that transmits pain to the brain. In patients, cayenne has reduced significantly the number of cluster headaches suffered. The reduction in headaches usually lasts for over a month's time. A double-blind study that used cayenne through the nose twice a day during a week of cluster headaches found that patients had far less pain and it lasted for 15 days. [*Cephalalgia* 1993;13:114–6]

Ginkgo Biloba: This herb, known throughout the medicine world, may be effective in relieving cases of migraine headaches. An extract has been linked to stopping the "platelet-activating factor" that is thought to play a role in the onset of migraines. [*Lancet* 1987;i:248–51] Two small studies in France have also alluded to ginkgo's potential in relieving migraine's painful effects, although no major clinical study has looked into the issue just yet.

For specific causes of headache and how to remedy them, see the **Anxiety** and **Depression** chapters.

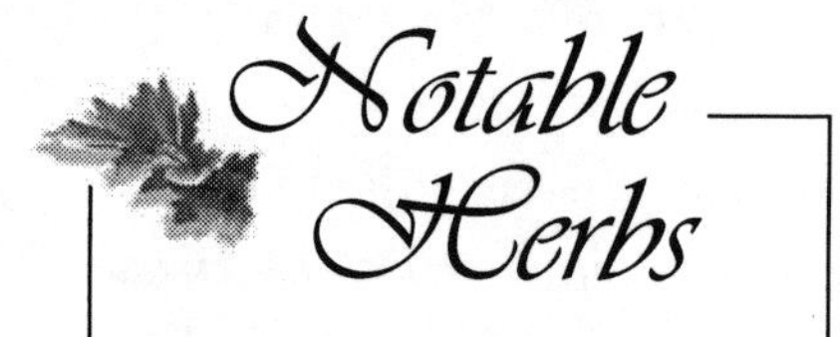

Feverfew

Peppermint Oil

Cayenne

Ginkgo Biloba

Other Nutraceuticals That May Work:

Riboflavin (vitamin B-2)

Magnesium

Heart Disease

Also See Congestive Heart Failure

Heart Disease is a primary cause of death in North America. Heart disease often starts with arteriosclerosis, hardening and thickening of the arterial walls, and then progresses to chest pain, dyspnea, irregular heart beat, tachycardia, murmur, and ultimate heart failure. The three primary causes are obesity, cigarette smoking, and elevated cholesterol levels. As expected, there is an abundance of research into all ways to help the heart. Many herbs and other supplements are noted for their ability to help improve circulation, prevent arteriosclerosis, regulate heart rate, and have an anti-inflammatory affect on the vascular system.

HERBS TO TRY:

Hawthorn: *American Family Physician* says this is a "highly promising" herb. High in flavonoids, hawthorn may work by widening the arteries and thus improving the flow of blood – an action otherwise known as "dilation." That theory was backed up by the results of one study out of Germany [*Arzneirninelforschung* 1995;45:842-845]. Because of these cardiovascular health benefits, hawthorn is one of the most prescribed natural remedies in Europe. A study in 1994 found the herb effective in treating patients with congestive heart failure (CHF). [*Phytomedicine* 1994; 1: 17-24] In a 1996 review of literature, German researchers concluded that clinical trials have shown hawthorn to be beneficial in symptoms of stage II CHF. [*Fortschr Med* 1996;114:27-9] Hawthorn has been linked to better blood pressure and a higher quality of life and mental well-being.

Coenzyme Q_{10}: Of course not a herb, this coenzyme (that occurs naturally in the body) is nonetheless a supplement with much promise against congestive heart failure. Evidence is not all agreeable though, with some studies refuting others. Some of the beneficial results include a 1999 study that showed 22 patients who had an increased stroke index at rest and at work and a decreased pulmonary capillary wedge at rest when taking coenzyme Q_{10}. It concluded that those with congestive heart failure may benefit from supplementation with Q_{10}. {*Biofactors* 1999;9:285-9] This and several other studies have prompted *American Family Physician* to believe Q_{10} may have a beneficial role in CHF, but that it so far appears "modest."

Garlic: This herb is well known for its cardiovascular and circulation-improving traits. A major study by the American Heart Association reported that garlic can maintain the elasticity of aging blood vessels, which tend to lose their ability to stretch with time. [*Circulation* 1997;96(8):2649-2655] Garlic helps widen blood vessels as a result of relaxing the muscles that surround the walls, which is why it's a major herb for hypertension. Its effect on blood vessels signals why it may be appropriate for patients with heart disease.

Turmeric: What makes curry yellow may also treat inflammation. Turmeric is part of the ginger family and has proven in animal studies to reduce inflammation, a belief held for centuries in India. The spice, taken internally, may work by inhibiting the production of prostaglandins, which are inflammatory chemicals. It reduces inflammation by lowering histamine levels and perhaps by boosting the production of cortisone by the adrenal glands. [*Ind J Med Res* 1971;59:1289–95] Its main ingredient is curcumin, is primarily responsible for this histamine-lowering ability. The herb has been found to prevent platelets from clumping up, which guards against atherosclerosis and improves blood circulation. [*Thromb Res* 1985;40:413–7]

Cayenne: Also known as capsaicin, the spicy cayenne is well known for its benefits to the circulatory system. It's traditionally used as a central ingredient in circulatory tonic. It has the ability to open up capillaries that allow blood to reach areas previously restricted because of poor circulation.

Boswellia: This Ayurvedic herb can defend against inflammation and restore blood vessels in connective tissue. It can improve circulation to parts of the body, especially joints that are inflamed due to arthritis. It's the boswellic acid, in particular, is thought to reduce inflammation. A review of unpublished studies into this herb found double-blind trials deduced that is was effective in relieving rheumatoid arthritis symptoms. [*Phytomed* 3(1): 67–70, 1996]. A number of scientific studies have confirmed the effectiveness of boswellia.

Soy Protein: Soy has isoflavones whose effects reduce the risk of atherosclerosis. The FDA has reported that it accepts soy protein, at 25 grams a day when taken within a diet low in saturated fat and cholesterol, as a legitimate way to reduce the risk of heart disease. It is also linked to reduced LDL cholesterol and raised HDL cholesterol.

Green Tea: Although much research is preliminary, there is evidence that green tea can fight against atherosclerosis. When there is oxidative damage to LDL cholesterol in the blood, the risk for atherosclerosis becomes greater. In this respect, green tea increases the body's antioxidant activity, which then protects against the artery-thinning disease, as a Japanese study found out in 2000. [*Ann Epidemiol* 2000;10:401–8]

Omega-3 Fatty Acids: There's a bundle of evidence into the health benefits of this supplement. It is believed that increasing the amount of omega-3 in your system helps prevent cardiovascular complications – including slowing the growth of an arteriosclerotic plaque. The American Heart Association recommends, on the basis of this cardiovascular evidence, that everyone should have two servings of fish a week. You can also find these fatty acids in flaxseed and walnuts – and their respective oils. [*Circulation* 2002;106(21):2747-2757]

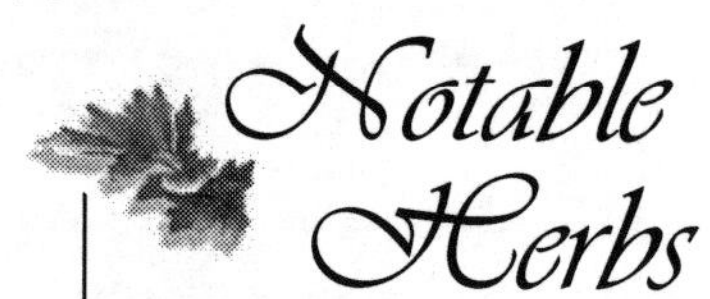

Hawthorne

Coenzyme Q_{10}

Garlic

Turmeric

Cayenne

Boswellia

Soy Protein

Green Tea

Other Nutraceuticals That May Work:

Omega-3 Fatty Acids

Vitamin E

Folic Acid

Vitamin C

Heart Rhythms

In this section, we can include such cardiac problems as heart arrhythmia, irregular heartbeat, and ventricular premature beats – essentially anything that means your ticker isn't beating to its normal rhythm. Irregular heart rhythms can range from being entirely non-serious all the way to life-threatening. It is certainly not a condition to take mildly, and before any self-appointed herbal therapies are started, a doctor should always be consulted first to give the go-ahead or other suggestions. Irregular heart beats don't result in symptoms per say, but many patients report having increased anxiety, dizziness, lightheadedness, or have the unusual sensation of being more aware of the heartbeat. Other symptoms that may occur include: chest pain, hypotension, shortness of breath, perspiration, and reduced urine flow. First things first: avoid caffeine. Herbal remedies aim to reduce the frequency of abnormal heart beats or avoid arrhythmia altogether.

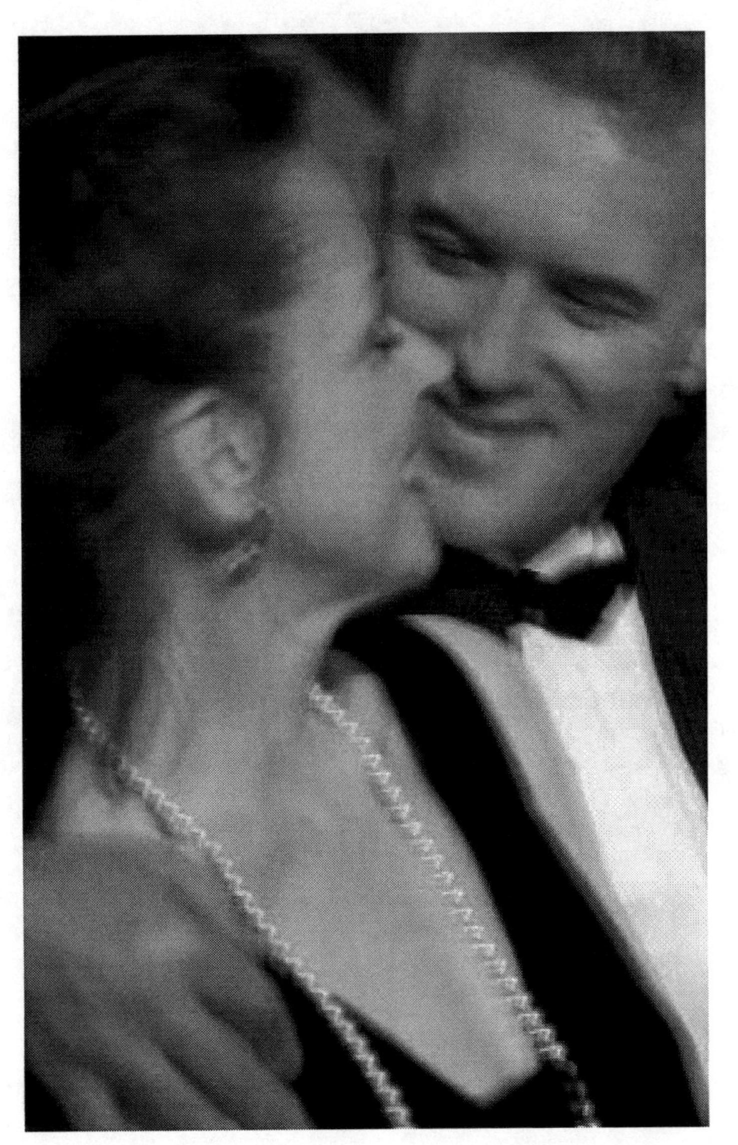

A preliminary study found that people with a particular kind of arrhythmia had reduced arrhythmia when they took dl-THP.

HERBS TO TRY:

Hawthorn: Again, this herb is linked to most things to do with the heart. There isn't much human evidence yet to suggest it could help with heart rhythm, but it has (for what it's worth) been used traditionally for this purpose. In a very experimental

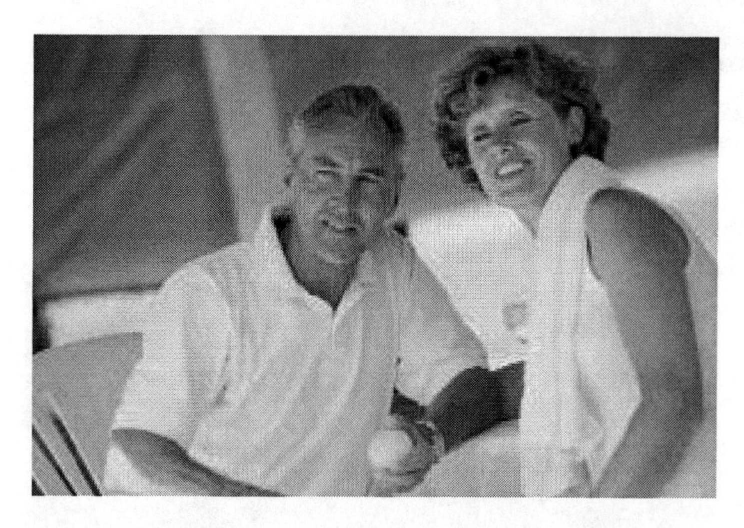

Fish oil – high in omega-3 – helps keep the heart ticking properly.

animal study in 1999, hawthorn extract significantly reduced heart arrhythmias that were purposely induced. [*Basic Res Cardiol* 1999;94:71–7]

Fish Oil: For four months, patients with "ventricular premature complexes" (a type of arrhythmia) received either a tablespoon of fish oil each day or safflower oil that acted as placebo. Those on fish oil found they had far less abnormal heartbeats, with 44% of them having at least a 70% reduction in the frequency of those abnormal rhythms. [*Am J Cardiol* 1995;76:974–7] This would suggest fish oil – high in omega-3 – helps keep the heart ticking properly.

Corydalis: This Chinese plant is historically known to invigorate blood when it's used for medicinal purposes. One of its main ingredients is "dl-THP." This is possibly the reason why this herb may prevent any heart arrhythmia. This herb needs far more research, but a preliminary study found that people with a particular kind of arrhythmia ("supraventricular premature beat") had reduced arrhythmia when they took dl-THP. [*J Xi'An Med Univ* 1998;10:150–3]

Notable Herbs

Hawthorn

Corydalis

Other Nutraceuticals That May Work:

Fish Oil

Magnesium

Hepatitis

Hepatitis is a disease that is transmitted sexually or through other bodily fluids, including blood. It is characterized by inflammation of the liver. It is most commonly caused by a virus. Viral hepatitis is classified as either Type A, Type B, or Type C. Type A is caused by transmitting fecal material on unwashed hands and eating contaminated food and water. Type B transmitted by an injection of contaminated blood through intravenous drug use, as well as through sexual activity. Type C is transmitted through blood transfusions, IV drug use, and sexual activity.

Common symptoms mirror those seen with the flu, and include: fever, fatigue, nausea, and vomiting. There also may be weight loss, dark urine, colorless stool, and tasteless cigarettes. Different forms of the disease do exist, including a chronic, autoimmune disorder. Vaccinations are quite reliable in preventing the disease. Herbal treatments decrease the inflammation and help the liver. Most research into herbs for hepatitis has occurred in Asia, where far more people have contracted the virus.

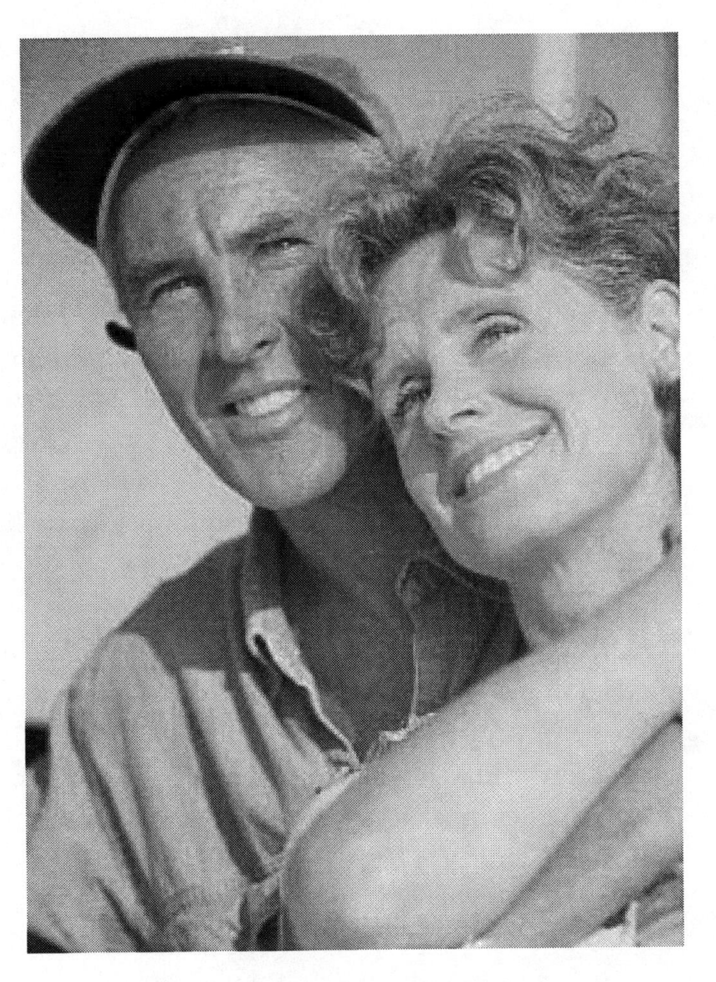

Vaccinations are quite reliable in preventing the disease.

HERBS TO TRY:

Milk Thistle: The folklore appears to be right about this herb – it does help combat liver disorders. Europeans have used milk thistle for centuries in treating liver disorders and now clinical studies have firmly back up that claim – silymarin, the herb's main ingredient helps to stimulate certain enzymes that allow the liver to neutralize toxins. Milk thistle certainly won't cure hepatitis, but it will help the liver. In 2002 there was a literature review that focused on 14 studies into this herb's effect on liver disease. They found milk thistle to be safe and well-tolerated as a treatment. [*Am J Med* 2002;113(6):506-15] Milk thistle might even stimulate the production of new liver cells and improve any scarring.

Chinese Herbs: Plants found in China are on the forefront of hepatitis treatment, and a recent review of studies has concluded that they can play a role in helping the body dispose of the hepatitis B virus. In 27 studies, patients who took a mixture of Chinese herbs either alone or in combination with the disease's conventional medicine – interferon alpha – experienced twice the benefit that those only taking interferon alpha had. Chinese herbs helped reduce the hepatitis B virus to nearly undetectable levels. [*Liver* 2001 Aug;21(4):280-6]

Licorice: In Japan particularly, licorice root is sometimes used as an injected therapy for hepatitis B and C. There begins the herb's link to hepatitis. The main ingredient, glycyrrhizin, has proven to block the hepatitis A virus from mutating when studied in a test tube. For humans, a preliminary study found 2.5 grams of licorice, taken three times a day, was more effective than a leading drug in helping those with viral hepatitis. Licorice needs a whole lot more research, but so far so good (so to speak). Definitely consult your doctor before trying this, as glycyrrhizin has been linked to high blood pressure.

Phyllanthus: This member of the Ayurvedic school of herbal medicine (India) has been studied in people who have hepatitis B. In a month-long trial, phyllanthus helped kill the hepatitis B virus in 60% of patients. [*Lancet* 1988;2:764–6] A few years later, though, another *Lancet* study showed that the herb failed to eradicate the virus, signaling a promising, but frustrating herb. What may work best is the species that grows in West India – at doses of 900 to 2,700 mg a day, it has led to far better and significant effects on the liver and hepatitis B. [*J Lab Clin Med* 1995;126:350–2]

Red Peony: This small flower that grows wild in China may have medicinal value, particularly in its roots. And, it's Chinese researchers who have looked into it. One of the most recent of many preliminary studies found that an extract of red peony root helped relieve cirrhosis in patients with chronic hepatitis. [*Chung Kuo Chung Hsi I Chieh Ho Tsa Chih* 1994;14:195,207–9]

Notable Herbs

Milk Thistle

Chinese Herbs

Licorice

Phyllanthus

Red Peony

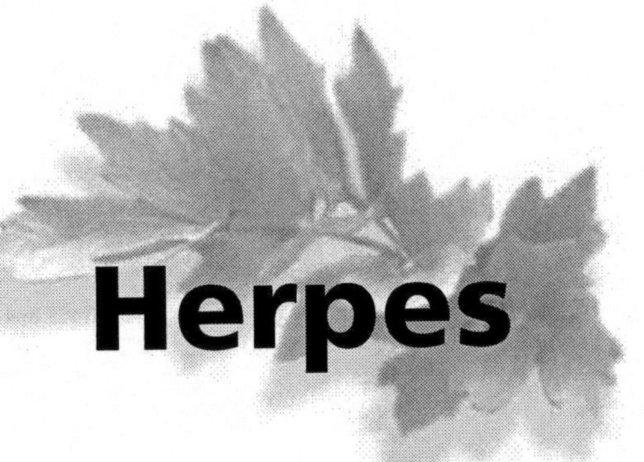

Herpes

Herpes is a highly contagious, viral, inflammatory group of viruses that affect the skin, causing burning, swelling, tingling, and the formation of cold sores, open wounds, and vesicles. There are two main kinds. The best known is herpes simplex, which causes painful blisters and sores around the genitals and the mouth. The other is herpes zoster, better known as chickenpox or shingles. Most herbal remedies are aimed at herpes simplex, so it's important to know which type is present. There is no cure for herpes, but some medicines are known to help. Herbal medicines soothe the irritation of herpes and help to cure the disease by fighting the virus and reducing inflammation.

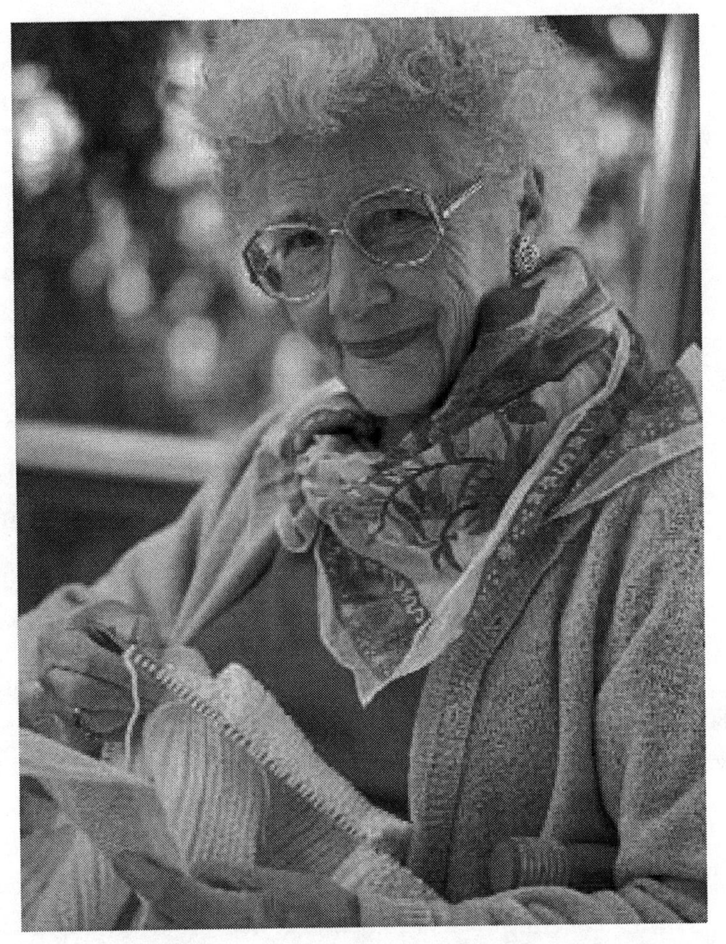

Herbal medicines soothe the irritation of herpes and help to cure the disease by fighting the virus and reducing inflammation.

HERBS TO TRY:

Lemon Balm: Used as an ointment, lemon balm is effective in healing cold sores that occur because of *herpes simplex*. In one double-blind study, a cream that contained lemon balm helped heal far more blisters and symptoms of herpes than a placebo cream. [*Phytomedicine* 1994;1:25–31] It is usually applied two to four times a day, and results are noticeable about a week later. Lemon balm is known to treat and prevent cold sores and genital herpes. Compounds within the herb bind to the virus and stop it from spreading. It also limits any itching, swelling, and burning.

Astragalus: This Chinese herb is known to have *anti-herpes s*implex activity. In a 1998 study, researchers tried a line of therapy on people with herpes simplex that included astragalus and a drug, interferon alpha. Results showed that those patients who used the combination did substantially better than those who only used interferon alpha. The researchers went on to "suggest" astragalus in the treatment of herpes simplex. [*Zhonghua Shi Yan He Lin Chuang Bing Du Xue Za Zhi* 1998;12(3):269-71]

Aloe Vera: This topical cream, used for so many medical conditions, may help heal *herpes simplex* sores that appear on the skin. One study examined 60 men with genital herpes who either applied a placebo cream or aloe cream three times a day for five days. The herbal remedy sped up healing and led to more healed patients than placebo. [*J Dermatol Treat.* 1997;8:99-102] Another study enrolled 120 men with genital herpes and came up with the same result: aloe proved to be most effective. [*J Eur Acad Dermatol Venereol.* 1996;7:294-295]

Witch Hazel: This shrub contains "proanthocyanidins" – a big bumpy word that has proven to be an antiviral that can fight the *herpes simplex* virus. A revealing double-blind study involved people with cold sores who rubbed on a cream that had just two percent witch hazel bark extract in it, six times a day for eight days. By the end, those using witch hazel extract had a hugely significant reduction in both the size of the cold sores and their spread. [*Z Allerg Med* 1998;74:158–61]

Common Selfheal: A strange name for a plant surely, but it's due to the traditional thought that it can "heal all." In 1998, Canadian researchers identified an ingredient in common selfheal (a.k.a. *prunella vulgaris*) that they tested against *herpes simplex*. It wound up showing extremely significant decreases in the virus, prompting them to conclude that the ingredient can specifically target herpes simplex in a way no other substances have. [*Antiviral Res*. 1999;44(1):43-54]

Evidence for supplements that help fight herpes zoster is weak and inconclusive. It's been noted that these might help fight the virus: proteolytic enzymes, vitamin E, vitamin B-12, and adenosine monophosphate.

Notable Herbs

Lemon Balm

Astragalus

Aloe Vera

Witch Hazel

Common Selfheal

Other Nutraceuticals That May Work:

Lysine (an amino acid)

Vitamin C

Vitamin E oil

Zinc/Glycine (topical treatment)

Proteolytic Enzymes

Vitamin E

Vitamin B-12

Adenosine Monophosphate.

High Blood Pressure/Hypertension

As its name suggests, this ailment is characterized by abnormally elevated blood pressure, especially in the arteries. Blood pressure is the force against artery walls that the blood creates when it is pumped through the body. A "normal" reading for blood pressure is about 120/80 mmHg. You are diagnosed with hypertension if your blood pressure exceeds 140/90 mmHg. A new category is "prehypertension" – this means you have a reading somewhere in the middle of those two. It is meant to be a warning signal. It is often called the "silent killer" because you may not have any symptoms until major damage is done to organs such as the heart, kidney, and brain.

Hypertension can be caused by any number of factors including obesity, stress, a disease or illness, pregnancy, or a family history of high blood pressure. It is a risk factor for heart disease, kidney disease, and stroke. Risk factors of hypertension include: diabetes, obesity, a sedentary lifestyle, stress, too much salt intake, alcohol use, and a family history. The first steps to take upon diagnosis is to eat a low-fat diet full of fruits and vegetables, cut back on salt intake, cut down on alcohol, lose weight if necessary, and exercise. But there are also herbal therapies meant to reduce blood pressure and improve circulation in the body. They can also act as a sedative or tranquilizer to slow the heart rate.

HERBS TO TRY:

Hawthorne: High in flavonoids, hawthorn helps widen the arteries and improve the flow of blood – an action otherwise known as "dilation." This theory was backed up by the results of one study out of Germany [*Arzneirninelforschung* 1995;45:842-845]. Because of its cardio benefits, hawthorn is one of the most prescribed natural remedies in Europe. Overall, it appears to be perfectly safe for the old ticker. The Germans are really on top of this herb, as another study showed that hawthorn tended to mildly lower blood pressure in those who took it [*Fortschr Med* 1993;111:352-354]. Hawthorne is a small shrub, a member of the rose family, and its berries, flowers, and dried leaves have shown benefits to the heart.

Yarrow: Also containing flavonoids, the plant has been found effective in lowering high blood pressure. The herb is found all over the world, anywhere from meadows and pastures to the side of highways on a small embankment. One study had 120 people aged 40 to 60, one group receiving 15 to 20 drops of yarrow twice a day for six months. What happened? LDL cholesterol and triglycerides decreased, HDL cholesterol increased, and blood pressure was significantly decreased after only two months. [*Drugs Exp Clin Res* 2000;26:89-93.] The herb's antispasmodic and mildly diuretic action help in this hypertensive effort, improving the circulation. For this purpose, it is taken as a tonic.

Garlic: These potent cloves are a historical remedy for a number of cardiovascular conditions including, hypertension. A chain of events occurs linking it to reduced blood pressure, all to do with the widening of blood vessels as a result of relaxing the muscles that surround the walls. Beyond this, it is not exactly known why garlic works for high blood pressure. One pilot study took a large dose of garlic preparation (about 2,400 mg) for nine patients with severe hypertension. Amazingly, only five hours elapsed before systolic pressure fell on average of seven mm and diastolic pressure 16 mm. The latter continued on a significant decrease for up to 14 hours after the dose with no side effects [*Pharmacotherapy* 1993;13(4):406-7]. Despite this, experts still remain on the fence. The main ingredient in garlic that would heal so well is allicin, a sulfur compound that escapes when you chew or crush garlic. If you take supplements, ensure allicin is listed.

Evening Primrose Oil: This herb is a native of North America and the oil with medicinal qualities is taken from the tiny red seeds. It is about three-quarters "linoleic acid" and one-quarter "gammalinolenic acid", which is part of the omega-6 group. It may have beneficial effects for the treatment of hypertension and heart disease. In two studies from Canada (performed on animals), the oil was found to significantly reduce blood pressure. Experts believe that certain processes – such as relaxing the blood vessel walls – are involved in the potential use of this oil. A few animal studies have shown positive results, but human studies are needed in order to recommend this oil for treatment against high blood pressure.

Olive leaf: Extracts from this plant, including a number of phytochemicals and flavonoids, comes from its leaves. And, it may just help to lower blood pressure *and* prevent angina attacks. It's a strong supplement: it has shown effectiveness against any virus or bacteria on which it's been tested. As for hypertension, olive leaf has been studied for a couple of decades. One study, on 12 patients coming to the doctor for the first time and 18 patients already undergoing conventional treatment, found that there was a significant decrease in blood pressure for *all* patients. Side effects? None. [*J Pharm Belg* 1996;51:69-71]

Stevia: This natural agent is isolated from the plant *Stevia rebaundiana,* it is more potent than sugar as a sweetener, and has been used as such for a few decades in Japan and Brazil. Preliminary studies found that this sweetener might come with a sidenote: an antihypertensive effect. Could it be? A 2003 study set out to see if stevia could be effective in 174 people. For two years they charted the course of the patients and marked their hypertension ratings. In the end, those on stevia had a far lower percentage of people with problems in the left ventricle than did people on placebo. Taken orally, the sugar substitute significantly decreased both systolic and diastolic blood pressure without any adverse effects.

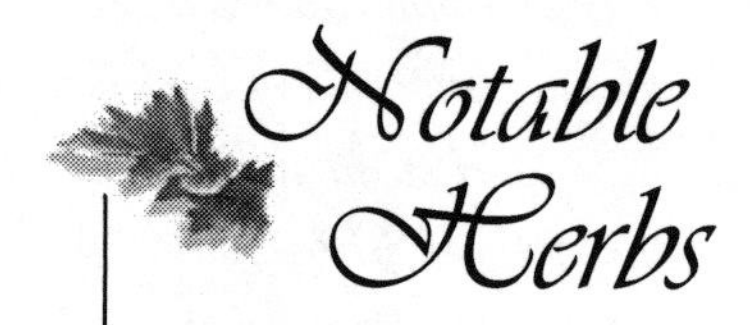

Hawthorne

Yarrow

Garlic

Evening Primrose

Olive Leaf

Stevia

Other Nutraceuticals That May Work:

Calcium

Potassium

Magnesium

Vitamin C

Fish Oil

Coenzyme Q_{10}

Infections: Ear

The most susceptible part of the ear to infection is the middle ear – it contains delicate bones essential for hearing. Infections there cause inflammation and fluid build-up that lead to what an ear infection is clinically known as: otitis media. Ear infections are quite frustrating and they can cause irritability, sleeping problems, runny nose, fever, loss of balance, ear pain, and hearing difficulty. If they are left without treatment, ear infections can lead to permanent hearing problems. All evidence into herb and supplemental therapies is anecdotal – meaning no clinical study has tested them out on humans. (This doesn't mean they don't work, but that if you tried them, they would likely be considered experimental.)

HERBS TO TRY

Garlic: This potent herb is a well-known killer of bacteria. Relating specifically to ear infections, researchers from the Boston University School of Medicine found that garlic was as effective as a common antibiotic in killing 14 different bacteria that have been linked to recurrent infections of the ear. As well, garlic killed some bacteria that antibiotics failed to. [*Your Health* April 1994:53]

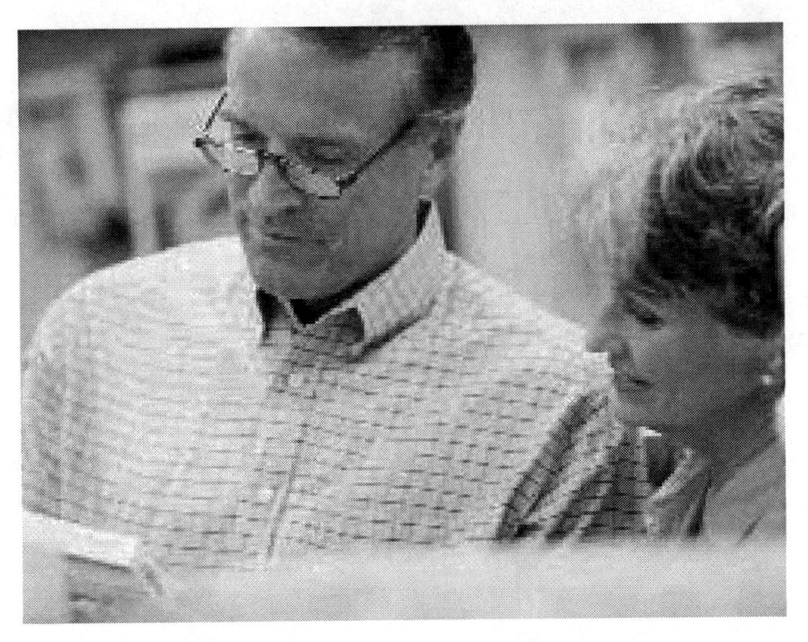

Ear infections are quite frustrating and they can cause irritability, sleeping problems, runny nose, fever, loss of balance, ear pain, and hearing difficulty.

Echinacea: This herbal remedy is tied to maintaining a healthy immune system that can fight off ear infections. This treatment has really just been studied in children, who are the most likely segment of the population to get ear infections. Medical textbooks suggest that children might

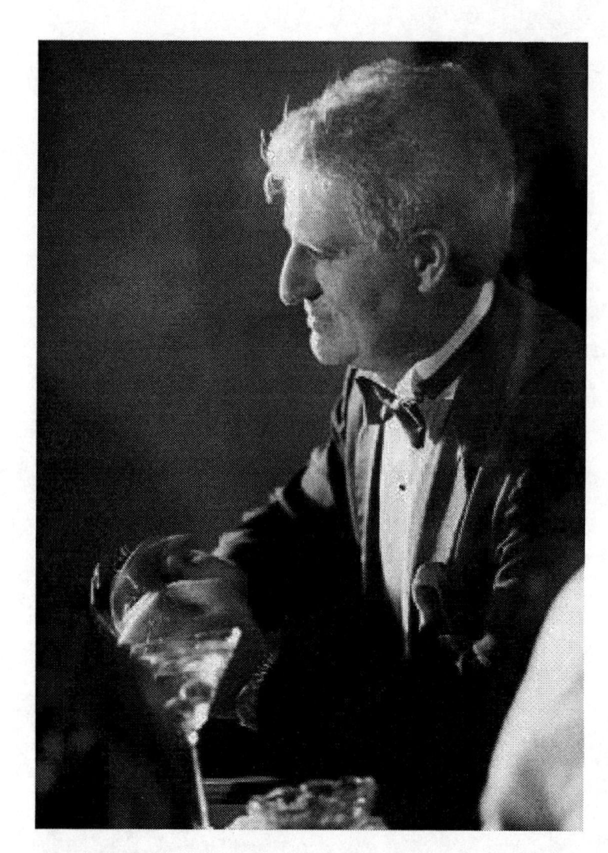

Although there is no evidence to support taking goldenseal, it nonetheless may help in clearing an ear infection.

benefit from echinacea tincture taken at least three times daily. There lacks research to back this up.

Goldenseal: This herb has the same type of effect as echinacea, as it is a strong antibacterial (just like Garlic). Although there is no evidence to support taking goldenseal, it nonetheless may help in clearing an ear infection. It also is an immune system booster.

Vitamin C & Zinc: These two supplements are grouped together because they are both purported to stimulate the immune system to fight infection. Several studies have documented this ability. They have never been distinctly tied to ear infections per say, but still some doctors recommend taking supplements of both (no more than 25 mg a day for adults).

Notable Herbs

Garlic

Echinacea

Goldenseal

Other Nutraceuticals That May Work:

Vitamin C

Zinc

Insomnia

Insomnia is characterized by continual sleep problems. It can cause you to have trouble falling asleep, cause you to wake easily and have trouble falling back asleep, and it can weaken your immune system. The condition is not linked to a specific number of hours a person is sleeping, because people vary in their sleep needs. If you have any of these symptoms you could be diagnosed with insomnia: Trouble falling asleep; waking up frequently during the night and trouble returning to sleep; waking up too early; unrefreshing sleep. Insomnia can occur in almost everyone from time to time, but for some people it is a constant, chronic struggle. It can be a side effect of medication, it can be caused by stress, or it can be a symptom of a more serious condition, like major depression. Other causes include, night work, jet lag and substance abuse – coffee, alcohol, drugs, stimulants, decongestants, or long-term sedative use. It can cause fatigue, difficulty concentrating, irritability, and a lack of energy. Herbal medicines can be quite effective in treating insomnia, and most act as sedatives or mild tranquilizers.

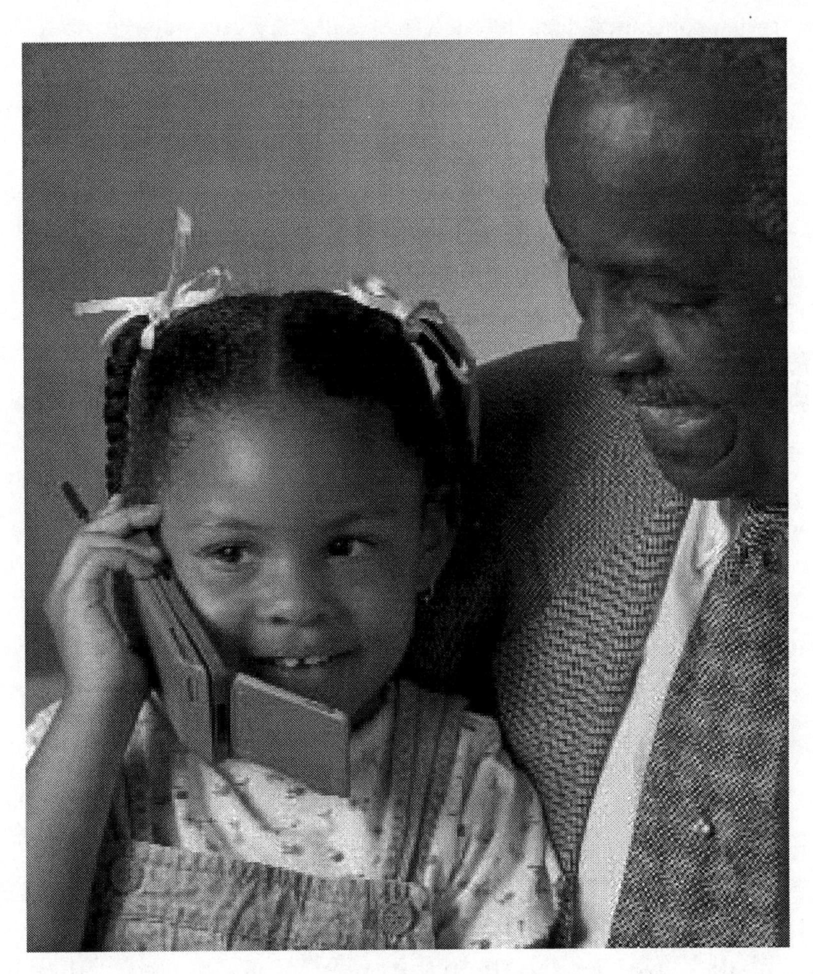

Insomnia can cause fatigue, difficulty concentrating, irritability, and a lack of energy.

HERBS TO TRY:

Valerian: This herb's root is a traditional remedy for sleep and has been studied many times over for its effect. Results are both promising and inconclusive, meaning valerian needs a rigorous trial to see just how effective it can be. In 1992, a study found valerian root helped improve patients' sleep and the time required for them to fall asleep without leaving them lethargic in the morning. [*Psychopharm.* 1992;108:248-255] A review concluded that, although test results vary a bit, valerian does improve sleep when it's taken every night for one or two weeks. [*Am Fam Physician.* 2003;67(8):1755-8] It is a safe sedative and the best herb for insomnia.

Kava Kava: This herb is well known and well-researched as a treatment for anxiety, and these calming traits mean it may be effective for sleep disturbances as well. Kava may help target stress and psychologically help you sleep better. In 24 patients who suffered insomnia due to stress, (on average for the last 15 years!) kava was given for six weeks and valerian for another six weeks. By the end patients reported that not only had their insomnia significantly decreased, but so had their overall stress. [*Phytotherapy Research* 2001;15:549-551]

Lemon Balm: This herb has been looked at in combination with valerian for improving sleep. When compared to a popular drug that aids sleep, this herbal mix was effective over a two-week period, just as effective as the drug, and resulted in less difficulty concentrating the next day. [*Psychopharmakotherapie* 1996;6:32–40] Three years later, another study found that 360 mg of valerian and 240 mg of lemon balm taken before bed helped one-third of the people sleep better. [*Fitoterapia* 1999;70:221–8]

Lavender: Some caution should be taken with lavender flower oil when taken internally – although Germany's progressive "Commission E" has approved such use to treat insomnia. In North America, it's accepted that the aroma of lavender oil is calming and may provide relief from insomnia. In a study of elderly people who inhaled lavender oil, the results were as effective as if they took tranquilizers. [*Lancet* 1995;346:701]

If none of these prove effective, you may also try: Chamomile, Hops, Passion Flower, Scullcap, Catnip, or St. John's wort.

Notable Herbs

Valerian

Kava Kava

Lemon Balm

Lavender

Other Nutraceuticals That May Work:

Melatonin

L-trytophan
(an amino acid)

Vitamin B-12

Irregular Menstrual Cycle

An irregular menstrual cycle can be caused by a variety of factors, including long-term use of the birth control pill, a very active lifestyle, anorexia/bulimia, drastic weight loss or significant weight gain, and even stress. All women may experience a delayed period from time to time, but ongoing trouble with an irregular cycle should be considered as any other medical concern, and you should go see your primary health care physician to get a proper diagnosis. You could be pregnant, for instance. An irregular cycle can also be a sign of something more serious like endometriosis or uterine or cervical cancer. Having a regular physical examination is important in maintaining your gynecological health. Herbal treatments for an irregular cycle should only be used if pregnancy has been ruled out and you are not trying to conceive. Typically these treatments stimulate the uterus and balance hormonal levels, and there is little clinical evidence available to back up any herbs.

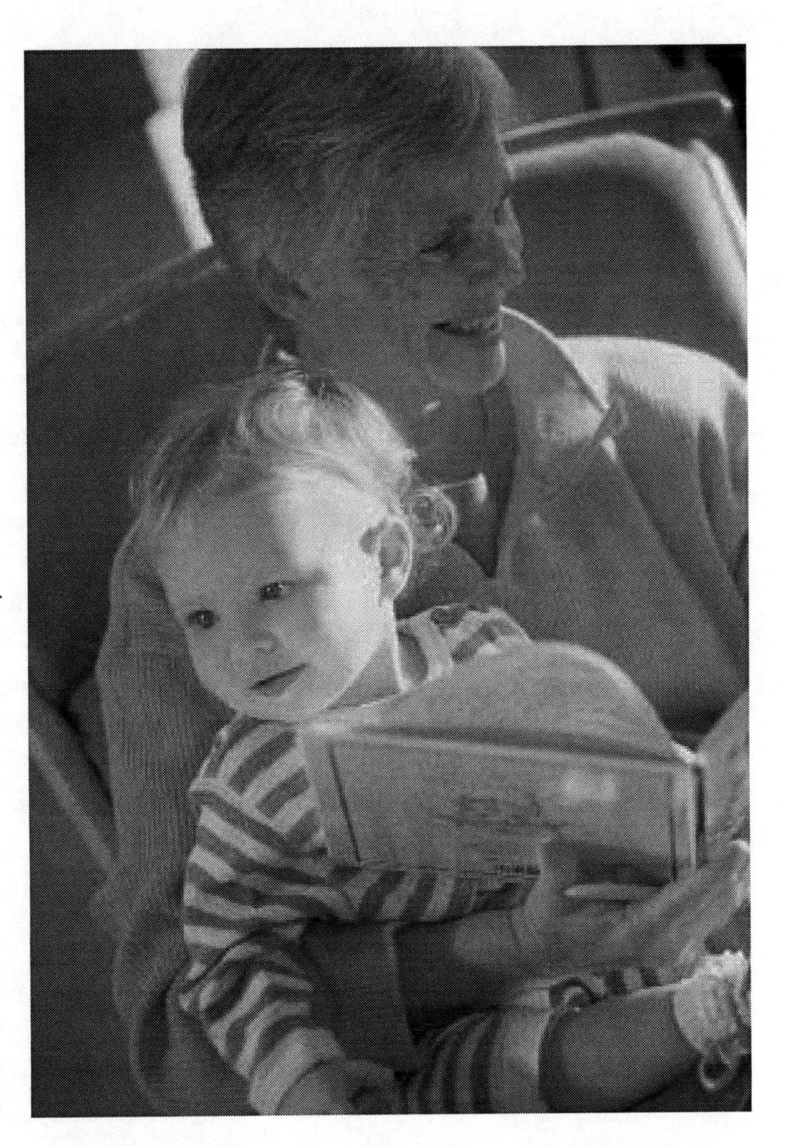

Having a regular physical examination is important in maintaining your gynecological health.

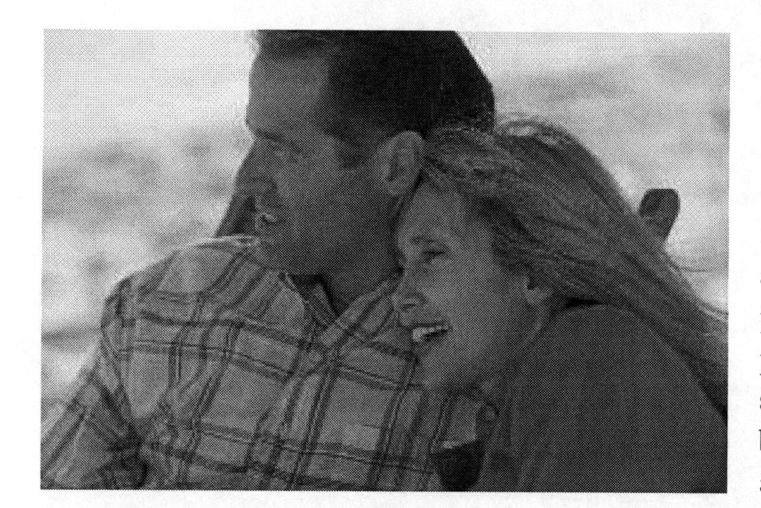

Black Cohosh is an increasingly popular treatment for menopausal symptoms such as hot flashes.

HERBS TO TRY:

Black Cohosh: According to tradition, Black Cohosh is used for "women's complaints." It is an anti-inflammatory, it lowers blood pressure, and acts as an antispasmodic. It also has sedative properties. It is an increasingly popular treatment for menopausal symptoms such as hot flashes. It has been the subject of some bad press, but a 2003 study found it unrelated to negative health risks, including cancer. [*Int J Oncol.* 2003 Nov;23(5):1407-12] The American College of Obstetrics and Gynecology supports the use of this herb for up to six months in female menstrual-related issues such as menopause.

Vitex: This herb, a.k.a. "chaste tree," is used sometimes as a treatment for infertility and amenorrhea (when a woman's menstrual cycle is absent). It has been shown to reduce the level of prolactin, which when at high levels can lead to amenorrhea. A German trial found that women had normal prolactin production when they took three months of vitex treatment. [*Arzneimittelforschung* 1993;43:752–6] Vitex has also been shown to help with "luteal phase defect" – a condition that can cause menstrual cycle abnormalities. Research is not completely firm here, but one study did find that 10 out of 15 women with amenorrhea had a normal period after taking drops of vitex for half a year. [*Gynäkol Praxis* 1990;14:489–95]

Other herbs that are used, but not tested (thus not recommended for women) include: Blue cohosh, yarrow, rue, and motherwort.

Notable Herbs

Black Cohosh

Vitex

Irritable Bowel Syndrome

Irritable Bowel Syndrome is a functional disorder. It is, in the simplest description, when your bowels don't work as they should. IBS affects somewhere between 10 and 20% of adults, and is thought to be the cause of more than three million visits to physicians every year. The syndrome's many uncomfortable symptoms include bloating, gas, diarrhea, constipation, and cramps. A swollen abdomen and a constant feeling that you have not moved your bowels combine for an unpleasant situation that is only relieved when the bowls do indeed finally move. There may be pain and it can stretch from the abdomen—which may be tender to the touch—up to the chest, and even cause heartburn. The intensity of IBS symptoms will vary, as will the length of time they last. A well balanced diet, full of whole grains, fruits, and vegetables, is very important. Most symptoms can be abated with herbal medicines, which soothe and regulate an inflamed digestive system and provide pain relief.

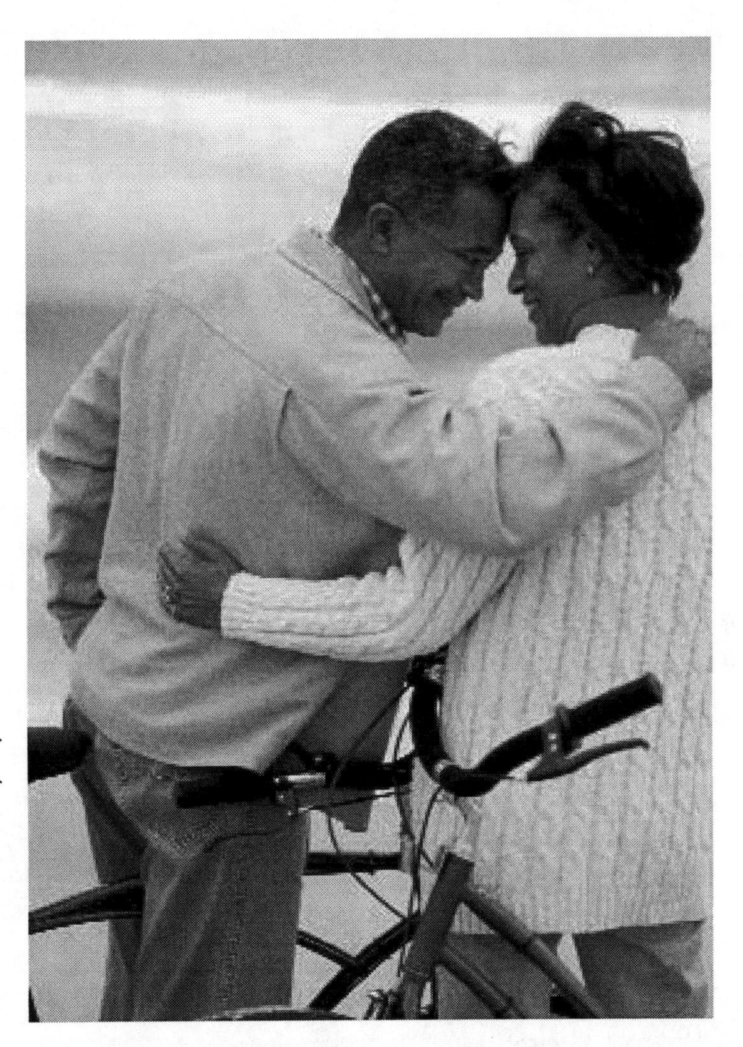

A well balanced diet, full of whole grains, fruits and vegetables, is very important in treating irritable bowel syndrome.

HERBS TO TRY:

Psyllium: This seed is extremely high in soluble fiber and is the main ingredient in such laxatives as

Metamucil. Double-blind trials have found it to be effective in relieving symptoms of this nagging condition. [*Gastroenterol Hepatol* 1990;5:507–13] Inside the psyllium seed is a gel that bulks up the intestinal tract because it is not digested. Combined with water, it swells up and provides lubrication. In a study of more than 170 patients with chronic constipation, psyllium was a superior treatment to a regular over-the-counter laxative called docusate sodium. [*Aliment Pharmacol Ther*. 1998;12(5):491-7] Another study found that psyllium – also known as ispaghula husk – to be highly effective in relieving simple constipation, it also resulted in less diarrhea and abdominal pain than the laxative it was tested against. [*Curr Med Res Opin.* 1998;14(4):227-33]

Artichoke Leaf: Extract from this plant is principally used to help treat dyspepsia, a condition that shows abnormal symptoms in the upper gastrointestinal tract. But there are symptoms of this condition that are also seen in IBS, giving rise to artichoke leaf being studied for its effect on irritable bowel syndrome. For six weeks, the herb was studied on a group of patients. Nearly all of them (96%) reported that artichoke leaf was better or at least equal to any previous therapy they had gone through. It showed no adverse effects, meaning artichoke leaf has good potential in relieving IBS. [*Phytother Res*. 2001;15(1):58-61]

Aloe Vera: The aloe plant helps clean mucus from colon walls and acts as a laxative to help improve bowel function and quell the diarrhea effects of colitis. It was proven in a study of 35 men and women randomized to a treatment that combined aloe vera with psyllium – otherwise known as fiber, the well known laxative. Those on the aloe vera combination had more frequent bowel movements with softer stool. It showed aloe vera was an effective laxative. [*Digestion* 1991;49(2):65-71] However, aloe vera does not appear to reduce abdominal pain.

Peppermint: A natural antispasmodic, it is known to relax intestinal muscles, reduce gas, and help relieve any cramps. You can take peppermint oil, or "enteric-coated" pills. A study of 42 children with IBS found that 75% of those taking peppermint oil pills had less severe symptoms – particularly the abdominal pain – and nearly half reported they were feeling "much better." For adults, two controlled trials have shown evidence that peppermint oil relieved symptoms of IBS when taken in enteric-coated pills. [*Am J Gastroenterol* 1998;93:1131–5]

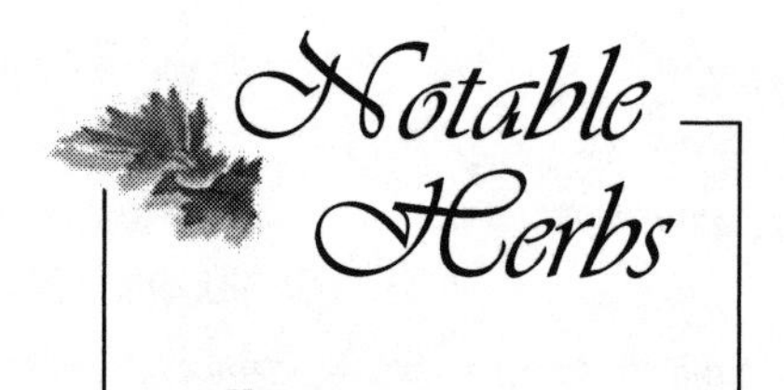

Psyllium

Artichoke Leaf

Aloe Vera

Peppermint Oil

Other Nutraceuticals That May Work:

Probiotics

Kidney Disorders

Our kidneys filter our blood, purging it of waste materials and toxins and making sure all nutrients are available. They siphon salt and water to maintain a chemical balance. They release hormones, keep blood pressure intact, produce red blood cells, and keep bones healthy. Kidney diseases affect the degree to which the filtering process works. Disorders of the kidney cause toxicity and damage to other organs that depend on blood, like the heart, blood vessels, and skin. Nearly half a million people in the U.S. have Polycystic Kidney disease, one of the top causes of kidney failure.

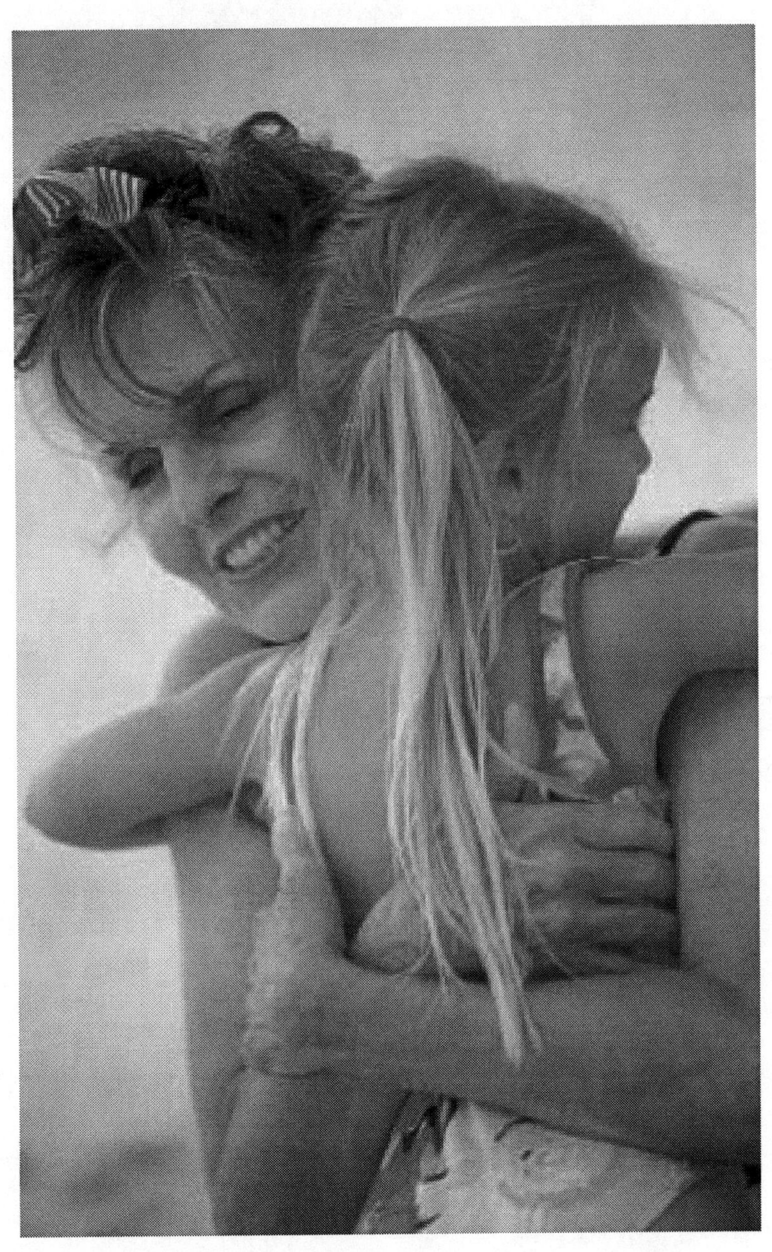

Nearly half a million people in the U.S. have Polycystic Kidney disease, one of the top causes of kidney failure.

HERBS TO TRY:

The best herbal remedies for kidney problems are ones that help prevent those problems in the first place. And the best way to approach that is to look at the leading causes of kidney disease, and try herbal cures to beat those before they take significant tolls on your kidneys.

Please see the **Diabetes** chapter. It is the leading cause of kidney failure.

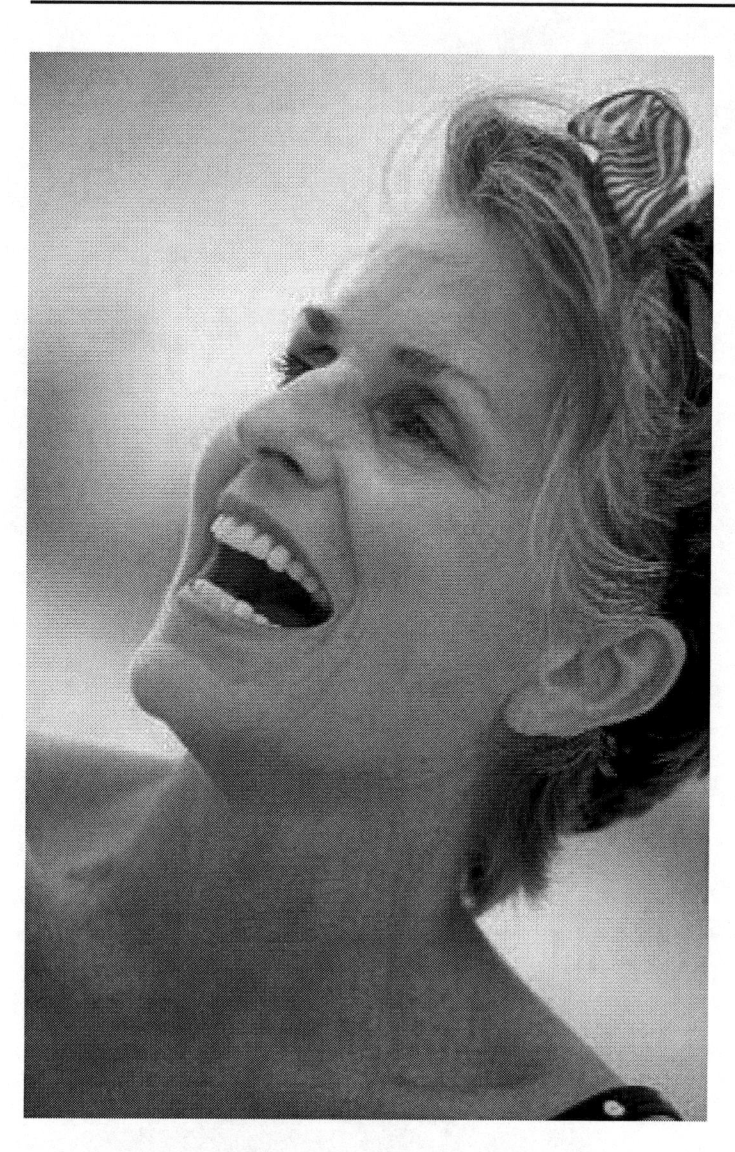

The best herbal remedies for kidney problems are ones that help prevent those problems in the first place.

Please see the **High Blood Pressure** chapter. It is the second leading cause.

Please see the **Benign Prostate Hyperplasia** chapter.

Please see the **Urinary Tract Infections** chapter.

Liver Problems

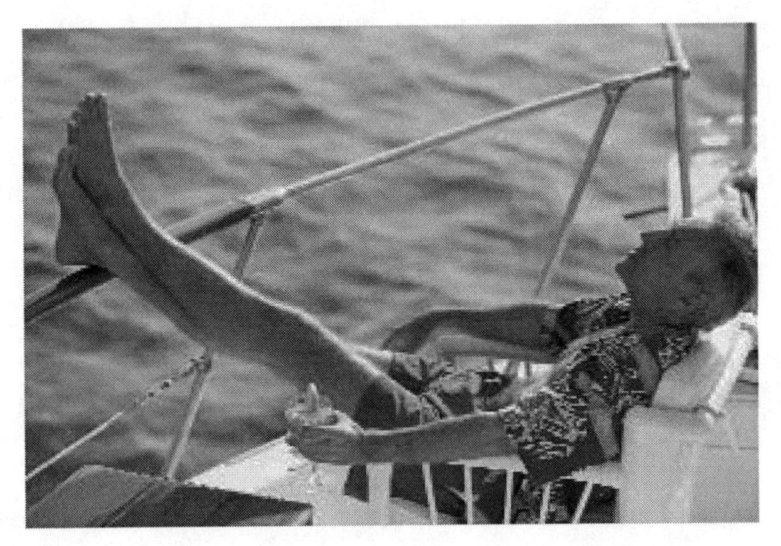

The most common cause of liver cirrhosis is alcoholism – 10 to 15% of alcoholics will develop this disease.

The liver has multiple functions in the body. It acts as both a filter for toxic substances and a storage unit for essential vitamins, sugars, fats, and other nutrients. Dozens of disease states can affect the liver, ranging from cirrhosis to cancer and hepatitis to autoimmune disorders. Liver cirrhosis involves severe damage that impairs the liver's ability to function normally. Symptoms related to cirrhosis include: jaundice, weight loss, abdominal pain, testicular atrophy, irregular menstruation, and swelling in the abdominal area. The most common cause of liver cirrhosis is alcoholism – 10 to 15% of alcoholics will develop this disease. Lesser causes include: drug use, toxins, infections, heart disease, and inherited diseases. Diseases that affect the liver are serious, as levels of waste materials that have not been properly filtered by the liver can build quickly, causing toxicity and death. It is important to note that regular and prolonged use of NSAID pain relievers can invoke liver damage. Herbs can act to aid liver function and reduce related inflammation and pain.

HERBS TO TRY:

SAMe: Not a herb, but this acid (a.k.a. "S-adenosylmethionine") may be able to improve liver function in people whose organ is severely damaged. This is especially true for alcohol-related liver cirrhosis – patients with this condition had a significantly overall death rate and need for a liver transplant when they took SAMe every day for two years. A large amount of SAMe was needed. [*J Hepatol* 1999;30:1081–9] Several other studies in the 1990s have shown it improved the outlook in cases of liver cirrhosis, helped stop an antioxidant important for liver function from being depleted, and was beneficial in relieving blockage of bile in the liver.

Milk Thistle: The folklore appears to be right about this herb – it does help combat liver disorders. Europeans have used milk thistle for centuries in treating liver disorders and now clinical studies have firmly back up that claim – silymarin, the herb's main ingredient helps to stimulate certain enzymes that allow the liver to neutralize toxins. In clinical trials, silymarin has proven to boost liver function and protect is against toxic damage (especially relating to alcohol). [*J Hepatol* 1997;26:871–9] In 2002, a literature review that focused on 14 studies into this herb's effect on liver disease, found milk thistle to be safe and well-tolerated as a treatment. [*Am J Med* 2002;113(6):506-15] Milk thistle might even stimulate the production of new liver cells and improve any scarring.

Licorice: In Japan particularly, licorice root is sometimes used as an injected therapy for hepatitis B and C. It is an antiviral, an anti-inflammatory, and an antioxidant. The main ingredient, glycyrrhizin, has proven to block the hepatitis A virus from mutating when studied in a test tube. For humans, a preliminary study found 2.5 grams of licorice, taken three times a day, was more effective than a leading drug in helping those with viral hepatitis, which damages the liver. Licorice needs a whole lot more research, but so far so good (so to speak). Definitely consult your doctor before trying this, as glycyrrhizin has been linked to high blood pressure.

Phyllanthus: This member of the Ayurvedic school of herbal medicine (India) has been studied in people who have hepatitis B. In a month-long trial, phyllanthus helped kill the hepatitis B virus in 60% of patients. [*Lancet* 1988;2:764–6] A few years later, though, another *Lancet* study showed that the herb failed to eradicate the virus, signaling a promising but frustrating herb. What may work best is the species that grows in West India – at doses of 900 to 2,700 mg a day, it has led to far better and significant effects on the liver and hepatitis B. [*J Lab Clin Med* 1995;126:350–2]

Red Peony: This small flower that grows wild in China may have medicinal value, particularly in its roots. It is Chinese researchers who are looking into the health benefits of this herb. One of the most recent of many preliminary studies found that an extract of red peony root helped relieve cirrhosis in patients with chronic hepatitis. [*Chung Kuo Chung Hsi I Chieh Ho Tsa Chih* 1994;14:195,207–9]

Notable Herbs

Milk Thistle

Licorice

Phyllanthus

Red Peony

Other Nutraceuticals That May Work::

SAMe

B Vitamins

Digestive Enzymes

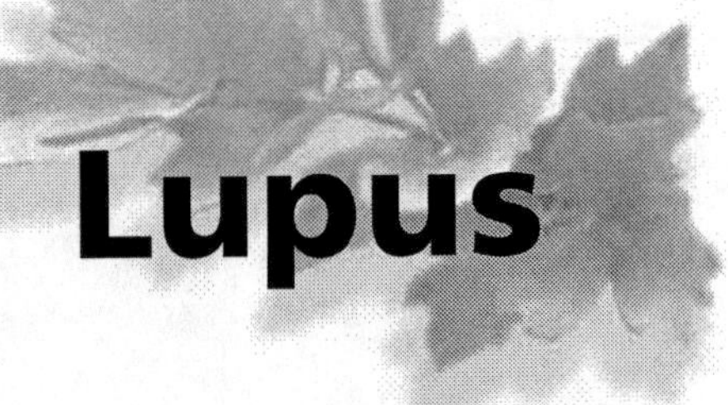

Lupus

As you may have heard in the media, Lupus is described as "the disease with a thousand faces." This is because it affects everyone differently and it is very hard to diagnose. From what doctors and researchers understand about this disease, and it's not that much, Systemic Lupus Erythematosus is generally thought to be an inflammatory connective tissue disease of unknown cause. An autoimmune disorder, lupus is a relative of rheumatoid arthritis. It is one of the many diseases that for some reason cause the body's immune system to overact and attack tissue as if it was a foreign invader.

Both hereditary and environmental factors such as viruses and UV light may play a role in lupus. It affects mostly women, and symptoms include fever, skin rash, arthritis, acute hemolytic anemia, small hemorrhages in the skin and mucous membranes, inflammation of the pericardium, and, in serious cases, disorders of the kidneys and central nervous system. Patients may experience malaise, fatigue, weight loss, nausea, and vomiting. Herbal treatments are mostly anti-inflammatory in nature.

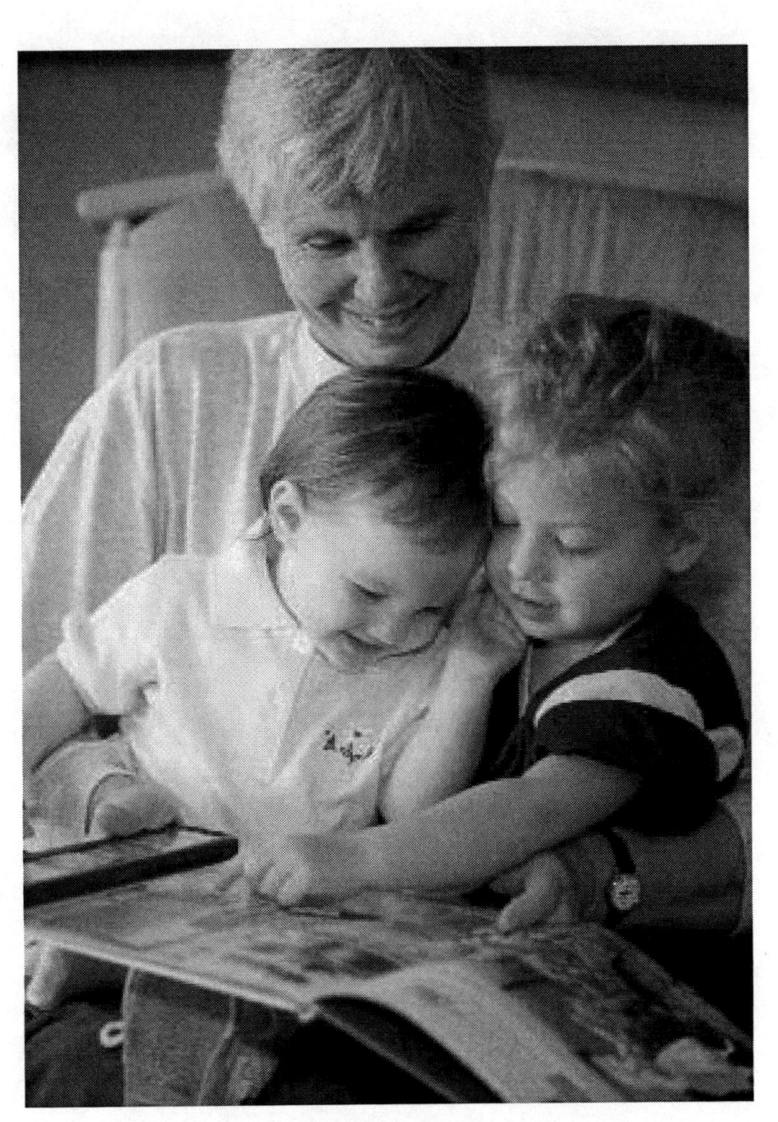

Lupus affects everyone differently and it is very hard to diagnose.

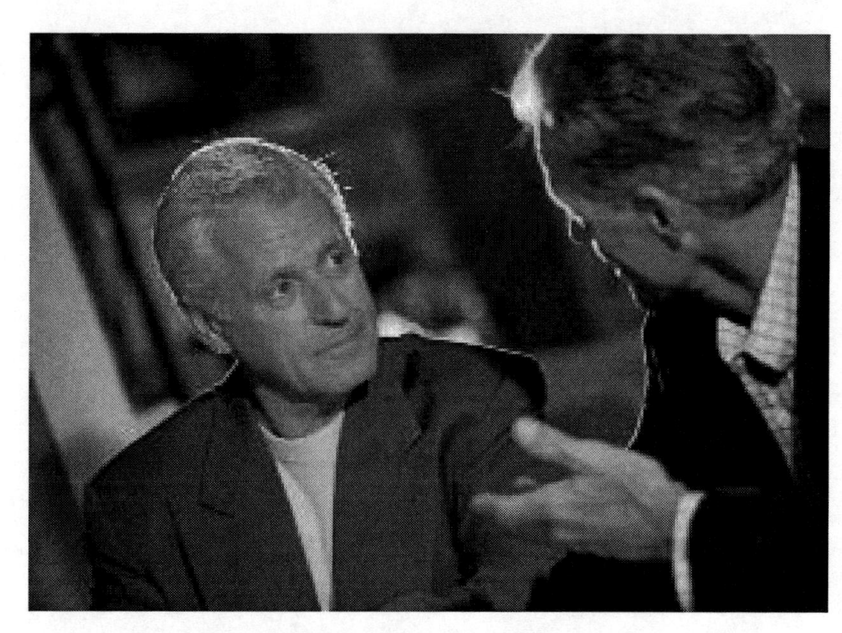

Both hereditary and environmental factors such as viruses and UV light may play a role in lupus.

HERBS TO TRY:

Astragalus: The Chinese are again at the forefront of testing herbal remedies (close runner up: Germany) and late in the 1990s they looked to see if astragalus may play a beneficial role in people with systemic lupus erythematosus. Understanding that plenty more research is required before this herb can be recommended, initial signs are bright: astragalus appeared to lower the overactive immune function in patients in a preliminary trial, meaning less tissue damage. [*Alt Med Alert* 1999;Nov:125–8]

Evening Primrose Oil: The central ingredient in this oil, culled from plants with a yellow flower that grow worldwide, is behind its health benefits: gamma-linolenic acid, or "GLA." Evening primrose contains about eight to 14% of this fatty acid. GLA is known to benefit patients with lupus and rheumatoid arthritis because of its strong anti-inflammatory effects. GLA seems to be a building block for the body's stockpile of "prostaglandins" – compounds that block inflammation.

For other potential herbs, see **Autoimmune Disorders** chapter.

Notable Herbs

Astragalus

Evening Primrose

Other Nutraceuticals That May Work:

Vitamin E

Vitamin A

DHEA

Menopause

As we all know, menopause is not a disease. It is a natural change of life for every woman. However, just because women should embrace this natural cycle doesn't mean they have to like the symptoms that come along with it. Hot flashes, spotting, night sweats, cold hands and feet, frequent urination, insomnia, and vaginal symptoms (dryness, itchiness, bleeding after intercourse) are common complaints for women going through menopause. Women should take note that osteoporosis and coronary heart disease are most likely to appear in menopause and postmenopausal periods. Fortunately, herbal cures can help by balancing out hormone levels in a natural way and reducing uncomfortable symptoms.

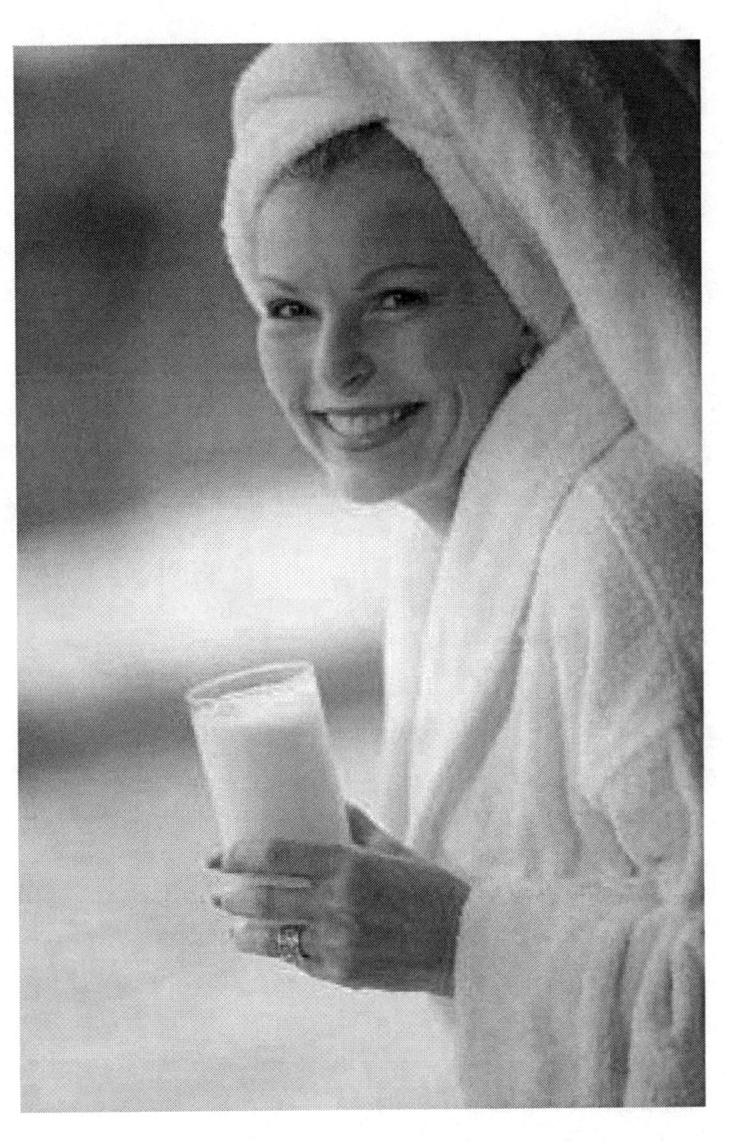

Just because women should embrace menopause doesn't mean they have to like the symptoms that come along with it.

HERBS TO TRY:

Black Cohosh: According to tradition, Black Cohosh is used for "women's complaints." It is an anti-inflammatory, it lowers blood pressure, and acts as an antispasmodic. It also has sedative properties. It is an increasingly popular treatment for menopausal symptoms such as hot flashes. It has been the subject of some bad press, but a 2003 study found it unrelated to negative health risks, including cancer. [*Int J Oncol*. 2003

Nov;23(5):1407-12] The American College of Obstetrics and Gynecology supports the use of this herb for up to six months in female menstrual-related issues such as menopause.

Dong Quai & Chamomile: This concoction, known commercially as "Climex," has been tested in menopausal women as therapy for related symptoms. The former is China's favorite herbal remedy for female-only conditions and of course, chamomile is a popular soothing tea. Together, in a 12-week study on 55 postmenopausal women, the two herbs led to a significant decrease in the frequency and intensity of hot flashes compared to placebo. This combination comes in chewable tablets, with women taking five a day. [*Clin Exp Obstet Gynecol.* 2003;30(4):203-6]

Kava: Extract of this herb may reduce anxiety and other symptoms that arise when a woman enters menopause. [*Fortschr Med* 1991;119–22] In a 2001 study, researchers found that kava was an effective aid in hormone replacement therapy in reducing anxiety in postmenopausal women. [*Maturitas* 2001;39:185–8]

Soy: Chalked full of vitamins and minerals, soy might also help limit menopausal symptoms in women. A couple of studies in 2002 and 2003 have only reached tentative conclusions, but they were both in the same vain: soy and particularly its "isoflavone" extract help reduce the number of hot flashes for women.

Herbal Mixture: None have much supporting evidence on their own, but taken together in a tincture licorice, dong quai, wild yam, motherwort, and burdock helped lower menopausal symptoms in a 1997 study. [*J Naturopathic Med* 1997;7(1):73–7] It also didn't appear to have an effect on hormone levels.

A Note on Red Clover: Red clover extracts are increasingly being used by women to treat their menopausal symptoms. Like many herbal remedies, there is more hope involved than definitive treatment. It's important to note that red clover does not conclusively help in treating menopause. Two double-blind trials found it ineffective in reducing hot flashes or other symptoms, and other research has concluded that the herb has "no demonstrable benefit for menopausal symptoms." Only one study, in 2002 seems to find a benefit in red clover. This study found it to significantly reduced hot flashes.

Notable Herbs

Black Cohosh

Dong Quai

Chamomile

Kava

Soy

Migraines

A migraine is a lot more than a bad headache! Migraines are vascular, painful, debilitating, chronic headaches. More than 23 million Americans suffer from bouts of migraine. The government reports an unexplained 60% rise in migraines over the last two decades. Symptoms include throbbing pain on one or both sides of the head, irritability, nausea, vomiting, constipation, diarrhea, photophobia, sensitivity to noise, and constriction of the cranial arteries. Many people experience a visual disturbance or "aura" before the onset of a migraine attack. Some patients experience numbness, tingling, and weakness in parts of the body. In addition to hereditary factors, certain foods, drugs, weather patterns, stress, abnormal blood circulation, and scents (perfume, cigarettes) can trigger these painful attacks. Herbal medicines treat migraines by reducing inflammation and pain.

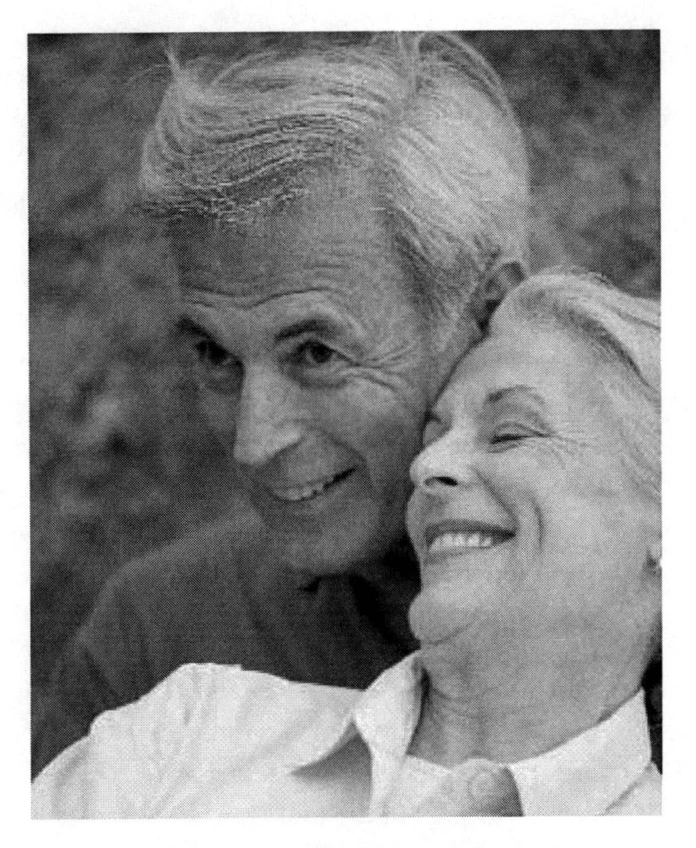

More than 23 million Americans suffer from bouts of migraine.

HERBS TO TRY:

Feverfew: This popular medicine for headaches acts as an antithrombotic and anti-inflammatory. Feverfew's effectiveness might lie in its ability to stop serotonin from secreting and also reduce the size of inflamed blood vessels in the brain (they cause the throbbing pain). In 2000, researchers reviewed clinical studies into the herb's ability to relieve headaches or migraines. [*Cochrane Database Syst Rev.* 2000;(3):CD002286] Four major trials were included in the review, and all were found to suggest feverfew was more beneficial than placebo in treating headaches. They led to less frequent, less severe, and shorter migraines. The only problem was that the largest and most focused trial found no significant difference between the herb and placebo. Still, there is much to suggest feverfew could work for you.

Ginkgo Biloba: This herb, known throughout the medicine world, may be effective in relieving cases of migraine headaches. An extract has been linked to stopping the "platelet-activating factor" that is thought to play a role in the onset of migraines. [*Lancet* 1987;i:248–51] Two small studies in France have also alluded to ginkgo's potential in relieving migraine's painful effects, although no major clinical study has looked into the issue just yet.

Peppermint Oil: Smoothing this oil across your temples might just help to relieve a tension-related headache. So said one preliminary study, as well as a double-blind one, which found that a 10% peppermint oil lotion rubbed over the temples three times every half-hour was more effective than Tylenol in relieving headache pain. [*Nervenarzt* 1996;67:672–81] Yet another study found that peppermint oils – including its central ingredient, menthol – were just as effective as over-the-counter pain medication, and also better than placebo. [*Aust Fam Physician* 1996;25(2):216-220]

Cayenne: This one should only be used with the guidance of a doctor, because it is inhaled through the nose. It's been found to relieve all types of headaches, including migraines. This regular member of the spice rack works by inhibiting substance P – the nerve chemical that transmits pain to the brain. A preliminary trial found that "intranasal" (as it's called) cayenne may be effective in reducing the pain associated with acute migraines. [*Headache* 1995;35:277] This herb needs to be substantiated.

Ginger: Not as well documented, ginger still might help relieve the pain of migraines. There is anecdotal evidence revealing that ginger can be used in migraine cases, especially for the side effect of nausea. [*J Ethnopharmacol* 1990;29:267–73] "Gingerols" located in the root may be responsible for relieving nausea and acting as a mild painkiller.

Notable Herbs

Feverfew

Ginkgo Biloba

Peppermint

Cayenne

Ginger

Other Nutraceuticals That May Work:

Magnesium

Vitamin B-2

5-HTP

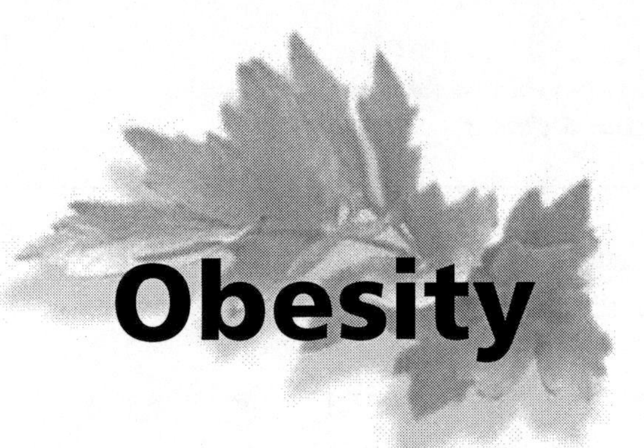

Obesity

Obesity is now considered the number one health problem in North America, affecting as many as one in three adults (in the U.S.). It is also a global epidemic. If a person is diagnosed as obese, it means they are significantly overweight, with about 30% body fat. The condition puts you at a higher risk for diabetes, heart disease, high blood pressure, stroke, arthritis, lung problems, and even premature death. Factors that can lead to obesity include: genetics, overeating, a sedentary lifestyle, certain drugs, and psychological problems (i.e. depression). Water aerobics, exercise, and proper nutrition are essential for weight loss and weight maintenance. Several herbs may help you beat the "battle of the bulge" as well by limiting fluid retention, decreasing appetite, and stimulating the metabolism. Obesity is a serious health risk and most decisions on ways to shed pounds should come after consulting a doctor.

HERBS TO TRY:

Psyllium: This form of soluble fiber is well-known to work with intestinal difficulties (it is the main ingredient in such laxatives as Metamucil). When people eat foods high in fiber, they get a much higher feeling of being "full." This is because fiber swells after ingestion, taking up more room. At the same time, it is easy to pass through the intestinal tract. By leading to a feeling of fullness, it prevents a person from overeating, which of course causes weight gain. A double-blind trial showed that women who took 20 grams of psyllium before a meal would end up with a lower fat intake and a higher feeling of fullness after the meal. [*Int J Obes Metab Disord* 1995;19:338–42]

Green Tea: The "thermogenic" effect of tea is usually attributed to the caffeine, but studies have found a green tea extract leads to thermogenesis of a far greater extent than could be explained by the caffeine content. This thermogenesis is key to a cellular process and stimulating it could be of value in helping manage obesity. [*Int. J. Obesity* 2000;24:252-258] In a study, young men who took six green tea pills were able to use up far more energy and burned more fat than those taking caffeine pills or placebo. [*Am J Clin Nutr* 1999;70:1040–5]

Goat's Rue: This is actually a noxious weed according to the authorities, but it has shown some powerful weight loss effects in animal studies. Its clinical name is *Galega officinalis*. The weed is known in the medical world for its hypoglycemic action, and is part of a mixture meant to treat diabetes. Use caution here, because results have only been shown in mice so far, but they are so revealing you should know about them. For a month, obese mice were treated with this herb. It was found that even when eating higher proportions of food, this herb may still stimulate weight loss. Its weight-reducing action is, thus, totally unrelated to dieting. How this works is still unclear, but the result is not: loss of body fat. [*J Pharm Pharmacol.* 1999;51(11):1313-9]

Chromium: Not a herb, but rather a mineral, this one should be noted as it is backed by some of the strongest evidence to date. Chromium basically helps the body use insulin – high insulin levels in the body are linked to obesity. One study suggested chromium can help those with both hypoglycemia and Type II diabetes. [*Int. J. of Bio. Med. Res.* 1989;11(2):163-180] Two years earlier, chromium was tested in 180 people in China with Type II diabetes. They found that high doses of the mineral normalized glucose and insulin levels in participants, results that the lead investigator called "spectacular." *[Metabolism: Clin. and Exp.* 1987;36(4):351-355] Results on weight loss in particular is not yet clinically proven.

5-HTP: Linked to serotonin, a neurotransmitter that regulates appetite, 5-hydroxytryptophan (or 5-HTP) has proven in a few smaller trials to promote weight loss and curb appetite. [*Am J Clin Nutr* 1992;56:863–7] One found that overweight women taking 5-HTP for three months lost far more weight than women on placebo. [*Adv Exp Med Biol* 1991;294:591–3] In terms of research, so far so good.

Note... Ephedra May Be Dangerous: If you are somehow getting your hands on ephedra to help lose weight, you should stop. It is a common ingredient is many herbal weight-loss mixtures, but this "herbal ecstasy" may in fact increase your risk of seizure, stroke, and heart attack. In late December 2003, the FDA decided to ban ephedra because of "unacceptable health risks" found by researchers at the University of California at San Francisco.

Note... Weight Loss Supplements Remain Unproven: A new study that looked at scientific literature going back decades identified about 50 supplements that have been promoted and researched into providing weight loss. There is a firm conclusion: more research needs to be done into this area. Everyone is primed and ready to achieve weight loss, and much fervor accompanies any new products that hit the shelf. You can certainly try any that you believe may work. But know this: "overall, herbal products and dietary supplements promoted for weight loss lack sufficient supporting evidence and safety data." [*J Am Pharm Assoc.* 2004;44(1):59-67]

Notable Herbs

Psyllium

Green Tea

Goat's Rue

Other Nutraceuticals That May Work:

5-HTP

Chromium

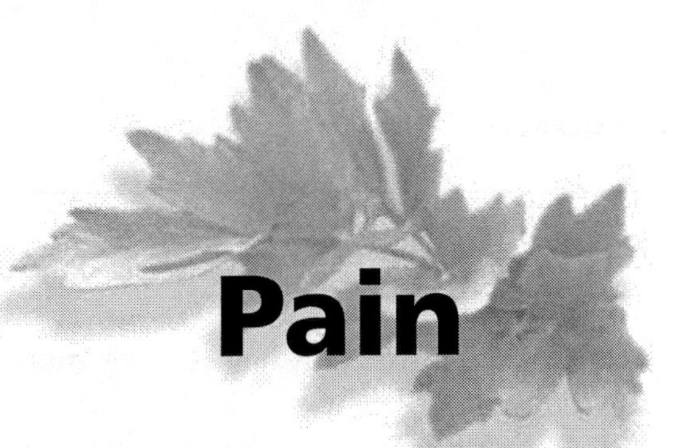

Pain

Pain is a developing issue or process. Nerve endings in your skin and other tissues send impulses through nerve connections to the spine. These electrical charges travel up your spine to your brain. It's your brain that causes you to "feel" the pain. There are many different kinds of pain. Arthritis suffers will tell you, cancer patients will tell you, surgery patients will tell you... we all suffer differently. We're all different and we all require different treatments for varying concerns. Treatments are available to reduce most pain. If untreated, pain can worsen other health problems, slow recovery, and interfere with healing. Don't let anyone say your pain is "in your head." Herbal pain relievers are often anti-inflammatories, as pain and inflammation often go hand in hand. Other pain relievers act as sedatives and tranquilizers to help you deal with and desensitize you to the pain you're experiencing.

HERBS TO TRY:

Cayenne: This red spice in your kitchen cabinet can be used as cream that is meant to provide short-term relief from pain, and is often used for arthritis. One of its primary ingredients is found in chili peppers—it's what makes them hot—and can lessen pain when put on the skin. Capsaicin works by decreasing the level of substance P, which is a neuropeptide that communicates pain sensations. With fewer impulses sent via substance P, you feel less pain. It needs to be applied three or four times a day. One study found that just a 0.025% capsaicin cream worked significantly better than normal cream for osteoarthritis of the knee. [*Seminars in Arthritis and Rheumatism* 1994;23:Suppl 3:25-33]. In another, 100 arthritic patients received capsaicin cream or placebo – those taking the chili pepper ingredient had significantly more relief from pain, 80% of them experiencing pain reduction after two weeks. [*Clin Ther*. 1991;13(3):383-95] In many clinical trials, capsaicin proves time and time again that it can decrease the pain of many disorders including shingles, neurologic pain, arthritis, and headaches. [*Clin J Pain* 1998;14:97–106]

Boswellia: This Ayurvedic herb (Indian medicine) can defend against inflammation and restore blood vessels in connective tissue. Used in arthritis, this herb causes no side effects while providing reasonable pain relief for sore joints. The boswellic acid, in particular, is thought to reduce inflammation. A review of unpublished studies into this herb found double-blind trials deduced that is was effective in relieving rheumatoid arthritis symptoms. [*Phytomed* 3(1): 67–70, 1996]. A number of scientific studies have confirmed the effectiveness of boswellia. In a study of 175 people with arthritis, four weeks of boswellia treatment helped 122 of them reduce pain and stiffness. It also seemed particularly effective in lowering back pain.

Ginger: This spice's effect on pain comes from its ability as an anti-inflammatory. Among the best studied herb for arthritis, researchers have found that ginger root may inhibit prostaglandins and leukotrienes, which are involved in inflammation and pain. Thus, the spice is an anti-inflammatory. It's been found to reduce knee pain in arthritis patients when standing or walking, as well as enhance the quality of life better than placebo. Patients receiving ginger extract had fewer gastrointestinal side effects and needed far fewer pain killers. [*Arthritis Rheum* 2001;44(11):2531-8] Ginger may work by slicing substance P levels. Some believe an oral dose of two to four grams of dry ginger per day is a good idea; or a half-inch of sliced ginger root.

Lavender: This calming, soothing oil comes from the lavender plant's leaves and has been used in Iranian folk medicine for centuries as a remedy for inflammatory diseases. Can its soothing effect translate to pain relief? A 2003 study (on mice) used a mixture that included lavender oil to firmly back-up the traditional belief that lavender can quench pain. Researchers are calling for more investigations into lavender's active chemical ingredients. [*J Ethnopharmacol.* 2003;89(1):67-71] In the meantime, it's available at natural health stores and may be worth a shot – use only topically.

Marigold: Yet to be truly tested for effectiveness, the homeopathic remedy of Calendula cream – or Marigold – may be useful for surface wounds like grazes and scalds. It's perfectly suitable for the "family medicine chest." [*Prof Care Mother Child.* 1994;4(7):212-3]

Turmeric: What makes curry yellow may also treat osteoarthritic pain and inflammation. Turmeric is part of the ginger family and has proven in animal studies to reduce inflammation, a belief held for centuries in India. This spice, taken internally, may work by inhibiting the production of prostaglandins, which are inflammatory chemicals. Some doctors use this broad-leafed shrub specifically for rheumatoid arthritis. Its main ingredient is curcumin, which is said to reduce inflammation by lowering histamine levels. The Arthritis Foundation reports that one small human study reduced pain by using a concoction of turmeric, boswellia, and zinc in osteoarthritis patients. Although never studied on its own in humans, turmeric should still be considered mildly effective on pain due to inflammation.

TWHF: The Chinese herb with one of the most awkward names — Tripterygium wilfordii Hook F possess anti-inflammatory and immunosuppressive traits. Its main ingredient, triptolide, is said to have these properties and has been shown to protect neurons from injury and thus pain. [*J Neuroimmunol.* 2004 Mar;148(1-2):24-31] TWHF has been used for over 2,000 years in Chinese medicine. Western medicine has finally recognized it for the treatment of rheumatoid arthritis and leprosy. Researchers believe it is promising and should be studied for autoimmune diseases and all kinds of inflammation.

Note on Willow Bark: Maybe you know, maybe not: aspirin originally came from the bark of the willow tree. You might see willow bark supplements in a natural health store, but you should probably avoid them. It's said that the bark can help decrease pain by interfering with inflammation and nerves in the spine that carry pain signals. But no study has been performed on humans, and many experts are skeptical that humans can actually absorb any of its pain-relieving ingredients. Plus, the pain relief of willow bark is typically slower than aspirin. And it's probably even more expensive. For what it's worth, stick to aspirin over this one.

For head pain see the **Headaches** and **Migraines** chapters.

Notable Herbs

Cayenne
Boswellia
Ginger
Lavender
Marigold
Turmeric
TWHF

Parkinson's Disease

Made famous, or infamous rather, by Muhammad Ali, Michael J. Fox, and Pope John Paul II, Parkinson's is a chronic and progressive nervous disease. It's linked to decreased dopamine production and characterized by tremor, weakness, confusion, a shuffling gait, stiff and rigid limbs, very slow movement, and eyes that will close involuntarily. It belongs to a group of conditions called "movement disorders." What occurs is a group of cells in the brain that produce dopamine (a neurotransmitter that links the brain to movement and coordination) start to malfunction and eventually die. Thus there is less and less dopamine available.

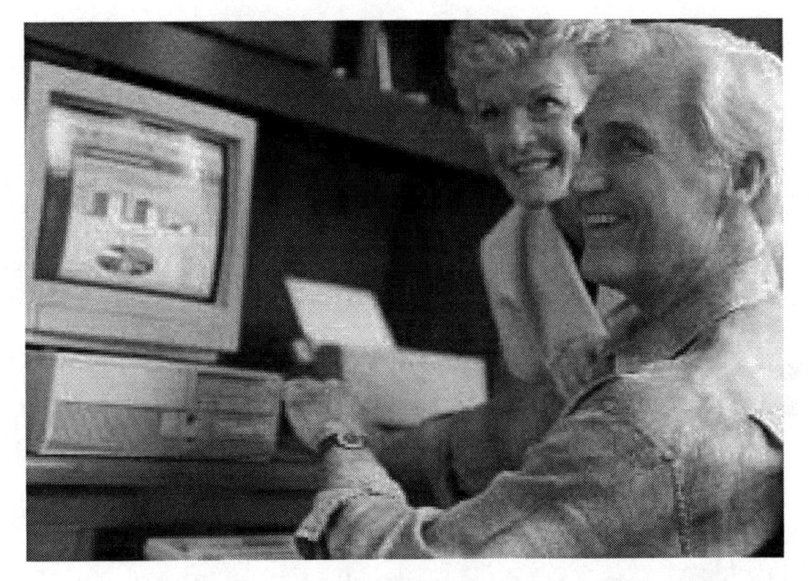

Parkinson's has no cure and doctors are always learning more about this serious and debilitating disease.

Factors that may cause the disease include: genetics, aging, toxins, or a virus. Parkinson's has no cure and doctors are always learning more about this serious and debilitating disease. There is very little evidence to suggest that herbal medicines work because of the complex nature of the disease. It is also difficult to raise antioxidant levels in brain tissue. So far, there are only a few preliminary trials. Certain supplements can have adverse effects or even worsen symptoms, so it is very important to consult your doctor first.

HERBS TO TRY:

TWHF: The Chinese herb with one of the most awkward names — Tripterygium wilfordii Hook F anti-inflammatory and immunosuppressive traits. Its main ingredient, triptolide, is said to have these properties and has been shown to protect neurons from injury and thus pain. [*J Neuroimmunol.* 2004;148(1-2):24-31] TWHF has been used for over 2,000 years in Chinese medicine. The hopeful note on Parkinson's comes from a 2003 study in rats. Research always has to begin with animals. They found that "tripcholoride," which also comes from the herb, significantly prevented the decrease of dopamine – therein showing its potential for Parkinson's. It also increased the chances of survival for those neurons; thus avoiding the disease. [*Exp Neurol.* 2003;179(1):28-37]

HP-200: This is otherwise known as the herb, *Mucuna prurient*. Preliminary research suggests it could be beneficial against Parkinson's. In patients with the disease, researchers found that HP-200 treatment led to a significant reduction in symptoms all the way from the beginning to the end of the trial. [*J Altern Complement Med* 1995;1:249–55]

Psyllium: More preliminary research, because that is all there is so far, has found that the husks of psyllium seeds improve constipation and bowel function in Parkinson's patients. Psyllium is a well known laxative, but it might be particularly useful in this disease because movement, even bowel movement, is disrupted in people with Parkinson's. [*Mov Disord* 1997;12:946–51] Typically, three to five grams of psyllium seed husks each night with a few glasses of water is recommended.

SAMe: This supplement has been tested to see if it can reduce depression in patients with Parkinson's disease who are taking one of the more popular drugs: levodopa. Long-term use of levodopa may deplete the level of SAMe in the brain, which might bring upon the onset of depression because SAMe is known to have an antidepressant effect. So, in 21 patients taking levodopa, researchers found that 72% of those given SAMe supplements felt their depression improved compared to just 30% of placebo patients. [*Curr Ther Res.* 1990;48:154-160] *Caution: Only use SAMe for this purpose under the guidance of a doctor. It might interfere with levodopa's intended effect.*

Note... On Parkinson's Treatment: Some supplements – including vitamins C and E – have shown to be effective in preliminary trials

Notable Herbs

TWHF

HP-200

Psyllium

Other Nutraceuticals That May Work:

SAMe

Coenzyme Q_{10}

CDP-choline (a.k.a. "citicholine")

Vitamin E

Vitamin C

5-HTP

Pelvic Inflammatory Disease

Pelvic Inflammatory Disease is often a symptom of other pelvic diseases and is second only to AIDS as the most common and serious complication of sexually transmitted diseases. Simply put, it is an infection of the uterus and the upper genital tract. It is characterized by inflammation, and can be caused by gonorrhea, chlamydia, ovarian cystic disease, or postpartum infections. It is extremely painful. About one million women in the U.S. have an episode of PID every year, and over 100,000 become infertile every year because of it. Herbal medications may help reduce the inflammation and act as pain relievers, but none have been tested specifically on PID.

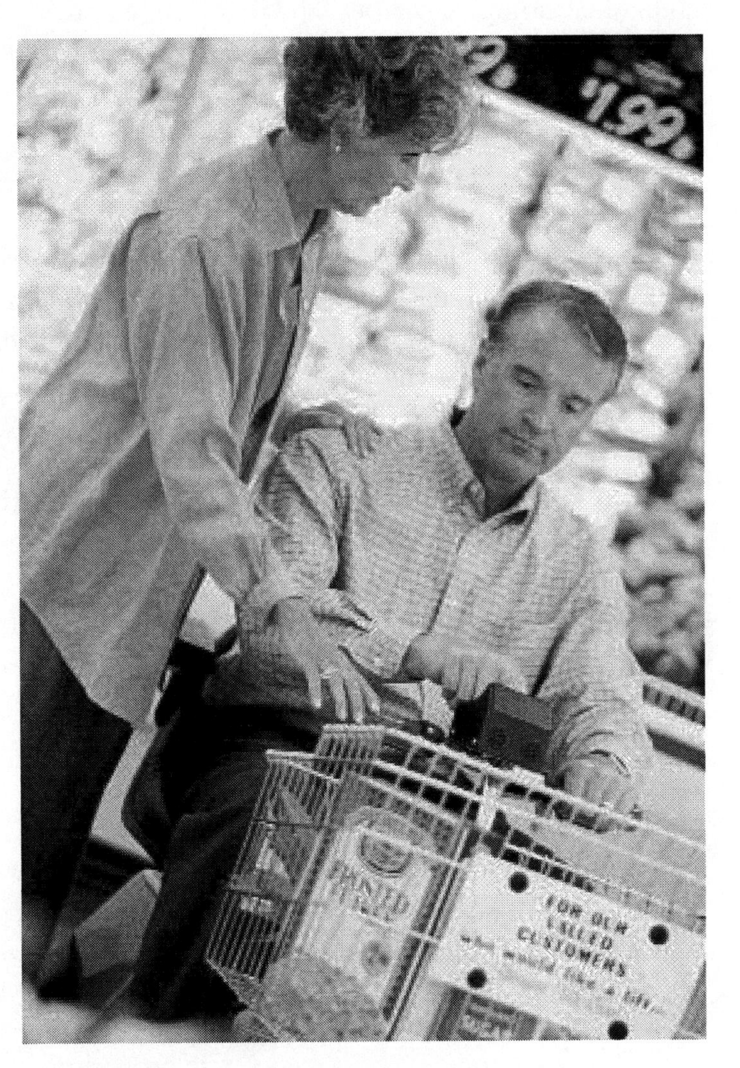

About one million women in the U.S. have an episode of PID every year, and over 100,000 become infertile every year because of it.

HERBS TO TRY:

Turmeric: What makes curry yellow may also treat pain and inflammation. Turmeric is part of the ginger family and has proven in animal studies to reduce inflammation, a belief held for centuries in India. The spice, taken internally, may work in this way by inhibiting the production of prostaglandins, which are inflammatory chemicals. Its main ingredient is curcumin, which is said to reduce inflammation by lowering histamine levels. The herb's anti-inflammatory effects are such that it may be useful in treating PID.

Ginger: Ginger is reputed to help relieve abdominal pain and soothe the digestive tract. Stimulating digestive enzymes, it is an aid in moving food through the body. It also helps relieve diarrhea and it has known anti-inflammatory qualities.

Greater Celandine: This herb's been found to relieve – significantly more than placebo – abdominal cramping, nausea, and that feeling of being full as a result of indigestion. [*Comp Ther Med* 1993;1:189–93] *Caution: This herb has been linked since then to an increased risk of hepatitis.*

Peppermint: A natural antispasmodic, it is known to relax intestinal muscles, reduce gas, and help relieve any cramps. You can take peppermint oil, or "enteric-coated" pills. Not studied for pelvic inflammatory disease, it has been studied for irritable bowel syndrome (IBS) – both conditions have abdominal pain as an effect. A study of 42 children with IBS found that 75% of those taking peppermint oil pills had less severe abdominal pain. Nearly half reported they were feeling "much better." For adults, two controlled trials have shown evidence that peppermint oil relieved symptoms of IBS when taken in enteric-coated pills. [*Am J Gastroenterol* 1998;93:1131–5]

Boswellia: This Ayurvedic herb can defend against inflammation and restore blood vessels in connective tissue. Tested for this ability in arthritis (the king of inflammatory diseases), this herb causes no side effects while providing reasonable pain relief. The boswellic acid, in particular, is thought to reduce inflammation. A review of unpublished studies into this herb found double-blind trials deduced that is was effective in relieving rheumatoid arthritis symptoms. [*Phytomed* 3(1): 67–70, 1996]. A number of scientific studies have confirmed the effectiveness of boswellia. In a study of 175 people with arthritis, four weeks of boswellia treatment helped 122 of them reduce pain and stiffness.

Goldenseal: This herbal antibiotic is traditionally used to fight infections. Its main ingredient, "berberine," has been shown to slow the growth of a bacteria that causes many conditions in the pelvic and intestinal areas of humans, *H. pylori.* [*Biol Pharm Bull* 1998;21(9):990–2]

Notable Herbs

Turmeric Ginger
Greater Celandine
Peppermint
Boswellia
Goldenseal

Premenstrual Syndrome (PMS)

Symptoms of premenstrual syndrome vary from woman to woman, but generally they encompass emotional, physical, psychological, and mood disturbances that occur after ovulation and end with the onset of the menstrual flow. They are caused by the hormonal changes of the menstrual cycle, and they can include cramping, palpitation, tender breasts, sweating, depression, a tendency to cry, aggravation, short temper, bloating, headache, or any number of physical and emotional concerns. PMS can be very mild or very serious, and it is important to see your health care provider for a proper diagnosis and examination. Herbal medicines can be quite effective with this syndrome. For those with serious cases, herbal therapy can ease symptoms and help them cope with this often misunderstood and socially stigmatized condition.

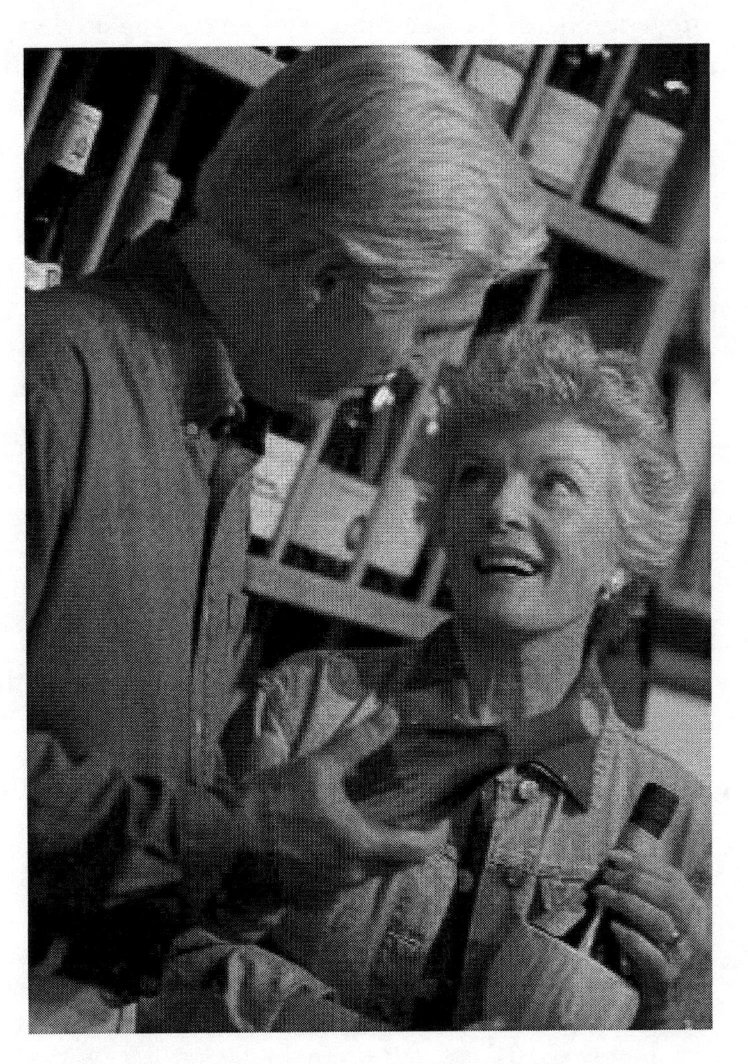

For those with serious cases, herbal therapy can ease symptoms and help them cope with this often misunderstood and socially stigmatized condition.

HERBS TO TRY:

Black Cohosh: According to tradition, Black Cohosh is used for "women's complaints." It is an anti-inflammatory, it lowers blood pressure, and acts as an antispasmodic. It also has sedative properties. It is an increasingly popular treatment for menopausal symptoms such as hot flashes. It has been the subject of some bad press, but a 2003 study found it unrelated to negative health risks, including cancer. [*Int J Oncol.* 2003 Nov;23(5):1407-12] German health authorities have approved it for use in PMS symptoms. The American College of Obstetrics and Gynecology supports the use of this herb for up to six months in female menstrual-related issues.

Vitex: This herb (a.k.a. "chaste tree") is used sometimes as a treatment for infertility and amenorrhea (when a woman's menstrual cycle is absent). It helps balance estrogen and progesterone. It has been shown to reduce the level of the hormone prolactin (especially right before a women's period), which at high levels can lead to amenorrhea. A German trial found that women had normal prolactin production when they took three months of vitex treatment. [*Arzneimittelforschung* 1993;43:752–6] Vitex has also been shown to help with "luteal phase defect" – a condition that can cause menstrual cycle abnormalities. A major double-blind study found that vitex extract led to significantly less PMS symptoms in women who used it for three months. [*BMJ* 2001;20:134–7]

Evening Primrose: Follow this trail of thought: Women with PMS may have difficulty converting linolenic acid to *gamma*-linolenic acid (GLA). Thus, it's possible to assume a lack of GLA may have something to do with PMS, so evening primrose oil – very high in GLA – has been looked at as a way to reduce symptoms. It may be best to use this oil over a few menstrual cycles. In double-blind trials in the 1980s, evening primrose led to beneficial results in women with PMS. [*Rec Adv Clin Nutr* 1986;2:404–5]

Ginkgo Biloba: French researchers found an extract of this herb, taken at 160 mg a day, helps eliminate congestion and psychological disturbances caused by PMS better than placebo. [*Rev Fr Gynecol Obstet* 1993;88:447–57]

Notable Herbs

Black Cohosh

Vitex

Evening Primrose

Ginkgo Biloba

Other Nutraceuticals That May Work:

Calcium

Magnesium

L-tryptophan (amino acid)

Psoriasis

Psoriasis is a persistent skin disease characterized by inflammation and most notably by red, dry, and thickened patches of skin most often seen on the elbows, knees, lower back, and scalp. It ranges from mild to severe (from unnoticeable to covering the entire back) and each form of psoriasis differs in every factor including how the scales appear on the skin. The most common form is "plaque psoriasis" which begins with small red bumps and escalates to larger red areas and scales. Some patients may experience joint pain as well. Researchers have found that certain people have a genetic predisposition to psoriasis, although it can also be caused by environmental factors, a faulty immune system, acidic foods, drugs, sunburn, infections, obesity, alcohol use, hormonal changes, and stress. Contrary to what it looks like it, psoriasis is not contagious and about two percent of the population has the disorder. Herbal treatments reduce the inflammation, redness, and pain associated with the disease.

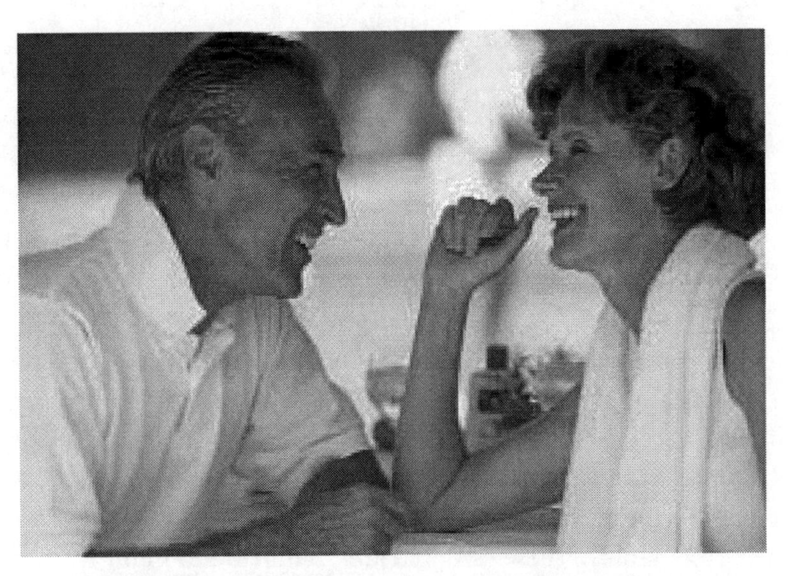

Researchers have found that certain people have a genetic predisposition to psoriasis, although it can also be caused by environmental factors, a faulty immune system, acidic foods, drugs, sunburn, infections, obesity, alcohol use, hormonal changes, and stress.

HERBS TO TRY:

Oregon Grape Root: This plant is abundantly found in North American forests and is known also as "Mahonia." Some of mahonia's properties may be effective in battling some of the body's internal causes that brings about psoriasis, not the least of which is too many "keratinocytes." In Germany, more than 440 patients with acute and chronic psoriasis were treated with ointment made from this plant. The results: 81% had improved symptoms or were completely healed. This promising plant dropped the number of people who had severe psoriasis from 30% to less than six percent in just three months of treatment. [*Germ. J. of Derm. Treat.* 1995;6/1:31-34] One year later another study found that in four weeks of treatment, Oregon grape root significantly reduced symptoms in patients taking it. The treatment was labeled a success. ["*Phytomedicine* 1996;3(3):231-235]

Capsaicin: Also known as cayenne, this cream made from a spicy pepper is a proven powerful pain reliever when it's rubbed onto the skin around sore joints and muscles. Capsaicin cream has been looked at in treating psoriasis, another dermatologic disease that leads to itchy, red skin. The idea is that itching follows the same pathway as pain – thus if the cayenne pepper helps relieve pain, it will do so for itching too. It was proven in a study of 200 patients with psoriasis that even a 0.025% capsaicin cream significantly reduced itching, scaling, thickness, and redness compared to the effects of a plain cream.[*Journal of the American Academy of Dermatology*, Sept. 1993;29:438-42]

Omega-3 Fatty Acids: These help promote wound healing, and are sometimes used for people who have suffered burns to their skins. For psoriasis, some research has shown that people taking supplements of these essential fatty acids (found in high amounts in flaxseed and evening primrose oils) had reduced symptoms of psoriasis than if they had only used traditional medications. A *Lancet* double-blind study found that 10 grams of fish oil (high in omega-3) improved psoriasis skin rash. [*Lancet* 1988;i:378–80] In another trial, a fatty acid lessened the severity of the skin disease when it was used for two months. *[Dermatologica* 1991;182:225–30] Omega-3 is widely known to have anti-inflammatory properties.

Aloe Vera: This herb that has cut such a wide swath through the medicinal world, might also be mildly effective in relieving psoriasis symptoms as well. A review of the herb in clinical trials determined that it may be useful for patients with the skin disorder, when used topically on the skin. [*Br J Gen Pract.* 1999;49(447):823-8]

Notable Herbs

Oregon Grape Seed

Cayenne

Aloe Vera

Other Nutraceuticals That May Work:

Omega-3 Fatty Acids

Vitamin D (prescription only)

Shark Cartilage

Milk Thistle

Sinusitis

Sinuses are hollow air spaces in the human body – if they are infected or inflamed, you have come down with a case of sinusitis. The acute kind lasts up to three weeks; the chronic kind lasts up to two months (or longer) or the recurrent kind, the most miserable kind, strikes a few times a year. Here are the potential symptoms, depending on which sinuses have been inflamed: headaches in the morning, pain in your jaw and teeth, swelling and pain in the eyes, earaches, and neck pain. Other common symptoms of sinusitis include fatigue, fever (in half of patients), cough, sore throat, loss of smell, runny nose, and very bad nasal congestion. Common causes include: physically injuring the sinuses, a common cold, allergies, swimming, or even an infected tooth. Every year, about 37 million Americans contract the condition. Below, herbal remedies may help clear up mucus congestion, but they lack clinical evidence. It's either these unproved remedies, or a steroidal nasal spray.

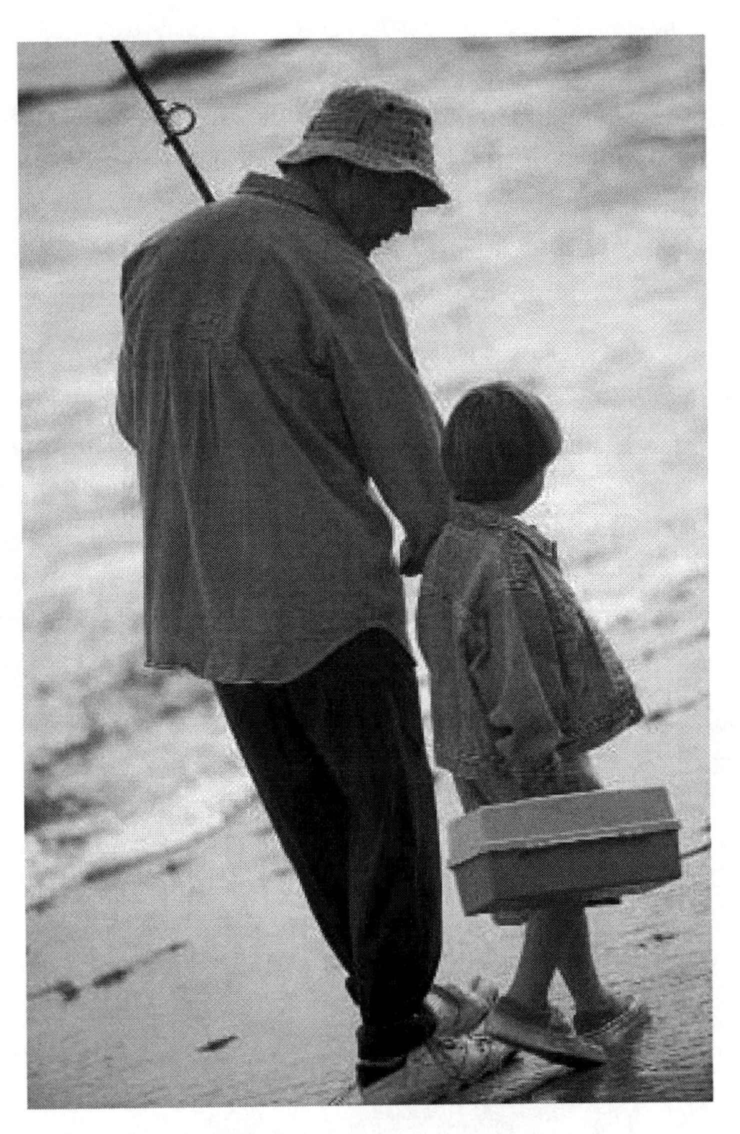

Every year, about 37 million Americans contract sinusitis.

HERBS TO TRY:

Peppermint: This is a strong antibiotic oil, and can stop bacteria and some viruses in their tracks. It may be helpful in relieving mucus congestion in the sinuses as well as lungs. The component of peppermint, menthol, is the working ingredient in question. Much of this is anecdotal, as there lacks any hard evidence to back it up. In Germany, peppermint oil is approved for mucus congestion. If you want to try it, try inhaling it, or adding it to a humidifier.

Eucalyptus oil: This is thought to work just the same as menthol, clearing sinus congestion when inhaled. It may have an effect on membranes in the nasal passage and cut down on nasal stuffiness. It actually is a main ingredient in "Vaporub."

Horseradish: There aren't any definitive studies per say, but this potent herb is well-known for its ability to dissolve mucus, which in turn can relieve congestion. One of its components, "allyl isothiocyanate," works – as you can tell when you eat it – to stimulate nerves in the nose, possibly make you shed tears, and thins out mucus. Try grating fresh horseradish root and taking three grams of it at a time, up to three times a day.

Bromelain: Not a herb, but an enzyme found in pineapples, this is nevertheless notable in terms of helping ease cough, congestion, sinusitis, and allergies that hit the sinuses. It is still mentioned quite a bit as a natural supplement to combat sinusitis, as bromelain reduces inflammation and fluid build-up in the nasal passage. The most successful study isn't to recent, taking place in the 1960s, but here it is: 87% of patients who took the enzyme reported either good or excellent results (68% of placebo did the same). [*Headache* 1967;7:13–7] This anti-inflammatory enzyme may be the trick for you.

Notable Herbs

Peppermint Oil

Eucalyptus Oil

Horseradish

Other Nutraceuticals That May Work:

Bromelain

Smoking Cessation

While smoking isn't a disease in and of itself, it has been proven to be a leading cause of disease and the number one preventable cause of death. Smoking is a serious addiction. Some people can quit smoking cold turkey, but others need help. The decision to quit smoking is one of the best decisions you could ever make. Herbal medicines can help calm your nerves and help you fight the urge to light up. None of these are proven.

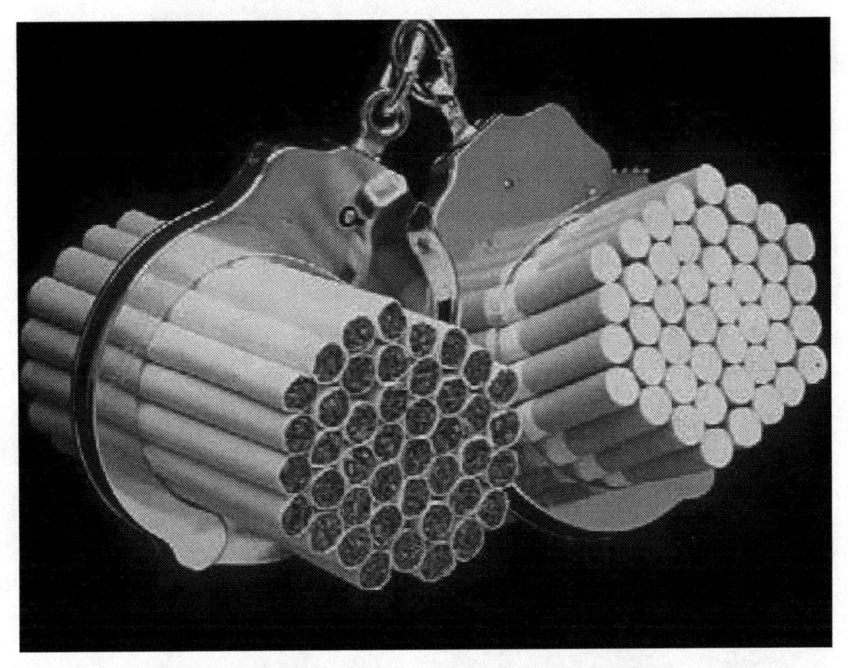

The decision to quit smoking is one of the best decisions you could ever make.

HERBS TO TRY:

Lobelia: This annual flowering herb has a long history of helping remedy respiratory conditions and because of its ingredient "lobeline" it is used to prevent the urge to smoke. People wishing to quit may benefit, as this ingredient affects the nervous system in a way similar to nicotine, and acts like dopamine in the body. It has even been studied and found effective in treating people to withstand stronger

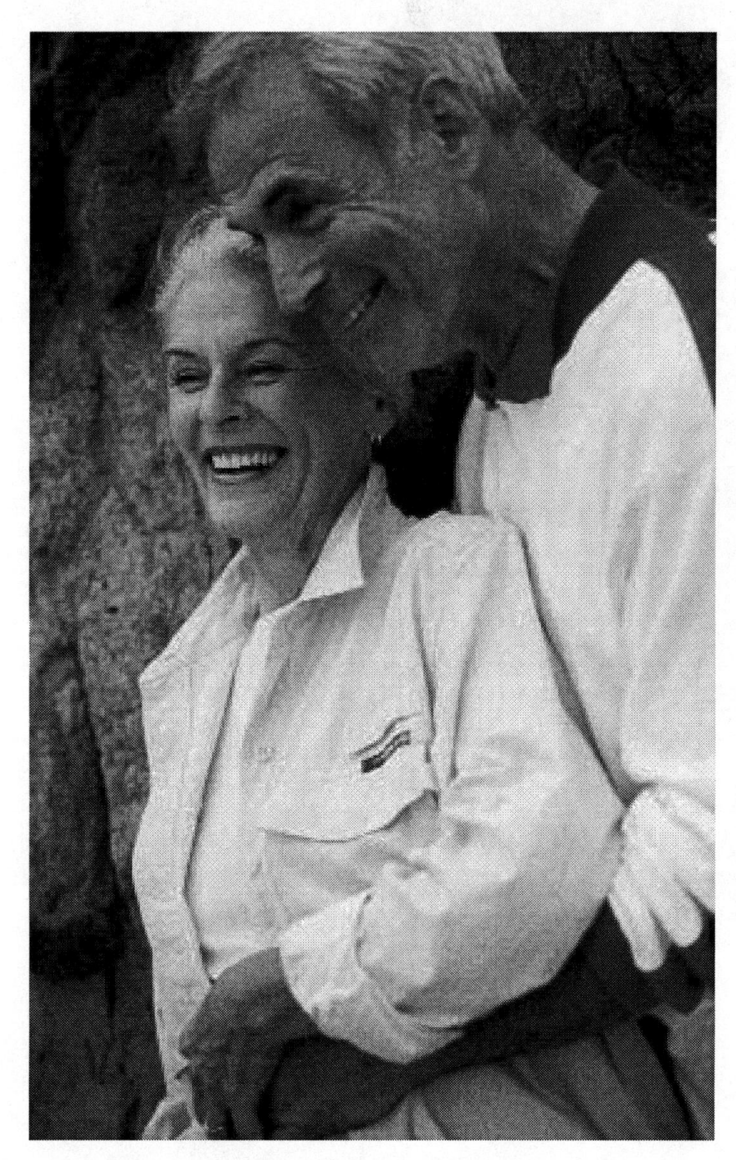

Lobelia plant may help stymie those nicotine cravings.

urges as well: amphetamines and methamphetamines. It was found effective in helping treat psychostimulant abuse. [*Biochem Pharmacol.* 2002;63(2):89-98] This plant may help stymie those nicotine cravings.

Wild Oats: Also known as "*Avena sativa*" this herb is the only other herb to be looked into clinically as a potential therapy for addiction to nicotine and tobacco. Those studies appeared in the 1970s though, and when you look at all the evidence, it would suggest that wild oats is not nearly as effective as lobelia. [J *Pharm Pharmacol.* 1975;27:92-8]

If you're willing to take a chance on herbal help, these herbs are considered possibilities, but have not been tested: Licorice, passionflower, skullcap, alfalfa, eucalyptus, hops, and gotu kola.

Notable Herbs

Lobelia

Sore Throat/Tonsillitis

A sore throat can stem from a viral infection, allergy, or simple irritation. It can be difficult to swallow and your throat and glands can swell uncomfortably. Herbal treatments help combat the swelling, and soothe an irritated throat.

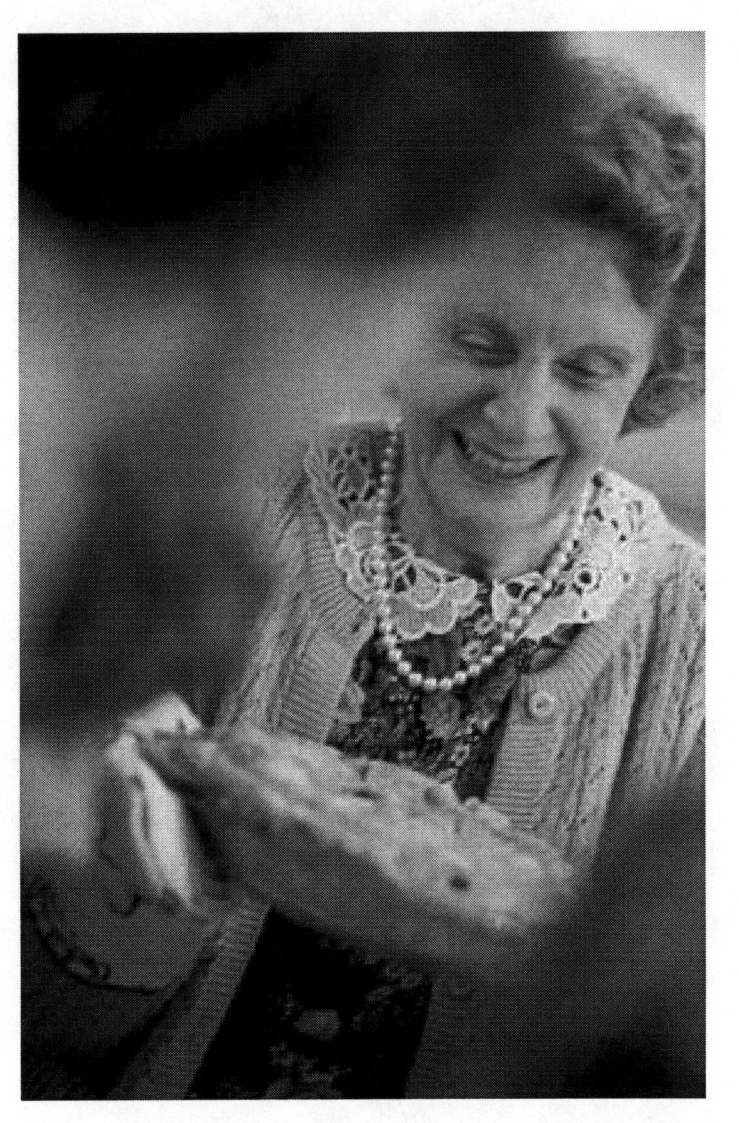

Herbal treatments help combat the swelling, and soothe an irritated throat.

HERBS TO TRY:

Goldenseal: This herb used to fight colds and flu contains berberine and canadine, two alkaloids that are proven to have antimicrobial and some immune-stimulating effects. However, due to the small amounts of alkaloids occurring in the root, it is unlikely these effects would occur outside the test tube. Goldenseal soothes irritated mucous membranes in the throat making it potentially useful for those experiencing a sore throat with their cold.

Berries with Tannins: Astringent tannins are found in blueberries, blackberries, and (red) raspberries. They are known to be beneficial in soothing sore throats, although modern research doesn't yet support this claim.

Slippery Elm: The FDA considers slippery elm a safe and reasonably

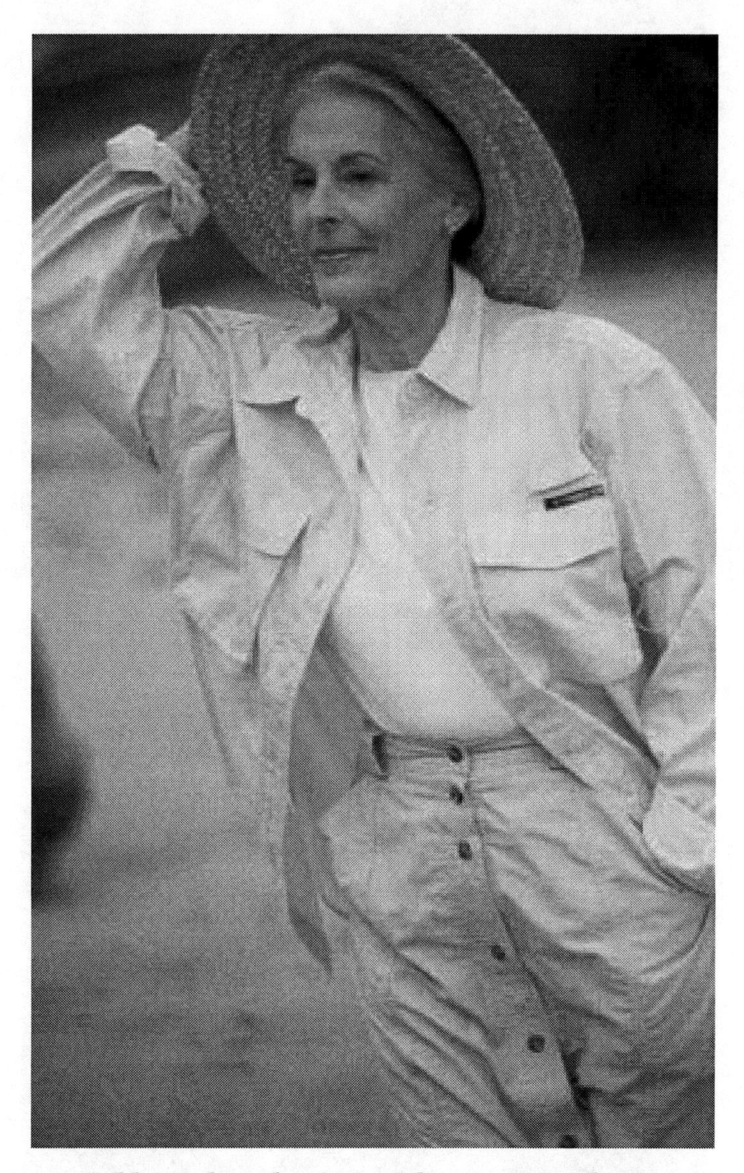

Goldenseal soothes irritated mucous membranes in the throat making it potentially useful for those experiencing a sore throat with their cold.

effective way to relieve sore throat and cough – it is even available in the form of throat lozenges.

Astragalus: The Chinese have long used this root to boost the immune system, strengthening the body against bacteria and viruses. Astragalus has been linked to the growth of active immune cells as well as increasing the number of stem cells in bone marrow. It also might boost interferon in the body, which can prevent or shorten a bout of cold or flu. No controlled studies on humans have confirmed its effects, but basic science and animal studies suggest its effectiveness.

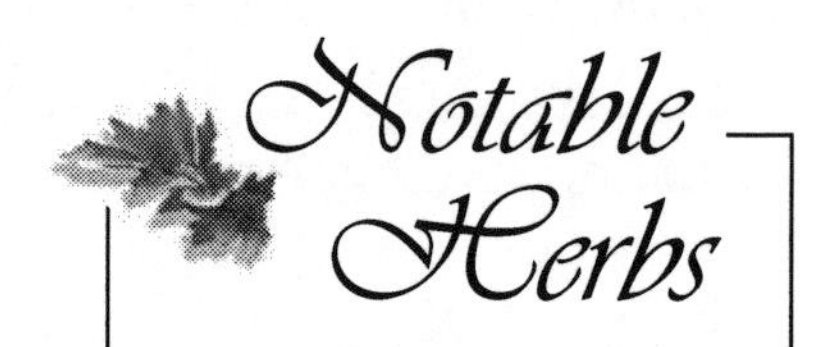

Goldenseal

Slippery Elm

Astragalus

Other Nutraceuticals That May Work:

Blueberry, Red Raspberry, Blackberry

Vitamin C

Zinc

Stroke

A stroke is a medical emergency. It is caused by a sudden lack of blood reaching the brain, leaving tissue without oxygen and nutrients. There are two major types of stroke. Ischemic incidents make up about 80% of all strokes, and are caused by a blocked artery leading to the brain. The leading cause of this blocked artery is the disease arteriosclerosis. The other major stroke type is a hemorrhagic stroke, and occurs when a blood vessel in the brain ruptures. A common cause is high blood pressure that leaves arteries susceptible to cracking. Perhaps the worst kind of hemorrhagic stroke is a "subarachnoid" incident that is usually felt by a massive and immediate headache more severe than anything else. Half of people who get this don't survive. In all, strokes are considered the third leading cause of death behind cardiovascular and cancer-related mortality. The numbers: about 160,000 of 750,000 stroke victims die because of the event. Most strokes now are not fatal, but they can cause paralysis, speech and visual problems, and dementia.

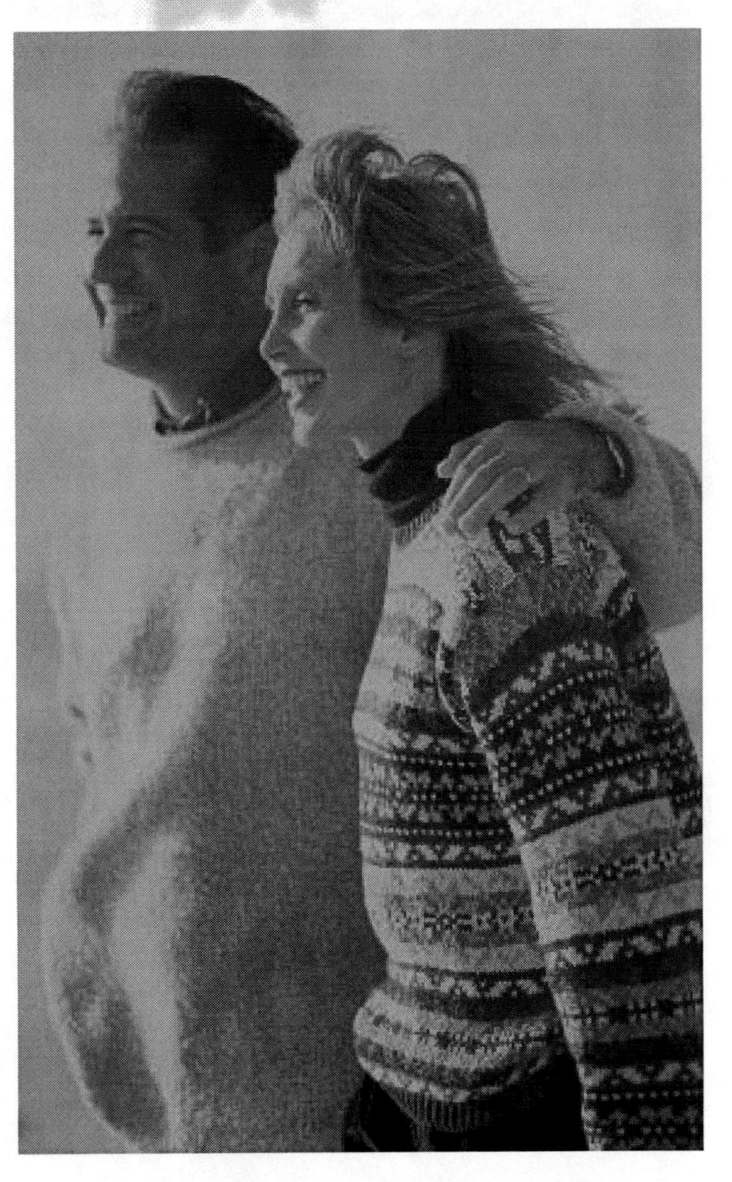

Most strokes now are not fatal, but they can cause paralysis, speech and visual problems, and dementia.

HERBS TO TRY:

The only thing to do is to avoid the possibility of a stroke. Once it hits, herbal remedies are not going to do a great deal of good. Turn to the chapters on these conditions for herbal

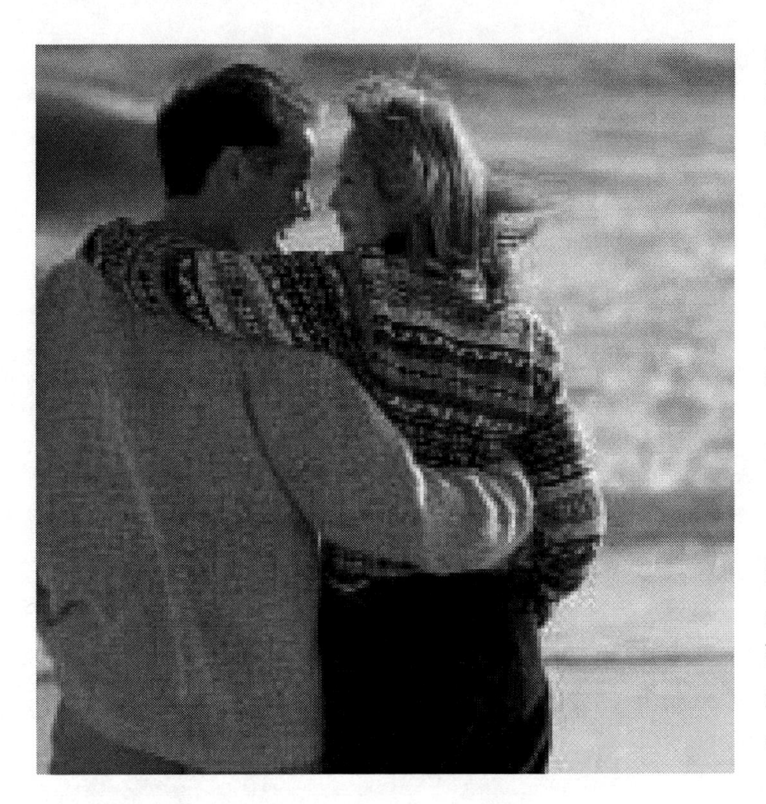

The only thing to do is to avoid the possibility of a stroke. Once it hits, herbal remedies are not going to do a great deal of good.

possibilities that will help keep your blood flowing and your artery walls strong:

Please see the **High Blood Pressure** chapter.

Please see the **Arteriosclerosis (Arthrosclerosis)** chapter.

Please see the **Diabetes** chapter.

Note: Several studies have looked into whether antioxidant vitamins might be able to prevent strokes because of their ability to scavenge free radicals and prevent LDL cholesterol from oxidizing. These include vitamins E and C. The main point: there is no evidence to suggest this works. These vitamins likely do not protect against the possibility of a stroke.

Ulcers/Gastritis

Simply put, an ulcer is an open sore. An ulcer can appear in the gastric system, in the mouth, or in the intestinal system. A peptic ulcer occurs in the lining of the duodenum (at the beginning of the small intestine) or the stomach. They often cause pain usually after eating. Its causes include: the H. pylori bacteria, drugs, and certain diseases such as alcoholism. Gastritis is basically an inflamed stomach lining. Sometimes gastritis will deteriorate the lining and cause bleeding, other times it does not damage it at all. There isn't a specific cause. Symptoms include: indigestion, nausea, loss of appetite, abdominal pain, dark vomit, and stool. When an ulcer occurs in the mouth, it's also known as a canker sore, which differs from a cold sore in that it occurs in the soft tissue and is not contagious. In general, ulcers can be located in the skin or mucous membrane, and lead to pain, loss of surface tissue, disintegration, and death of epithelial tissue, inflammation, and fluid discharge. It can be caused by stress, other diseases, or even ongoing use of NSAID pain relievers. An ulcer needs to be taken seriously so it can be healed as quickly as possible. Herbal treatments reduce inflammation, assist in healing, and decrease pain.

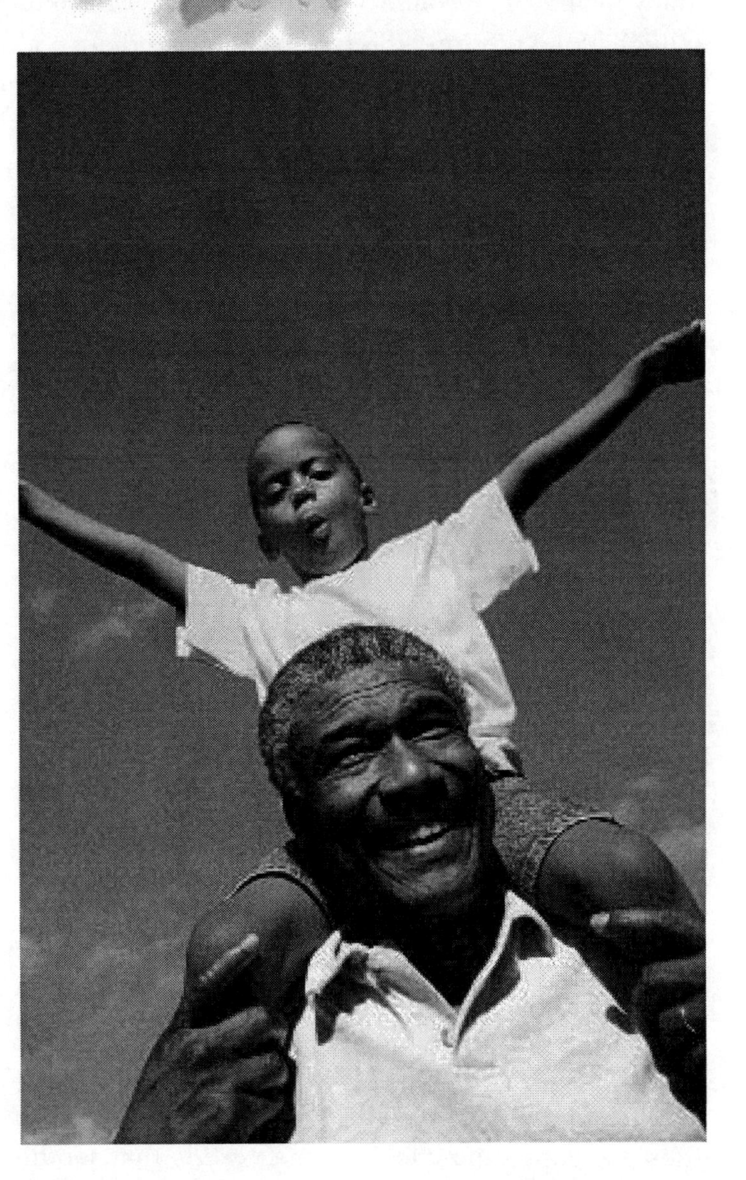

Ulcers can be caused by stress, other diseases, or even ongoing use of NSAID pain relievers.

HERBS TO TRY:

Licorice: In particular, "deglycyrrhizinated" licorice (or DGL) can be useful in stomach ulcers. Many people are recommended this extract. Unlike regular licorice root, which has been linked to high blood pressure, this type has an ingredient – glycyrrhizin – removed. Chewable DGL has proven useful in healing stomach, duodenal, and even canker sores [*Gut* 1985;26:599-602... *Lancet* 1982;ii:817... *J Assoc Physicians India* 1989;37:647]. Two double-blind trials found that a drug very similar to a main ingredient of licorice was effective against acid reflux [*Curr Med Res Opin* 1978;5:637-44... *Scand J Gastroenterol* 1986;21:1098-104]. In fact, one of them found it was 50% faster in curing acid reflux than placebo, and was 82% successful. This is about as close as medical studies have come to proving this type of licorice helps with the esophagus and movement of stomach acid. For canker sores, or ulcers of the mouth, try mixing licorice in warm water and swish it around.

Aloe Vera: The herb commonly found in skin creams can also be of help when taken internally. Make sure you're using a purified gel extract or capsules and not the bitter aloe latex or juice, which is a strong laxative. Since it is normally used as a cream, there is little substantial evidence into how it can help you internally. But in some preliminary research, Japanese investigators gave juice to 18 patients with peptic ulcers. All but one found relief. Other trials in Japan show that certain ingredients in aloe vera help limit the secretion of stomach juices and the formation of lesions. *Caution: Consult your doctor before trying aloe vera internally for this reason.*

Chamomile: This herb has shown an ability to stop inflammation and even act an as antispasmodic. It is commonly prepared as tea, best when taken many times a day. Clinical studies into its effect on heartburn are lacking, but what is known is that drinking the tea can relieve esophageal irritation because of its soothing nature on all gastrointestinal tissues, thus preventing ulcer formation. It exerts that soothing effect on mucous membranes, which is why it often recommended for canker sores and mouth irritations.

Other potential herbs that lack definitive studies include: butterbur, cat's claw, and marshmallow.

Notable Herbs

Licorice

Aloe Vera

Chamomile

Other Nutraceuticals That May Work:

B Vitamins

Zinc

Glutamine

MSM

Vitamin A

Selenium

Vitamin C

Colostrum

Urinary Tract Infection

A urinary tract infection can be very disruptive and quite painful. It is characterized by the frequent, urgent need to urinate, burning sensations during urination, and the sensation of an inability to urinate. Blood can appear in the urine and abdominal cramping is common. A urinary tract infection is a bacterial infection that inflames the bladder. A weakened immune system, due to antibiotic treatment, auto-immune disease, diabetes, or pregnancy is an ideal breeding ground for the bacteria that causes urinary tract infections. If not treated early enough, the infection can spread to the kidneys. Herbal treatments help kill the bacteria that causes the condition, strengthen the immune system, and relieve symptoms.

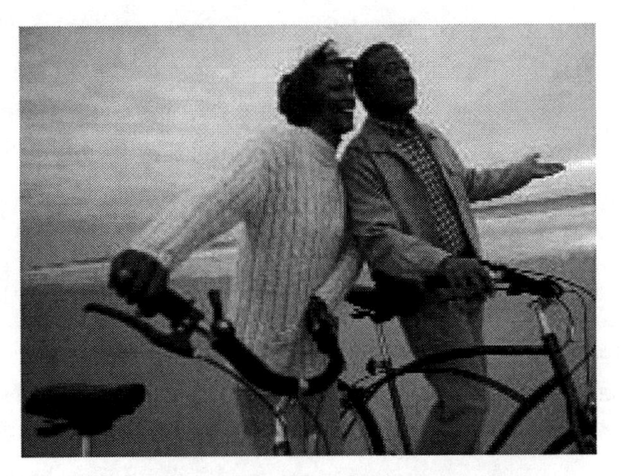

A weakened immune system, due to antibiotic treatment, auto-immune disease, diabetes, or pregnancy is an ideal breeding ground for the bacteria that causes urinary tract infections.

HERBS TO TRY:

Cranberry: Long used to treat urinary tract infections, these small red berries may be useful in alleviating symptoms of this condition. In one study, 16 ounces of cranberry juice a day led to beneficial effects in 73% of people with urinary tract infections. [*The Healing Power of Herbs*, 1992]. Of those who stopped drinking the juice, 61% had a recurrence of infection. Cranberries appear to prevent bacteria from "adhering" to the lining of the bladder and urethra. Many believe cranberry to be effective in preventing E. coli from attaching to bladder walls and causing infection. In a study of elderly residents at a nursing home, 120 ml of juice or six capsules of concentrated cranberry led to a 25% decrease in urinary tract infections in just over a year. [*J Am Geriatr Soc* 1997;45:S53] Fresh berry juice has been shown in several studies to be linked to a lower risk of getting infections and recurring infections.

Parsley: Folk medicine has held that parsley exhibits a diuretic effect on the urinary tract system. A study claims to have provided "substantial evidence" that this is true, as well as finding out how exactly it works. The study, on rats, found that those given a parsley seed extract to drink with water urinated a significantly larger volume compared to those drinking only water. When they used a specific kidney technique, the results were the same: the animals' urine flow was much higher with parsley seed. [*J Ethnopharmacol.* 2002;79(3):353-7]

Saw Palmetto: Many doctors, in the east and west, prescribe this herb to relieve infections of the urinary tract because it can be so beneficial. It is a bushy plant that typically grows in sandy soil in southeastern U.S., the Caribbean, and in the Mediterranean. Its partially dried black berries are the source of the plant's medicinal properties. It is known for its urinary antiseptic abilities, and is used for a variety of urinary tract ailments. The mechanism by which this herb helps with urinary problems remains unknown. In one double-blind study, the herb led to a statistically significant improvement in urinary symptoms in men over the age of 45 who had lower urinary tract symptoms. [*Urology* 2001;58(6):960-4]

Pygeum: Traditional African medicine dictates that sipping tea made from this tall evergreen tree, native to Africa, will control urinary disorders in men. Since the 1970s, it's been approved for treating mild to moderate benign prostate hyperplasia in Europe. Pygeum has been found to be safe and effective for this treatment, and studies have typically used 50 to 100 mg of extract twice a day. [*Curr Ther Res* 1995;56:796–817] The herb contains compounds that have a diuretic action, anti-inflammatory activity, and a unique ability to dispose of any built-up cholesterol deposits.

Nettle: Nettle root contains compounds that inhibit the action of sex hormones, thought to stimulate prostate tissue growth. It helps with urine flow as well, assisting the bladder's ability to empty itself in men with early-stage BPH. [*Urologe* 1994;334:90–5] Nettle helps increase urinary volume and flushes bacteria out. It's approved in Germany as part of treatment.

Goldenseal: One of this plant's active ingredients, "berberine" is known to stimulate the immune system, help kill the chlamydia bacterium and help the urinary tract (disturbed by chlamydia). It has been shown to be helpful in preventing bacteria from building on the bladder wall and resolving bladder infections. [*Antimicr Agents Chemother* 1988; 32:1274–7] Most recently, researchers found that berberine was an effective agent in protecting the urinary tract against toxicity and against "cystitis" – a type of infection. [*Pharmacol Toxicol.* 2001;88(5):232-7]

Notable Herbs

Cranberry

Parsley

Saw Palmetto

Pygeum

Nettle

Goldenseal

Other Nutraceuticals That May Work:

Vitamin C

Vitamin A

Probiotics

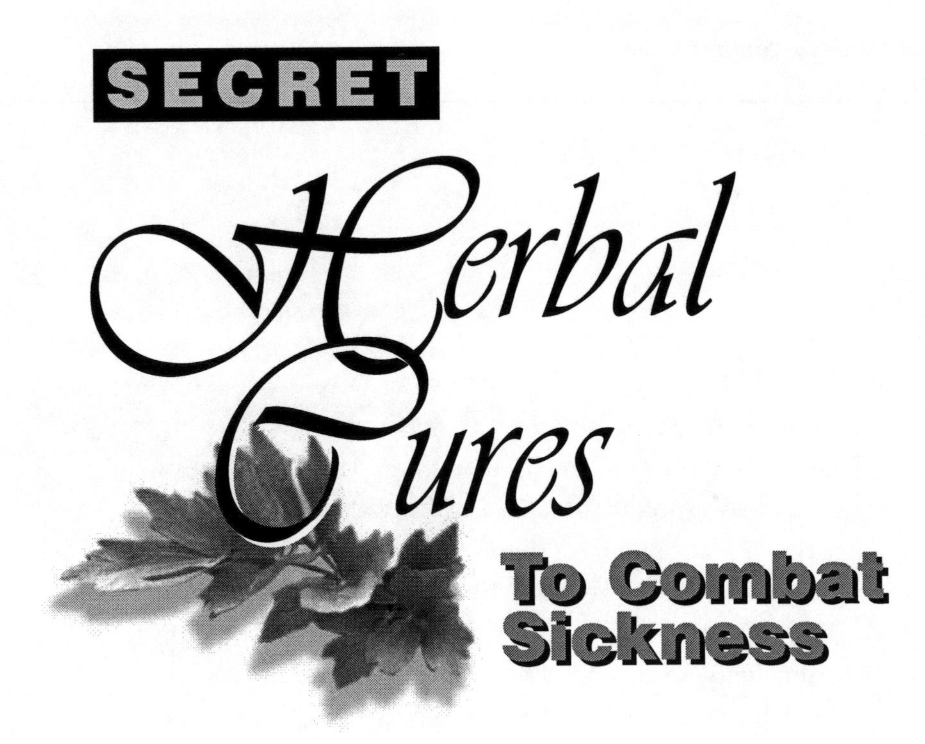

Part Three

INDEX OF HERBS

Briefly:

Over the course of writing this section, a few warning signs came up continually in regards to what kind of drugs and supplements may be affected by any of these herbs. There is much "theoretical" and "preliminary" evidence floating around the medical world because 98% of herbs (a rough estimate) have yet to be extensively studied. There are just some areas, involving risk of bleeding and blood sugar levels that should not be taken lightly. You should first consult your doctor before trying any herbal remedy if you are taking any of the following drugs:

- Anticoagulants or antiplatelets: these include aspirin, heparin, Ticlid, Pletal, and Lovenox.
- Warfarin: also known as Coumadin.
- Insulin
- Any drugs used to treat diabetes
- Any drugs used to treat high blood pressure
- H2-Blockers

Aloe Vera

Overview: Aloe vera has been in continuous use since the days of ancient Egypt. It's mentioned in the Bible. It was carried by explorers on their ships. Aloe is one of the most common herbal cures of our time and is also used in shampoos and lotions. Many people grow aloe as an attractive houseplant…and cut off a leaf when they need to use it.

Benefits: Aloe juice, taken orally, treats constipation. Powdered gel extract is taken orally to treat intestinal problems, including ulcers, diverticulitis, and inflammatory bowel disease.

The gel from the succulent aloe leaf is used to treat cuts, scrapes, and skin irritations, again, reducing pain and promoting healing. Research indicates aloe vera has antifungal, antibacterial, and antiviral properties.

Aloe is an effective treatment for psoriasis. One of the most recent studies found that over 80% of those who applied aloe to affected areas experienced substantial improvement (vs. six percent improvement in the control group).

Topically, aloe is used to treat first degree burns (typically sunburns) and minor second degree burns. It reduces pain and inflammation and promotes healing. In one study, people who used aloe vera healed in an average of 12 days, whereas those who treated the affected areas by covering them in gauze required six additional days to heal.

Considerations: Aloe vera has not been shown effective for treating deep wounds or promoting healing after surgery.

Do not take aloe vera juice if you are pregnant or breast feeding. Aloe should not be used as a long-term laxative. Don't take it in conjunction with other laxatives. Use caution with other supplements or drugs that might lower blood sugar levels.

Side Effects: While there are rare cases of people being allergic to aloe vera (evidenced by skin reactions – itching, rash, swelling), topical aloe vera is considered very safe. Taken orally as aloe vera juice, the only problems reported are due to a poorly processed product. If you experience cramps, stop taking the juice immediately. After your stomach returns to normal, buy a fresh supply of juice.

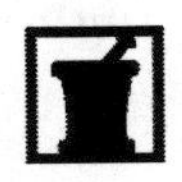

Dosage: Topically, apply about three to four times a day. Orally, take ½ cup of liquid gel extract or two pills after a meal.

Arnica

Overview: Arnica is a European perennial plant with a bright yellow flower similar to a daisy. The flower is commonly used in homeopathic medicine. The plant contains sesquiterpene lactones (which reduce inflammation and pain), thymol (an essential oil), flavonoids, inulin, carotenoids, and tannins.

Benefits: Arnica is used topically to treat eczema, acne, arthritis, and muscle pain. It has both antibacterial and anti-inflammatory properties.

Considerations: Do not take arnica orally. It can cause rapid heart rate, nervous reactions, weakness, and/or vomiting.

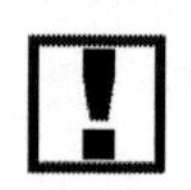

Side Effects: As a topical ointment, arnica is generally well tolerated. If used in too high a concentration or used for too long, though, it may cause skin irritation.

Dosage: Use the topical ointment on affected areas of skin.

Artichoke

Overview: Artichoke is actually a member of the daisy family. We eat the flower head of the globe artichoke, but it's the leaves that contain the higher medicinal value. "Cynarin" is the most studied ingredient and it is found in the leaves.

Benefits: Artichoke serves as a digestive stimulant. It helps to break down fats, stimulate growth of new liver cells, and reduce both cholesterol and triglyceride levels. It is also used to help relieve nausea, bloating, abdominal pain, and constipation.

Considerations: It may increase bile secretion. Consult your doctor before taking artichoke extract if you suffer from gallbladder or a bile duct condition. Artichoke leaves are not recommended for women who are pregnant or breast-feeding. Those allergic to daisies, marigolds, and ragweed might have reactions to artichoke. Don't take it with anticoagulants or anti-platelet herbs or supplements.

Side Effects: There are no concise side effects, but it can cause diarrhea, hunger, and nausea.

Dosage: The typical dosage of extract is 300 mg, two times daily (morning and night) for about six weeks. You can also use actual dried leaves, between one and four grams, three times a day.

Astragalus

Overview: While there are thousands of species worldwide, the medicinal variety of astragalus comes from central and western Asia. It's a perennial plant from the pea family, and the part used comes from the center of the root. Astragalus has been used in Chinese medicine for thousands of years, and it first came to the attention of Western medicine in the 18th century.

Benefits: It is used to boost the immune system (particularly in cancer and HIV patients). This well-documented herb may improve heart, kidney, and liver function, memory, and learning. Its reputed benefits include reducing the symptoms of fibromyalgia, stress, and chronic fatigue syndrome.

Considerations: None identified, but avoid using it with drugs that might decrease blood sugar levels.

Side Effects: At normal doses, there are no side effects reported in Chinese medical literature. Although, it remains insufficiently evaluated in Western research thus far because most studies have looked at a mixture of herbs rather than at astragalus in particular. It may decrease blood sugar levels, it could increase the risk of bleeding, and it might increase growth hormone levels.

Dosage: Astragalus is taken orally. You can buy the root in Asian markets or health food stores; it may also be called "huang qi." According to traditional Chinese medicine, you would drink a tea made with nine to 15 grams of the herb daily. For those who prefer Western delivery methods, take two to three 500 mg capsules daily or three to five ml of a tincture three times a day.

Basil

Overview: This member of the mint family may have originated in Africa and Asia, but it's now enjoyed in cooking the world over. The plant is an annual, and comes in a wide variety of flavors that delight chefs, cooks, and diners. It also has a diverse history of uses, apart from culinary, around the world.

Benefits: It contains beta-carotene, vitamin C and flavonoids. It may aid the digestive system by relieving constipation, alleviating gas, limiting cramps, and preventing vomiting. It promotes healing of minor injuries, and is sometimes used in skin ointments and acne treatments. In aromatherapy, basil is used to treat nasal congestion.

Considerations: It is recommended that children and pregnant or breast-feeding women not take basil supplements.

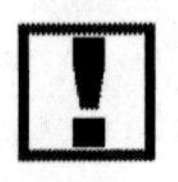

Side Effects: This extremely safe and tasty herb has no reported side effects. Although, prolonged use of the supplement is not recommended.

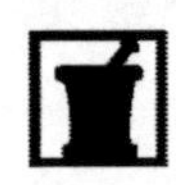

Dosage: Can be obtained in extract, oil, and ointment formulations for external use. Extract, leaves, tea, and tinctures are sold for internal use. Use as basil tea (one teaspoon of leaves in a cup of water), massage oil, or oil added to bath water for vapor.

Bilberry

Overview: Bilberry is in the same family as blueberries and cranberries, only it originated in northern Europe. The shrub is now grown in Canada, the U.S., and Asia as well. The berries are dark, wrinkly, and full of seeds. For medicinal purposes the leaves and berries are dried and used.

Benefits: Bilberries contain bioflavonoids called anthocyanosides and tannin. They are used to treat sore throats, vision problems including night blindness, and circulatory problems including arteriosclerosis. Some arthritis and gout sufferers take bilberry to relieve their symptoms.

Considerations: Only use dried bilberries to treat diarrhea as fresh ones may make the condition worse. High doses have led to anemia and wasting in test animals. Because it may lower blood pressure, avoid drugs or supplements that do the same. Avoid taking "quercetin" supplements at the same time as bilberry. Children should not take bilberry.

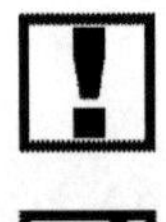

Side Effects: It may increase the risk of bleeding.

Dosage: For capsules, use between 240 and 480 mg of bilberry extract (standardized to provide 25% "anthocyanosides").

Black Cohosh

Overview: Also known as black snakeroot, black cohosh is a shrub-type plant native to North America. An attractive garden plant, the medicinal value comes from its roots and rhizomes.

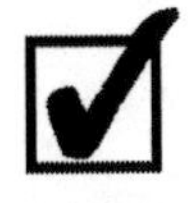

Benefits: Antispasmodic for nerves and muscles. Historically used for "female problems" – menopausal concerns in particular – black cohosh may reduce pain and swelling associated with rheumatoid arthritis, sciatica, osteoarthritis, or inflammation resulting from joint and muscle injuries. It needs more research, but it may also help with sore throats and persistent coughs associated with bronchitis and asthma.

Considerations: It should not be used by pregnant or breast-feeding women. It should also not be considered a substitute for hormone replacement therapy. Don't use it if you have a hormone-sensitive condition such as breast cancer or endometriosis. No known drug interactions, but don't use it with other drugs or supplements that might lower blood pressure. To be safe, don't use it with any herbs that might have estrogen-like effects.

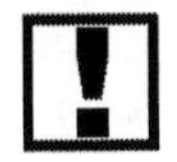

Side Effects: May cause occasional stomach upset, headache, lowered heart rate, and blood pressure. In a few studies, it has led to constipation, lack of bone mass, low blood pressure, nausea, vomiting, intestinal discomfort, and even irregular heart beat.

Dosage: Available in dried root, powdered extract, tablet, capsule, and tincture form. Its recommended dosage is 20 to 40 mg, twice a day, for up to six months.

Boxwood

Overview: This North American shrub is used traditionally as a medicine by native peoples. It's manufactured under the name of SPV-30, and it's the leaf that provides medicinal value in the extract.

Benefits: It is known as a tonic for the immune system. Boxwood is becoming increasingly popular as an AIDS treatment, due to a study that found leaf and stem extract delayed the progression of HIV.

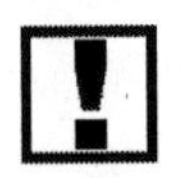

Considerations: When used as an HIV/AIDS medication, it should be done under the guidance of a medical professional. Don't eat the whole leaf, because it can cause life threatening side effects. Pregnant or nursing women should not use boxwood.

Side Effects: Taken orally, it can cause diarrhea or abdominal cramps. If used on the skin, it may cause contact dermatitis.

Dosage: In the HIV/AIDS study, researchers used 330 mg, three times a day. An important point to know is that exceeding this dose may reverse the effect: researchers found that doubling the dose actually decreased, not increased its effectiveness.

Butterbur

Overview: Butterbur is a plant from Europe and Great Britain with many interesting synonyms: langwort, umbrella plant, bog rhubarb, flapperdock, blatterdock, capdockin, bogshorns, butterdock. The shrub has huge leaves, up to almost three feet in diameter. It's the roots that are used for herbal medicine.

Benefits: Traditional uses include treatment for colds and fevers, asthma, migraines, and urinary problems (and historical records indicate it was used for the Great Plague as well). It is currently promoted as a cure for hay fever, based on a 2002 study that appeared in the *British Medical Journal.*

Considerations: Butterbur contains pyrrolizidine alkaloids, which are toxic and possibly carcinogenic. When it is processed, these compounds are removed. Therefore, only use extracts produced by a reputable supplier. Butterbur should not be used by children or women who are pregnant or breast-feeding.

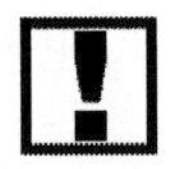

Side Effects: Possible side effects include itching skin, wheezing, stomach upset, headache, and fatigue. It may cause allergic reactions in those sensitive to ragweed, marigolds, and daises.

Dosage: The typical dose is 50 mg, twice daily with meals. Some recommend taking it for four to six months, then slowly tapering off.

Caraway

Overview: Native throughout Europe, Asia, and Africa, caraway is a biannual plant whose seeds have long been used as a flavoring. The dried fruit or seeds are also used medicinally – in fact, medicinal use dates back as far as 1,500 BC.

Benefits: Reliable scientific data exists showing that caraway, in conjunction with peppermint oil, is of value for treating irritable bowel syndrome. Some studies also indicate it may treat gingivitis and indigestion.

Considerations: Should not be used by very young children, and pregnant or breast-feeding women should not exceed the dosage below. To date, there are no known drug interactions.

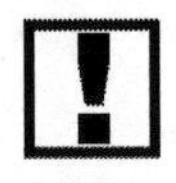

Side Effects: There are none indicated. If used on the skin, it can cause contact dermatitis.

Dosage: You can brew a tea (drink three times daily) from ¼ to ½ tsp of powdered caraway fruit in boiling water, or take up to four ml of a tincture three times daily. Enteric-coated volatile oil can be taken (up to 0.2 ml) three times daily, together with enteric-coated peppermint oil.

Cat's Claw

Overview: This plant hails from the rain forests of Peru's Andes Mountains. The roots are used in herbal medicine.

Benefits: Considerable evidence supports the use of cat's claw in the treatment of osteoarthritis. Anecdotal evidence or traditional medicine suggests it may be used to treat rheumatoid arthritis, gastric ulcers, and inflammation, and to boost immune function. It is an increasingly popular herbal treatment for HIV. The anti-inflammatory activity of cat's claw may be caused by the inhibition of TNF-alpha production. Cat's Claw water extracts have been shown to enhance DNA repair after chemotherapy-induced damage.

Considerations: Due to limited data, pregnant or breast-feeding women should err on the side of caution and avoid cat's claw. The herb may work against any antihypertensives taken as well as anticoagulants or antiplatelets. There are no established drug interactions. Patients with an autoimmune disorder should not take cat's claw. It has no known interactions with drugs or supplements.

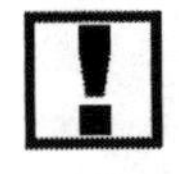

Side Effects: With very few trials carried out, cat's claw may cause headache, dizziness, or vomiting.

Dosage: In one study osteoarthritis patients took 100 mg per day of a freeze-dried preparation. You can also take up to a half a teaspoon of tincture twice daily, or 20 to 60 mg of dry, standardized extract once a day.

Cayenne (Capsaicin)

Overview: Cayenne plants originated as perennials in Mexico and Central America, but today they are grown as annuals the world over. They grow to three feet in height, have white or yellow flowers, and bear fruit in the form of peppers, which are used as both food and medicine. Capsaicin is what makes hot peppers hot. When you eat them your brain receives a "pain message" and responds by releasing endorphins, your body's natural painkiller. This also results in a hot pepper "high."

Benefits: The capsaicin/endorphin interplay results in a product that can be used topically to treat arthritis pain, psoriasis, shingles, and other nerve pain syndromes. These actions are well-documented. It's also used orally as a digestive aid.

Considerations: Some people are sensitive to capsaicin and will react with skin irritations. Test on a small area before general use. Wash your hands thoroughly after applying, and take extra precautions to ensure the cream never comes in contact with the eyes, nose, or mouth. Do not take it in conjunction with the asthma drug theophylline. Cayenne might reduce the effectiveness of some drugs: ACE Inhibitors, antacids, anticoagulants, and H2-blockers.

Side Effects: A burning sensation on the skin when you apply capsaicin is normal. Continue using it regularly and it should stop within one week. Avoid contact with the eyes. It is possibly unsafe to use it on a long-term basis as an oral supplement. Taken orally, it can cause upset stomach and sweating.

Dosage: Capsaicin creams are sold over-the-counter; follow package directions. Orally, unless you enjoy the taste of hot peppers, you can take one or two capsules up to three times daily.

Chamomile

Overview: The medicinal chamomile is of the German or Hungarian variety, different from the typical Roman or English chamomile. The dried flower is the part that gets used. Chamomile also has a long history of cosmetic use: for example, a strong brew of chamomile tea allowed to cool and poured over the hair after washing (don't rinse out) will lighten hair color when it's allowed to dry in the sun.

Benefits: This anti-inflammatory speeds healing of minor injuries and rashes. It also soothes indigestion, reduces stress, and helps you relax. It is sometimes used as a treatment for ulcers, insomnia, colds, and bronchitis. The active ingredients are flavonoids and essential oils.

Considerations: Chamomile is so safe it's accepted for use by children and pregnant or breast-feeding women. You should avoid contact with your eyes. However, it's recommended you not take it in conjunction with warfarin, heparin, or Trental because chamomile might increase their blood-thinning effects. It also may increase the drowsiness caused by some drugs.

Side Effects: None indicated among non-allergic people at recommended doses. Some people who have allergies to the daisy family may experience adverse reactions. Eating large quantities of flowers may result in vomiting.

Dosage: Topical ointments contain up to 10% chamomile. The product is also sold as bath salts and powders.

For internal use, purchase a commercial brand of chamomile tea and follow the manufacturer's directions, or steep two to three teaspoons of dried chamomile flowers in a cup of boiling water for 10 minutes. One teaspoon dried flowers equals one gram of drug. The recommended dose of chamomile is 10 to 15 grams.

Cinnamon

Overview: This age-old spice comes from the rolled up bark of a Sri Lankan evergreen laurel tree. There are many varieties of cinnamon, the most common found in the U.S. and derived from the *Cinnamon cassia* tree. The truest form comes from the *C. zeylanicum* tree. Despite being a delicious spice used in food, incense, oil, and perfume, this biblically mentioned herb has many medicinal properties.

Benefits: Use cinnamon to treat nausea, gas, menstrual cramps, diarrhea, diabetes, aid digestion, enhance appetite, and soothe pain from minor cuts. The herb can help produce saliva, break down fats, and produce bile. It acts as a gas-reducer and astringent and can even kill bacteria in the mouth – which makes it great for toothpaste.

Considerations: Taking cinnamon medicinally is not recommended for pregnant women, as effects have not been well studied. As well, people may have an allergy to this herb, so it is recommended you start by only taking small doses and gradually increasing them. Do not take cinnamon with any drugs used to treat diabetes and or blood glucose levels.

Side Effects: Cinnamon can cause allergic reactions. If so, stop right away. In prolonged use, cinnamon can cause an inflammation or sores inside the mouth. If taken at high doses, it might depress the nervous system. When used on the skin, it may cause a temporary burning sensation.

Dosage: For use in gastrointestinal problems, you may drink up to three cups of tea a day: boil ½ to ¾ teaspoons of cinnamon. Cinnamon tincture can be taken in ½ teaspoon, or two to three ml, three times a day. True cinnamon in volatile oil form is two or more times as strong as the U.S. available "Cassia." Even Cassia should only be used in a topical solution of just a few drops in a dilution of neutral oil, and for no longer than a few days. If taking cinnamon bark, the dose is two to four grams a day.

Corydalis

Overview: Also known as Yan Hu So, this yellow flowering plant is native to China, specifically the province Zhejiang. The useful part appears to be the fleshy knots below ground from where the roots shoot off.

Benefits: Studies have shown that this herb might be useful in insomnia, mild depression, tremors, and nerve pain. Less conclusive evidence shows it may have uses in controlling irregular heart beats (arrhythmia), peptic ulcers, and menstrual pain. The potent alkaloid inside this herb, "tetrahydropalmatine" (THP), has been found to produce sedative and pain-relieving effects. It also seems to help prevent stroke, lower blood pressure, and heart rates by affecting the cardiovascular system.

Considerations: People with liver problems may be more susceptible to liver damage (hepatitis), due to some toxicity in this plant. Pregnant and nursing mothers should also avoid corydalis.

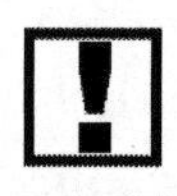

Side Effects: This herb seems to work well, and has few side effects compared to other sleep remedies. In some instances, though, it's been linked to nausea, vertigo, fatigue, and even hepatitis.

Dosage: A typical dose is between five and 10 grams of dried plant a day, or 10 to 20 ml of tincture daily.

Cranberry

Overview: This high vitamin C and antioxidant rich fruit is grown in the U.S. and has been used in the past to fight scurvy. These bright red berries traditionally found alongside a turkey dinner are great all year round. The plant is a close relative of the blueberry.

Benefits: The anti-adhesive and bacteria-blocking action of cranberries make them ideal in preventing urinary tract and bladder infections. Cranberry juice is a well-known defense against these frustrating infections. In the case of sexually active women with recurring UTI's, the potent juice may be able to reduce reoccurrences by as much as 50%. The berries seem to be equally effective in either juice or tablet form. It is also famed to help prevent kidney stones, to keep blood toxin-free, and to prevent gum disease.

Considerations: Cranberry juice and tablets seem to be safe for pregnant and breast-feeding women. Don't replace antibiotic treatment with cranberry juice, but rather take it after you finish your treatment to avoid a recurrence. People with a history of kidney stones should consult their doctor before taking cranberry tablets as it has not been well studied. By stimulating the kidneys, cranberry may reduce the effectiveness of any drugs you are taking (i.e. antidepressants, painkillers, alkaline drugs).

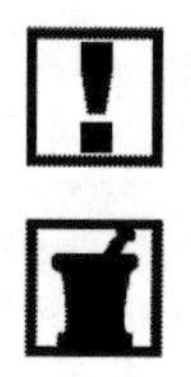

Side Effects: None have been recorded.

Dosage: Drink 300 to 400 ml of cranberry extract, or take a 400 mg tablet – twice a day. If you prefer juice, you can drink eight to 16 ounces a day for effectiveness.

Dandelion

Overview: This familiar yellow weed can be found on lawns everywhere despite our best efforts. You may find the leaves of this edible plant in your salad, and the root can be brewed into something like coffee. But these parts of the plant can also be used for medicinal purposes. Dandelion leaves are high in many vitamins, and most minerals.

Benefits: The leaves are used as a diuretic for water-retention, and can also be used in conjunction with the root for indigestion, heartburn, and postpartum and pregnancy support. Roots can be used independently for constipation, to control liver damage, and to aid digestion. It might be effective for urinary tract infections as well when used specifically with a "uva ursi leaf" extract – it lowered the recurrence rate in women.

Considerations: People with allergies to insulin should not take dandelion as it contains high amounts of this fiber. Also, dandelion should only be consumed under the advice of a doctor if you have gallstones, obstruction of bile ducts, ulcers (because of excess acid production), or water-retention. Don't use with any diuretic or hypoglycemic herbs.

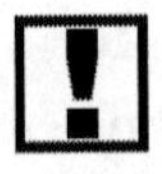

Side Effects: Dandelions may have a negative, hypoglycemic effect on people who are taking ciprofloxacin, thiazide, or loop diuretics, spironolactone, or triamterene. Those allergic to ragweed, marigolds, and daisies may be sensitive to dandelion as well. Those with diabetes, gallstones, and any gastrointestinal conditions should closely monitor their condition and stop using the herb if any negative effects are noticed. Despite this, dandelion is regarded as quite safe.

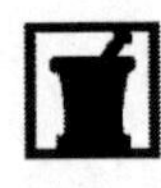

Dosage: For conditions requiring the root, try three to five grams dried root daily, or one to two teaspoons of tincture, three times a day. Alternatively, boil one teaspoon of dandelion root in water for a half an hour on low heat. Cool completely in a covered container. Take in one tablespoon doses, up to one cup per day. To make use of the leaves, pour one cup of boiling water over one to two teaspoons of dried leaves. Let steep for 20 minutes. Drink one to two cups per day, hot or warm. You can also have ½ to one teaspoon of tincture or add some fresh leaves to your salad.

Devil's Claw

Overview: This evil-sounding herb hails from South Africa. The name comes from its strange appearance. Its fruits are used medicinally after they are diced up and dried in the sun for a few days. It began as a remedy for pain and fever, and was a relatively popular arthritis treatment in Europe. It still is too – but the mechanism by which it acts is unknown. Some believe it is an anti-inflammatory.

Benefits: It is used for many types of joint pain, most notably the main types of arthritis: osteoarthritis, rheumatoid arthritis, and gout. It is a bitter herb known to stimulate appetite and help with an upset stomach.

Considerations: It may increase the risk of bleeding, and shouldn't be taken with warfarin. Since its effect is not well established, children, pregnant women, and people with liver or kidney disease should not use devil's claw.

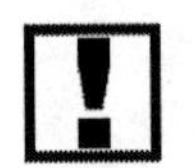

Side Effects: Other than mild stomach aches or intestinal distress, there are no reported side effects for devil's claw.

Dosage: Typically you take devil's claw at 750 mg doses, three times a day. An extract should be standardized to have three percent "iridoid glycosides."

Dong Quai

Overview: Also referred to as dang-gui and Chinese angelica, this celery relative has greenish-white flowers, but it is the root that is used as an herbal remedy. The root resembles the root of a carrot. It is one of the major herbs in Chinese medicine.

Benefits: This plant has been used primarily for blood flow problems. It can be used to treat irregular menstrual cycles, cramps, pain, premenstrual syndrome, menopause, as well as high blood pressure and liver disorders. It may also be used to treat inflammation, low-libido, rheumatism, and digestive problems.

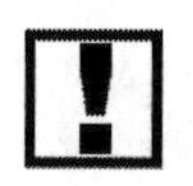

Considerations: This herb may have a negative effect if you are taking such drugs as heparin, ticlopidine, and warfarin. Use it cautiously if you are taking medications for blood pressure. Also, use caution if you are diabetic or have a glucose intolerance.

Side Effects: In people with very light colored skin, a sensitivity to sunlight may occur. In general people taking dong quai should avoid prolonged sun or UV exposure. Without reliable reports, it's possible dong quai could raise the risk of bleeding due to its anticoagulant effects. Traditionally, it's been linked to diarrhea, upset stomach, nausea, vomiting, loss of appetite or bloating (but research is limited). Other than this, side effects are rare and may exert mild stomach upset or allergic reactions.

Dosage: It is hard to self-prescribe this herb, so a proper dose should be recommended by a herbalist. A typical dose is three to four grams of powdered root taken in divided doses as a capsule or tablet, or a tincture taken in three to five ml doses three times daily. Also, you can take one standard pill three times a day.

Echinacea

Overview: Echinacea is one of the most popular over-the-counter herbs; the botanical names are *Echinacea purpurea, E. angustifolia* and *E. pallida.* The plant is native to the Great Plains and the southern United States; cultivated both there and in Europe. It is a purple "coneflower."

Benefits: Echinacea is the primary respiratory remedy in Germany for mild infections. The herb is an immune booster, and can either stave off or treat infections such as the flu. Powdered root of the plant can be used (alone or in combination with other herbs) to treat external open wounds. It may also help celiac disease, diverticulitis, chronic fatigue syndrome, bronchitis, ear infections, laryngitis, and cystitis.

Considerations: It loses effectiveness if taken year-round. Some herbalists recommend taking echinacea for two to three weeks, then resting for a week or two. Experts in Germany recommend not exceeding eight straight weeks of treatment. People with autoimmune deficiencies should seek a doctor's opinion before self-treating with echinacea. Also, people taking chemotherapy drugs, cisplatin, cyclophosphamide, docetaxel, Fluorouracil, methotrexate, paclitaxel should speak to a doctor to understand drug interactions. Echinacea may also decrease the effectiveness of econazole.

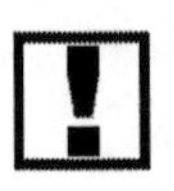

Side Effects: People with allergy to plants in the daisy family should avoid echinacea. The herb might cause increased urination and minor gastrointestinal symptoms, but they are very uncommon.

Dosage: It's best to start taking the herb right at the beginning of your cold, when symptoms are mild to stave off full infection. Take a three to four ml dose of tincture, or a 300 mg tablet three times a day. You can actually take this in double dose, or even every two hours on the first signs of infection, then reduce dose. Echinacea juice can be taken at two to three ml doses, three times a day.

Eucalyptus

Overview: You would probably recognize the powerful smell of this Australian plant. Now cultivated worldwide, this evergreen's leaves are used for many medicinal purposes.

Benefits: The potent vapors from eucalyptus are used in cold treatments in the same way as menthol. It is suspected to reduce nasal congestion and assist in breathing by affecting the receptors in the nose responsible for mucus. Thus it might be effective for sinusitis. It also seems to be an effective insect repellent, working almost as well as more commercial formulations.

Considerations: Eucalyptus oil shouldn't be used by people who have low blood pressure, liver problems, inflammatory disorders of the gastrointestinal tract or kidney, people with asthma, or by children under two or pregnant women (its effects on expecting mothers is unknown).

Side Effects: Drinking eucalyptus concentrations can result in nausea, vomiting, and

diarrhea, and if the oil is taken in large undiluted amounts, or even as little as a 3.5 ml amount, it could be fatal. If taken orally, this oil can have serious side effects that affect the mind and nervous system. Don't use orally with any sedatives.

Dosage: A dilution of 30 ml eucalyptus oil in 500 ml warm water can be used topically to prevent insect bites, or on the temples to prevent tension headaches. Just a few drops of eucalyptus oil can be put into a vaporizer or added to hot water and inhaled for nasal problems. A tea can also be made from 150 ml hot water and two to three grams of chopped leaves, or 0.05 to 0.2. ml of oil can be diluted with warm water and drunk to fight infection and low back pain.

Evening Primrose

Overview: A native of North America, this herb yields just leaves in its first year and yellow flowers with seeds in its second year. The second year is key, because it's the small reddish seeds that elicit the oil and thus the plant's medicinal effects. The oil is 60 to 80% linoleic acid and eight to 15% gamma-linolenic acid (GLA). The latter is one of the omega-6 fatty acids, and is used by the body to fight inflammation. Other than these, it contains a host of phytochemicals and nutrients.

Benefits: It is often used to help relieve the effects of eczema: skin itchiness, flaking, and inflammation. It's also taken for premenstrual syndrome. Its anti-inflammatory effects have made it useful in the treatment of rheumatoid arthritis as well. Some experts suggest taking evening primrose oil for a month or so to treat skin inflammation rather than starting a course of steroid medication. It helps to reduce hypertension and aids in weight loss.

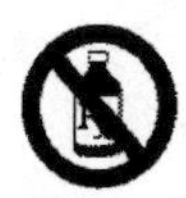

Considerations: This oil should not be used during pregnancy. Evening primrose oil promotes estrogen production, thus women who have been diagnosed with breast cancer as related to estrogen levels, should avoid or limit their intake. Those with a history of seizures or seizure disorders shouldn't take the oil. If taking blood pressure medications, check with a doctor first.

Side Effects: There is little evidence of side effects or health problems with this herb, when taken at recommended levels. Very high doses can lead to nausea, upset stomach, seizures, and headache.

Dosage: It's mainly taken in pill form. Look at the ingredients and choose the type with at minimum 40 mg of GLA per 500 mg of evening primrose oil. Daily dosage is about two to three grams of oil. But up to 360 mg of GLA may be needed if you are aiming to treat arthritis and very bad eczema, and researchers often use three to six grams of oil a day to achieve this level. Alternatively, you can take one teaspoon. of the plant with one cup of water.

Fennel

Overview: With a licorice-like flavor, fennel seeds have long been popular for spicing up food. This originally European plant is also cultivated in North America, Asia, and Egypt. In Greek mythology, this spice was told to give immortality. It is rich in beta-carotene, vitamin C, and a host of minerals.

Benefits: Much like anise, fennel oil helps relieve heartburn and indigestion by a few of its ingredients that keep some muscles – such as those involved in digestion – from spasms. This also makes it useful for treating stomach cramps and relieving gas pains. Fennel can also act as a diuretic and can be used to reduce fever, relieve pain, and fight bacteria, as well as to aid in bile production. The fennel oil and fruit also seem to contain a plant estrogen called estragole, which can treat bloating, breast tenderness, menstrual cramps, or aid in the production of milk in lactating mothers. Dosage of seeds in leaves should be increased by double or more for this purpose.

Considerations: Breast cancer patients or others with estrogen-related diseases should avoid large doses of fennel since its role as an "estragole" is not fully understood. These include uterine cancer, ovarian cancer, endometriosis and uterine fibroids. You should probably avoid fennel if taking these drugs: Cipro, any contraceptive, estrogen, or tamoxifen.

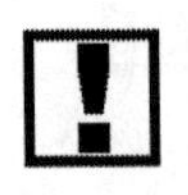

Side Effects: It is very uncommon, but an allergic reaction may occur. Side effects may develop if fennel seed is used for too long. It may cause a sensitivity to sunlight or ultraviolet light while using it.

Dosage: Taking fennel oil at 0.1 to 0.6 ml a day (not with food) can be effective. You could also try one to one and a half teaspoons of fennel seeds or a tea made from a half a teaspoon of crushed seeds (steeped for 15 minutes). Strain and drink up to three times a day. Or, try five to seven grams of the dried fruit or seed.

Feverfew

Overview: The leaves of feverfew – technically named, *Tanacetum parthenium* – are useful in alternative medicine. This plant is native to central and southern Europe and also grows widely across North America.

Benefits: Used topically, it disinfects minor wounds, relieves skin irritation, and repels insects. Feverfew also alleviates pain and inflammation from arthritis and other rheumatic diseases; but is best known for preventing or aborting migraine headaches. It works to relieve these headaches through it's abundance of sesquiterpene lactones, and most specifically (and also in largest amounts) parthenolide. It prevents platelets from clumping and stops the release of histamines and prostaglandins. Through this method it prevents swelling and inflammation and keeps away that throbbing pain from the passage of blood through the expanded blood vessels.

Considerations: This herb will not work immediately. It takes about four weeks before it becomes effective. It should not be used by pregnant or breast-feeding women or children under the age of two.

Side Effects: Chewing actual leaves is not recommended as doing so can cause mouth sores and gum bleeding. It doesn't really taste very good anyway, since the leaves are very bitter. Some minor stomach upset or nervous feelings may occur when taking this herb. It may cause allergies if sensitive to daisies, ragweed, and marigolds. Rarely, feverfew can lead to nausea, constipation, indigestion, bloating, and diarrhea.

Dosage: Look for 0.2 percent parthenolide, and take one capsule three times daily, with water, at mealtime. You can also get the same dosage from 125 mg of dried leaves. Tea can also be made from six to eight leaves.

Flaxseed (Omega-3)

Overview: If you aren't familiar with this omega-3 fatty acid containing food, you should be! The seeds taken from the three-inch fruit are rich in omega-3s which are gaining a lot of notoriety for their numerous medicinal benefits. It is the oil from these seeds that hold the potent medicinal value.

Benefits: These seeds contain soluble and insoluble fibers that aid in constipation and other intestinal problems. They also contain "lignans" that have been noted as prostate, colon, and breast cancer protectors. (The oil has no lignans in it.) Flaxseed oil can also be used to reduce skin inflammation, reduce LDL cholesterol, help relieve arthritis, reduce high blood pressure, and slow the onset of atherosclerosis.

Considerations: Although it is not quite as effective as fish oil, which is more easily absorbed by the body, flaxseed still has definite benefits and is a good alternative for people with seafood allergies. Alpha-linolenic acid, the main medicinal component of flax, has been indicated as having mutagenic effects (can indicate cancer) when heated, so the oil should be kept in a cool, dark place and should not be used in cooking. Those with abdominal pain and pregnant women shouldn't take it. For diabetics, it might delay the absorption of glucose. Speaking of absorption, flaxseed could hinder the effects of any vitamin or supplement taken orally. Use caution with any laxatives, blood pressure medication, or mood-altering herbs such as St. John's wort and valerian.

Side Effects: The side effects aren't well known, but because of the blood thinning quality of omega-3s, people on blood-thinning medications should speak to their doctor before taking flax. Taking vitamin E will also help to combat a loss of antioxidants. Flaxseed can alter a woman's menstrual period, so should be used cautiously for women with a hormone-sensitive condition. For men, a few studies have reported a raised risk of prostate cancer when taking flaxseed oil orally.

Dosage: The oil should be kept refrigerated and left in a dark, air-tight container. Take one tablespoon a day (which can be poured over salads or other veggies. If using the seeds, as a laxative or for intestinal problems, crush one tablespoon and take with a glass of water, three times daily. A gel capsule of 1,300 mg flax oil usually provides enough alpha-linolenic acid. You should try to get 1.1 to 1.5 g of omega-3s daily.

Garlic

Overview: In the U.S. about 250 million pounds of garlic is used in cooking every year. This smelly herb is part of the onion, chives, and leek family. Everyone knows what it looks like, and what they may not know is that it's been used for medicinal purposes for thousands of years. "Allicin" is the central compound, and is widely thought to be the source of garlic's health benefits. When you crush or cut cloves, it releases allicin. Another compound, "ajoene," appears responsible for reducing blood clots. It is easily one of the most studied herbs.

Benefits: This is what garlic can do: reduce LDL cholesterol while boosting the "good" HDL cholesterol. This can take two to four months to show. It can also help lower triglycerides and blood pressure. This can take anywhere from one to six months.

Garlic can help with circulation and enhance fibrinolysis, the process of removing blood clots. Germany has approved it as a dietary approach to managing cholesterol and ensuring the arteries stay clean. Garlic fights infections (external and internal). May help coughs (and other lung/throat infections), asthma, fevers, fungal infections, ear and sinus infections, and gastric upsets.

Considerations: Contraindications have been seen in patients taking anticoagulants, hypoglycemic drugs, those with allergies, and pregnant women. It can increase the anti-inflammatory actions of aspirin and interact with warfarin. Due to its antihypertensive actions, it can increase the potency of drugs taken for hypertension, but if taken with diuretics it can actually result in hypertension or diuresis. People with gastrointestinal irritation should use caution.

Side Effects: Mainly the odor. Ew! It can cause occasional heartburn and gastrointestinal problems or increase the body's number of white blood cells. May cause eruptions on the skin. Excessive amounts can lead to bleeding problems. Mostly, however, garlic is very safe.

Dosage: Cooking garlic will reduce its effectiveness by eliminating certain compounds. Either eat garlic cloves, anywhere from one to five cloves a day, or you can take about four grams of minced garlic a day. Try enteric-coated pills for best result, as they preserve these active compounds. Pills are also odorless, and you need about 4,000 mg a day.

Ginkgo Biloba

Overview: One of the most thoroughly researched herbs; from the leaf of the ginkgo tree. The tree, notably, is the oldest species in the world that survived the Ice Age. In traditional Chinese medicine the seeds are used to treat asthma and other respiratory conditions.

Benefits: Ginkgo stimulates circulation, particularly in the brain. It may help heart disease, angina, stroke, clogged arteries, depression, dementia, Alzheimer's disease, Raynaud's disease, Parkinson's disease, and tinnitus. It is known to improve cognitive function and memory in all ages, especially the elderly. It is known to possibly help with impaired circulation in the legs. Ginkgo is reported to improve sexual function in both men and women. (Note: may take one to three months to see results.)

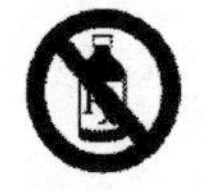

Considerations: Do not take ginkgo if you are on blood thinning agents (anticoagulants) such as warfarin or heparin, aspirin or non-steroidal anti-inflammatory drugs, or antidepressant drugs such as phenelzine sulfate or tranylcypromine. Do not take more than 240 mg of concentrated extract per day. Depressed patients should avoid combining St. John's wort with ginkgo. Don't use it if you have bleeding disorders, diabetes, epilepsy, or are undergoing surgery within two weeks.

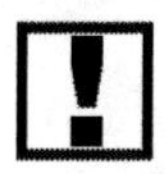

Side Effects: There are rarely any side effects to ginkgo. In studies, adverse effects included headaches, dizziness, and allergic skin reactions. There is a bit of concern that this herb can invoke seizures – those at risk should avoid ginkgo.

Dosage: Ginkgo comes in many forms, including capsules, tablets, and extracts. The standard dose is 120 mg per day (up to 160 mg), split into three 40 mg doses. Look for an extract at least 24% "ginkgo flavone glycosides" and six percent "terpene lactones."

Ginseng

Overview: This herb can be found in the root of three different plants, *Panax quinquefolius* (American ginseng), *P. ginseng* (Asian ginseng), and *Eleutherococcus senticosus* (Siberian ginseng). It serves as an "adaptogen," that helps boost the body's energy.

Benefits: Ginseng boosts energy and mood, and although it hasn't been completely proven, this could be a great herb for people with stressful lives. It is said to fight cancer, fibromyalgia, chronic fatigue syndrome, heart disease, impotence, stress, muscle soreness, low immunity, and depression. It may also improve stamina, and brain function.

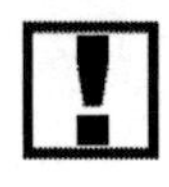

Considerations: Do not take ginseng if you have ischemic or vascular heart disease, thyroid disease, diabetes, or migraine. Consult your doctor first if you have a heart condition, high blood pressure, or an anxiety disorder. Theoretically, it could disrupt any antipsychotic or immunosuppressant drugs being taken.

Side Effects: It may cause insomnia, nervousness, or headaches. Mostly, it is very safe. Research continues in this area. Some believe there is a greater risk of hypertension if prolonged use of ginseng is combined with daily caffeine intake. Cut down on coffee if taking this herb.

Dosage: A typical dose is one to two grams daily of raw ginseng root or 100 to 200 mg of standardized extracts. (Commercial strengths vary; follow manufacturer's instructions.) Note: Quality of products available varies; seek out a trusted supplier.

Goat's Rue

Overview: Also known as French lilac, this wild European plant flowers in the peak of summer. It is picked then, and the leaves are dried out for medicinal purposes.

Benefits: Goat's rue can be used to aid diabetics, as it may help reduces blood sugar levels. Not yet studied in humans, it has shown a unique ability to assist with weight loss as well, perhaps being a possibility for obese patients.

Considerations: This should not replace insulin therapy, but a doctor should be consulted if you are currently on any diabetic treatments before you begin taking this herb to avoid potential complications.

Side Effects: It can cause hypoglycemia, increased sweating, nausea, vomiting, and intestinal problems. This herb should be monitored carefully because it may be unsafe for pregnant women. Consult your doctor about goat's rue.

Dosage: Drink twice daily a tea made from one teaspoon of dried leaves, letting it steep in boiling water for 10 to 15 minutes. You could also choose to take one to two ml of the tincture three times daily.

Goldenseal

Overview: Native to North America, this raspberry-look-a-like fruit bearing plant is being over-harvested for its medicinal properties. The root of the plant is used for creating tinctures, creams, ointments, and powders to be used topically.

Benefits: The alkaloids in goldenseal act as antibacterial and antiseptics. Taken orally, this herb can strengthen the immune system to help treat cold and flu symptoms, as well as help in stomach disorders such as indigestion and constipation, relieve muscle pain like sciatica, help skin conditions, and treat urinary tract infections.

Considerations: Do not take goldenseal if you are pregnant, have high blood pressure or an autoimmune disease such as multiple sclerosis or lupus, or if you are allergic to plants in the daisy family (i.e. chamomile). It shouldn't be used for longer than two weeks. It may also affect the drugs doxycycline and tetracycline (an antibiotic).

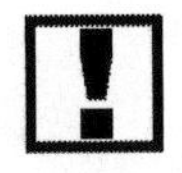

Side Effects: Side effects are usually only observed in high doses, which can cause gastrointestinal problems or nervous system problems. Even at high doses, this is rare.

However, one area should be noted: “cytochrome P450 3A4” a.k.a. CYP3A4. Many drugs are metabolized by CYP3A4, and they should not be taken in conjunction with goldenseal: Mevacor, Nizoral, Sporanox, Allegra, and Halcion are just a few. Consult your doctor if you have any questions.

Dosage: Look for an extract that contains berberine, the active ingredient. Orally, take 250 mg to 500 mg three times a day. For tea and gargling purposes, use up to one gram of goldenseal in boiled water. For topical cream, use as directed.

Gotu Kola

Overview: *Centella asiatica*, as this plant is officially known, grows in hot, tropical, swampy areas in India, Pakistan, Madagascar, Eastern Europe, South Africa, and Sri Lanka. It has red flowers and creates a fruit, but the leaves and roots are the good parts for medicine. It was accepted by France as a drug in the 1880s.

Benefits: It’s been long recognized as a treatment for psoriasis, leprosy, burns, and other skin conditions, as well as a healer of wounds. It is also used to treat symptoms of varicose veins, as well as a close relative, hemorrhoids.

Considerations: There are no known drug interactions. It may, however, interact negatively with drugs and herbs that have sedative properties.

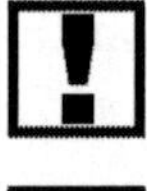

Side Effects: Rare allergic reactions or drowsiness may occur at very high doses.

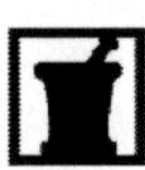

Dosage: Three cups of tea made with one to two teaspoons dried leaves, or 1/2 to one teaspoon of extract can be taken, or a tincture of two to four teaspoons. Look for a label that tells you how much “saponins” (triterpenoids) it has. A 100% content of these require only one to three 60 mg doses per day. A topical cream should have one percent gotu kola.

Greater Celandine

Overview: During flowering the leaves and little yellow flowers of this *Chelidonium majus* are collected and dried for medicinal use. This member of the poppy family was traditionally found in Europe and Asia, but Americans wanted a piece of the action, so now it’s being cultivated here too.

Benefits: The greatest evidence supports its use as a stomach-helper, it reduces indigestion and eases tummy troubles. It can also be used to ease gallbladder issues, decrease inflammation, and prevent cancers or infections. Its principle ingredient, chelidonine, has been linked to significantly helping with symptoms of gallstones.

Considerations: In the U.K., greater celandine is available only by prescription. People with liver damage should not take this herb unless recommended by their physician. You should avoid using any supplements that include greater celandine "dried above ground parts" as they have been implicated in hepatitis and have insufficient information behind them. Stick to greater celandine "rhizome" and root. It's best to consult your doctor first before trying this herb.

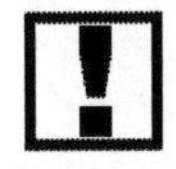

Side Effects: It can cause stomach upset if used in its fresh plant form. It may cause allergic reaction in some individuals. Children should not take this herb orally.

Dosage: The alkaloids are what give this plant its powers, so preserving them is most important. It's good to look for a listing of four mg chelidonine in each capsule of celandine. You can also take a tincture of one to three ml at least 10 minutes, and no more than 30 minutes before eating. Topical applications of the yellow latex can be applied to warts daily and left until dry.

Green Tea

Overview: Only in the past decade or so have scientists really started to look at the health benefits of green tea, an ancient drink. The preparation and harvesting is what makes all the difference. The unfermented form becomes green tea, which is becoming quite a popular social beverage as well as a medicinal one. It is chalked full of polyphenols, which have a slew of medicinal properties.

Benefits: This herb helps prevent and treat arteriosclerosis, high cholesterol, tooth decay, and leukoplakia. It also is thought to have some cancer-preventative benefits as well, and might help hepatitis, osteoporosis, and arteriosclerosis. It has great antioxidant and polyphenol content and is a good general health booster.

Considerations: This tea may also block iron absorption, so if you suffer from a deficiency, you may want to avoid green tea unless advised by your physician. It may create adverse effects with people taking any MAO inhibitors or warfarin.

Side Effects: While green tea contains half as much caffeine as coffee, it can still create nervousness and insomnia in high doses, so it's best not to drink it before bedtime. It may have adverse effects if you take contraceptives, antipsychotic drugs, Clozaril, or quinolones, but these are all theoretical.

Dosage: It is suspected that strong, bitter concoctions of tea are needed for the best effects, but it isn't certain how much is necessary for benefits to be reaped. It is suggested to be between three and 10 cups a day of one teaspoon dried green tea leaves to one cup of hot water, steeped only three minutes. This should provide you with 240 to 320 mg of polyphenols, which are the active medicinal ingredients in the tea. There are also pills whose typical dosage is 100 to 150 mg three times a day, but they are not as well documented as the tea.

Gymnema Sylvestre

Overview: Also known simply as gymnema, this tropical climbing plant is a great medicinal helper. The plant has also been named the "sugar destroyer" because the taste of sweet foods seems to be inhibited by the chewing of its leaves, which are the useful medicinal part.

Benefits: This drug is best known for its help in treating diabetes by lowering blood sugar gradually and raising insulin levels. It can improve glucose uptake while decreasing blood sugar levels.

Considerations: Diabetics and pregnant women should consult their doctor before taking gymnema as it may affect drugs like insulin, glipizide, and glyburide. For drugs that work on blood sugar levels, gymnema could make them work too well, causing hypoglycemia.

Side Effects: None have been found in healthy individuals. You should use it only under the guidance of a doctor because blood sugar levels are not to be toyed with.

Dosage: Doses of 400 mg of the water-soluble acids of the leaves have been used safely for up to two years with good effects in people with Type I and II diabetes. (It should be standardized to 24% gymnemic acid.) The powdered leaf can also be used in two to four gram doses.

Hawthorn

Overview: This tree, native to Europe, springs white blossoms and bright red berries in the summertime. Hawthorn is the source of many phytochemicals, which have health-promoting properties – including flavonoids, which hunt free radicals and reduce inflammation. They also give the berries the reddish-blue hue. Experts don't concur on which part of the plant is most beneficial to medicine, but the berries (fresh or dried), flowers, and leaves have all been alluded to.

Benefits: Hawthorn is believed to alleviate congestive heart failure in the early stages. It may improve blood circulation, increase the strength of heart muscles, and help reduce blood pressure by widening or "dilating" the blood vessels. It appears able to help patients with angina or heart failure by reducing blood pressure while increasing their capacity to exercise. It may also strengthen collagen, which makes up arteries and blood vessels. Essentially, any time a heart muscle has deteriorated, hawthorn may help. It can't reverse damage, but it can strengthen the heart and help with its vital function.

Considerations: The plant is a very safe herb, even over prolonged periods of time. It is of course never meant to be a substitute for medical intervention in the case of heart problems, but can complement a doctor's guidelines. This herb will not take action right away; it's been known to take six weeks before improvements are noticeable. Use caution if taking calcium channel blockers, any central nervous system depressants, nitrates, or Lanoxin.

Side Effects: Some adverse reactions include fatigue, sweating, rash on the hands, nausea, and stomach upset. Slightly worse effects can include headache, palpitations, dizziness, vertigo, nosebleeds, insomnia, and circulatory problems.

Dosage: The herb is sold in dried form in pills, fluid extract, solid extract, or tinctures. The most you should ever take is 900 mg a day, but doses can range as small as 160 mg a day. You don't take it all at once either, but rather two or three times a day to reach that number. It can also be used to make tea: drop a teaspoon into about a cup of boiled water for 15 minutes. Strain and drink. Alternatively, add one teaspoon of crushed hawthorn berries to a half-cup of cold water. Let stand overnight, then boil it in the morning, strain, and drink a teaspoon at a time. Take capsules with food or a tincture about 15 minutes before a meal.

Hemsleya Amabilis

Overview: This little-known herb is used for medicinal purposes only.

Benefits: It is used in Asia to treat cancer.

Note: Information published in the West on this herb is extremely limited. To learn about dosages, contraindications, and possible side effects consult a medical professional specializing in traditional Chinese medicine.

HP-200 (Cowhage)

Overview: An extract derived from the seed powder of the herb *Mucuna prurient*, this herb is also called "cowhage." It's used in Ayurvedic medicine, an ancient Indian medical tradition. Ayurvedic medicine is based on the principle of achieving a balance among emotions, bodily functions, lifestyle, and diet. Disease occurs when there's an imbalance in one or more areas.

Benefits: A 1995 clinical trial found significant improvement in Parkinson's when patients were treated with HP-200, which is actually the powdered formulation of the herb. It's sometimes used for anxiety, arthritis, and as a pain-reliever. What else? It's used to treat snakebites and the sting of a scorpion.

Considerations: Because Western research only features the one study, it's too early to tell whether there are contraindications. Avoid taking vitamin B-6 and Kava with this herb.

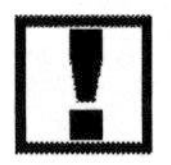

Side Effects: Some mild gastrointestinal upset was reported in the 1995 trial. Most commonly, there could be nausea and less commonly vomiting, dyskinesias, and insomnia.

Dosage: The amount used in the 1995 trial was 7.5 grams of the extract (dissolved in water) three to six times daily. Other information has a dose at 22 to 67 grams divided into two to five doses a day. Consult your doctor.

Huanglian

Overview: A commonly used herb in traditional Chinese medicine. Its Latin name is *Coptis chinensis;* another common name is Goldthread. The root of the plant is used. Medical elements of the herb are alkaloids: berberine (seven to nine percent), coptisine, urbenine, worenine, palmaline, jatrorrhizine, and columbamine.

Benefits: Huanglian is used in traditional Chinese medicine to treat gastrointestinitis, diarrhea, hypertension, and bacterial and viral infections. It shows promise as well for inhibiting growth of colon, gastric, and breast tumors. Currently there are no published reports of medical trials, although at time of this writing, a study is underway at the Memorial Sloan-Kettering Cancer Center.

Considerations: People with heart disease should only consider use of this herb under medical supervision.

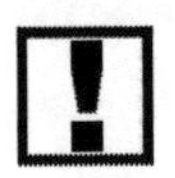

Side Effects: Possible side effects include nausea and vomiting. Toxic effects (i.e., from overdose) include seizures and heart failure.

Dosage: No standard dosage indicated at this time. Consult a medical professional skilled in this area.

Huperzine A

Overview: Huperzine A is an alkaloid from the Chinese moss *Huperzia serrata.* It is medicinally active, and is part of the alkaloids family. Although it comes from a plant, it is purified in labs and is a single chemical. It's very potent and it has a specific focus.

Benefits: Over the counter, it's sold as a supplement to improve cognitive skills, memory, and myasthenia gravis (an autoimmune disease). Huperzine A is used in traditional Chinese medicine for the treatment of schizophrenia and memory loss, specifically Alzheimer's. A 1999 study found beneficial effects when administered to adolescent students, with improvements identified in the memory test areas.

Considerations: High doses may be toxic. Patients with hypertension and liver or kidney disease shouldn't take huperzine A except with a physician's approval.

Side Effects: Possible side effects can include nausea, insomnia, dizziness, and cramps. (None were noted in the study of students.)

Dosage: Huperzine A is available in capsule and tablet form. Highly potent, doses should not exceed 200 mg twice a day.

Ivy Gourd

Overview: Ivy gourd (*Coccinia indica*) is a vine native to Africa, India, and Asia. However, in the last 20 years or so it has spread through Hawaii, where it is an invasive weed, spreading over trees and shrubs and killing them. The state government is working hard to eradicate it.

Benefits: Studies indicate that ivy gourd can help reduce blood glucose in Type II diabetes, but more research is needed. Used in Ayurvedic medicine to treat diabetes, bronchitis, and skin diseases.

Considerations, Side Effects, Dosage: Little information is available at this time. Consult a skilled medical professional.

Kava

Overview: From the South Pacific islands, where it is used socially to create a feeling of well-being, rather like alcohol is used in our culture. However, while it has soothing, relaxing effects, kava does not dull the mind. It's also not addictive.

Benefits: Kava is prescribed in Europe to treat insomnia, stress, and anxiety. It's also indicated for a long list of other conditions, including muscle aches, chronic pain, epilepsy, and/or anything where stress or anxiety plays a role.

Considerations: Antidepressants, psychiatric drugs (such as antipsychotics or buspirone), sedatives, and tranquilizers may cause excessive drowsiness when taken with kava. Do not combine kava and alcohol. However, kava combined with St. John's wort may help treat depression. Do not take longer than three months. Kava should be avoided by pregnant or breast-feeding women, or anyone with Parkinson's disease. Don't combine kava with any drugs or herbs that might increase the risk of liver damage.

Side Effects: Stomach upset. You may feel especially tired in mornings (though not "hung over") at the outset. High or prolonged doses can cause skin irritation. Very high doses can cause loss of appetite, shortness of breath, blurred vision, bloodshot eyes, difficulty walking, disorientation, and intoxication. If you experience these, discontinue kava use. There is concern that kava can be toxic to the liver. If taking this herb you should have a regular liver test.

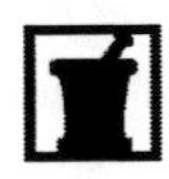

Dosage: Its available in a variety of formats, including tincture, tablet, softgel, liquid, dried herb/tea, and capsule. A quality extract will be standardized to contain at least 30% of the herb's primary active ingredient, kavalactones. A typical dosage for many ailments is 100 mg, three times a day; however, this medication should only be taken under professional supervision.

Note: After receiving reports of potential liver toxicity, in 2002 the Canadian government banned the sale of kava and all products in which it is an ingredient. As of this writing, kava is still available at health food stores in the U.S. In a recent Consumer Reports document, kava was listed as a "supplement to avoid." It is listed as a possible danger for abnormal liver function, with deaths reported. It is banned not only in Canada, but in Germany, Singapore, South Africa, and Switzerland.

Lavender

Overview: Lavender, famous for its smell, originated in the Mediterranean region, but is now cultivated around the world. Soaps, perfumes, and many other products take advantage of its powerful and appealing scent. The flowers are the part of the plant that is used medicinally—most specifically to extract its essential oil.

Benefits: Lavender is a natural antiseptic and astringent. Externally used for sunburn, insect bites, acne, and cuts and scrapes. It's taken orally to help relieve insomnia, restlessness, stomach upset, and irritable bowel syndrome. Historically used for depression, headache, and rheumatism, it is used extensively in aromatherapy and massage therapy. And what else? Possibly hair growth.

Considerations: No known drug interactions. However, since lavender has a mild sedative effect, avoid taking it in combination with other sedatives, such as tranquilizers.

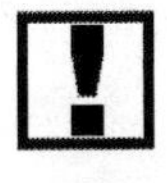

Side Effects: In rare cases, there may be an allergic skin reaction.

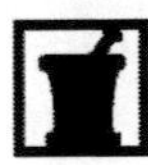

Dosage: Add one to two teaspoons of dried lavender flowers to boiling water to make a tea (steep for 15 minutes). Another way to take it orally is to mix up to four drops of tincture with a teaspoon of honey (use this method only under medical supervision).

Externally use the essential oil directly, or add it to bathwater. (Use on cuts interchangeably with aloe vera. Apply lavender oil two to three times a day.)

Licorice (Glycyrrhiza glabra)

Overview: Licorice is a shrub that has been used medicinally for centuries. It has also been heavily researched and studied. The key therapeutic element of licorice is glycyrrhizin, which is found in the rhizome (part of the root structure). Licorice also contains flavonoids and phytoestrogens that may be significant. In addition to its medicinal properties, licorice is often added to medications for its taste.

Benefits: Licorice is an anti-inflammatory. The evidence suggests it might help relieve peptic ulcers and hepatitis. It may help soothes coughs and asthma as well as boost the immune system. Also, it is thought to relieve chronic fatigue syndrome, fibromyalgia, shingles, eczema, and soothe PMS and menopausal symptoms in women.

Considerations: Take licorice orally as a medicine under a doctor's supervision. Do not take licorice if you are on medication for high blood pressure or diuretics, or if you are taking steroids. Avoid this kind of licorice if you have high blood pressure, glaucoma, diabetes, or diseases of the heart, liver or kidneys. Women who are pregnant or breast-feeding should not use licorice. Further, if you are taking licorice as medicine, avoid eating licorice candies and other food licorice products at the same time.

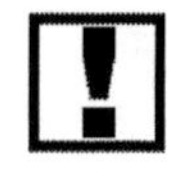

Side Effects: Licorice can raise blood pressure (while you are taking it). If you will be taking licorice for four weeks or more, get tested. High or prolonged doses of licorice can result in diverse side effects, including headache, swelling, stiffness, shortness of breath, upper abdominal pain, and lethargy.

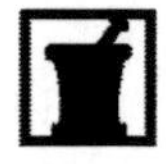

Dosage: Licorice is sold in a range of formats, including wafer, tincture, tablet, lozenge, liquid, dried herb/tea, cream, and capsule. A quality product will be standardized to contain 22% glycyrrhizic acid or glycyrrhizin. A typical dose of whole licorice is five to 15 grams a day. But the actual dosage will depend on your condition. Consult a trained medical professional. Licorice cream can be applied twice a day to affected areas of eczema, psoriasis, or herpes.

Licorice (deglycyrrhizinated)

Overview: A second form of licorice that is sold is deglycyrrhizinated, also known as "DGL" licorice.

Benefits: Coats and protects the digestive tract. Relieves ulcers, indigestion, and Crohn's disease.

Considerations: Take licorice orally as a medicine under a doctor's supervision. Do not take licorice if you are on medication for high blood pressure or diuretics, or taking steroids. Avoid this kind of licorice if you have high blood pressure, glaucoma, diabetes, or diseases of the heart, liver, or kidneys. Women who are pregnant or breast-feeding should not use licorice. Further, if you are taking licorice as medicine, avoid eating licorice candies and other food products at the same time.

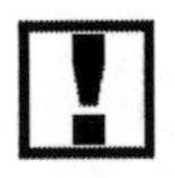

Side Effects: No side effects are associated with DGL licorice.

Dosage: Product should state deglycyrrhizinated or "DGL." Recommended from 200 to 500 mg or more before meals and at bedtime. Chew DGL wafers or tablets.

Lobelia

Overview: Lobelia is an annual plant that grows in North America. The leaves are used in medicinal preparations. The alkaloid "lobeline" provides the plant's health properties.

Benefits: Lobelia has traditionally been used to treat asthma, bronchitis, and coughs. Recently it has received attention for its role in smoking cessation. People wishing to quit may benefit, as this ingredient affects the nervous system in a way similar to nicotine, and acts like dopamine in the body. It has even been studied and found effective in treating people to withstand stronger urges as well: amphetamines and methamphetamines.

Considerations: Lobelia should not be taken by women who are pregnant or breast-feeding or by very young children. There may be potential hazards in mixing lobelia with nicotine alternatives. Consult your doctor.

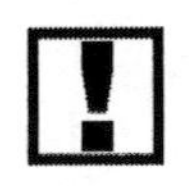

Side Effects: Causes nausea and/or vomiting at higher doses (anything over one ml). Any dose over 0.6 to one gram can be toxic.

Dosage: Apply lobelia ointments topically, several times a day, to relieve asthma and bronchitis. Take up to a maximum of one ml three times a day of a tincture made with vinegar, not alcohol.

Note: Lobelia was listed in a recent Consumer Reports document as a "supplement to avoid." They cite breathing difficulty, fast heartbeat, low blood pressure, diarrhea, dizziness, and tremors as related dangers. It is banned only in Bangladesh and Italy.

Marigold

Overview: Most of us are familiar with marigolds as they appear in our flower gardens. In their medicinal guise they are better known by their Latin name, *Calendula officinalis.* Marigold flowers have been used by healers in Europe and North America for centuries. Flavonoids make calendula an anti-inflammatory; other medical components are "triterpene saponins" and "carotenoids."

Benefits: Historically, calendula was used to treat wounds and promote healing, and as a treatment for skin conditions such as eczema. It may make a useful treatment for sunburn. It is currently being investigated as a possible treatment for cancer.

Considerations: There are no known drug interactions, but know that there is no evidence as yet completely supporting marigold. Pregnant or nursing mothers should avoid marigold because of its unproved effects.

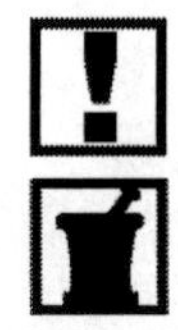

Side Effects: The only side effect is a skin rash in someone who is allergic.

Dosage: Use prepared ointments topically for skin conditions. A tea can be made, which some people take for peptic ulcer or ulcerative colitis: Use one to two teaspoons of flowers for one cup boiling water and steep 10 minutes. Drink three cups per day.

Milk Thistle

Overview: A member of the sunflower family. Interestingly, we have records of milk thistle being used to treat liver conditions dating back some 2,000 years. Today we have sound research from clinical trials that backs up its use. European doctors use it for liver conditions ranging from cirrhosis to hepatitis. The active compound in milk thistle is known as "silymarin" – a powerful antioxidant which is concentrated most heavily in the seeds of the plant.

Benefits: It's known to be beneficial for diseases of the liver and gallbladder, including gallstones. Milk thistle helps treats alcohol-related liver problems. It fortifies the liver—particularly important in patients undergoing chemotherapy.

Considerations: Milk thistle is generally safe and well tolerated. There are no known drug interactions, although it may reduce the effectiveness of any oral contraceptives. However, as an important note, any kind of liver condition should be checked out by a professional doctor.

Side Effects: On occasion, milk thistle may have a mild laxative effect, but this should clear up in about three days. It has very little toxicity. It is believed safe for nursing and pregnant women. Some people have a minor allergic reaction if they are sensitive to ragweed, marigolds, and daisies.

Dosage: You can buy milk thistle in several formats, including tincture, tablet, softgel, liquid, and capsule. Look for a supplement that is standardized to contain 80% silymarin. Dosage range is 400 to 600 mg standardized extract daily, divided into three doses. Take the supplement 30 minutes before meals. Milk thistle teas and products made with the leaf are not recommended, as concentrations of silymarin are too low to have therapeutic value. Experts also recommend consumers avoid tinctures made with alcohol. Improvement in a medical condition may take eight to 12 weeks. Fortunately, milk thistle can be taken safely over the long term.

Motherwort

Overview: Motherwort is a member of the herb family. It is grown in gardens in temperate climates. The flowers and leaves are generally used in medicinal preparations, although in China the seeds are used too.

Benefits: Motherwort is used to relieve menstrual problems, the symptoms of menopause and anxiety. It is also used to treat some heart conditions, especially those brought on by anxiety of stress. Interesting to note is that this herb is used the same way in both European folk medicine and traditional Chinese medicine, although Europeans additionally used it as a sedative. There is a lack of clinical evidence thus far.

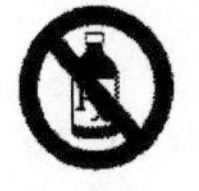

Considerations: Motherwort *must* be avoided during pregnancy, as it can cause a miscarriage. There are no known drug interactions.

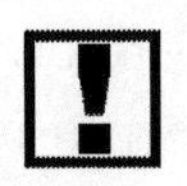

Side Effects: A high dose (three grams or more) can cause diarrhea, stomach irritation, and uterine bleeding.

Dosage: Use a teaspoon of dried herb in a cup of boiling water, steeped 10 minutes as a tea; drink three cups daily. Alternatively, use a tincture: ½ to ¾ teaspoonful, three times daily. German experts recommend a dose of 4.5 grams of dried herb daily.

Mullein

Overview: Mullein is a common wildflower that grows in much of Europe, Asia, and North America. It is also called "grandmother's flannel" because of its soft thick leaves. There are more than 300 species of the plant, but three in particular are prized for their health benefits. The leaves and flowers of the plant are used medicinally.

Benefits: Mullein is used primarily to treat respiratory conditions, including asthma, bronchitis, and coughs. A topical ointment is used to soothe skin conditions causing irritated skin and minor burns. It may also help with ear infections. There is a lack of clinical evidence so far.

Considerations: Safe for everyone, but because of a lack of evidence, pregnant or breast-feeding women should avoid it. There are no known drug interactions.

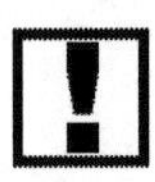

Side Effects: Rare reports of skin irritation in people who are allergic to the herb. For topical application buy a prepared product and follow package directions.

Dosage: Make a mullein tea by steeping one to two teaspoons of mullein in a cup of boiling water for 10 minutes; drink up to four cups a day. Squeeze mullein oil into the ear canal to help relieve the symptoms of an ear infection.

Nettle

Overview: Nettle—also often called "stinging nettle"—is a common weed in North America and Europe. Some people steam the leaves and eat them as a vegetable side dish or add them to soup. In traditional medicine the stem and leaves were used; today researchers are finding uses for the root as well.

Benefits: Current research indicates nettle root may be beneficial in treating benign enlarged prostate in men, both by slowing the growth of the prostate and relieving the symptoms of this condition.

Leaves and stems of nettle plants act as a diuretic, fight inflammation, and are an antihistamine. (Studies are examining whether nettle may be effective against hay fever.) Nettle was used in folk medicine to treat arthritis (all forms of joint pain), as well as acne and other skin conditions. There is research to support the use of nettle as a complement to conventional arthritis medications—that it makes them more effective. However, you should consult with a doctor before supplementing your medication in this way. There's preliminary evidence that it may be useful in treating hayfever too.

Considerations: If you take medication for diabetes or high blood pressure or take anticoagulants or medications that suppress the central nervous system speak to your doctor before taking nettle. Do not exceed the recommended dose. Nettle leaf may be safe for pregnant or breast-feeding women, but you should consult your doctor first.

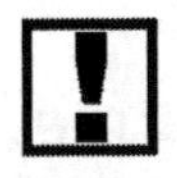

Side Effects: Nettle root may cause mild stomach upset, sweating, and allergic reaction (often on the skin). If you experience this, take your medication with food.

Dosage: Nettle is sold in tincture, liquid, dried herb/tea, and capsule format. Note that when you're buying nettle you must be clear on whether you want leaf or root: the two products treat different conditions and are used differently.

Dosage instructions vary depending on the specific condition. Here are two examples:

- For prostate problems: 500 mg standardized extract of nettle *root* twice a day. Combine with 160 mg two times daily of saw palmetto and 100 mg two times daily of *pygeum africanum* for maximum effect.

- For hay fever: 250 mg or 300 mg nettle *leaf* capsule containing the standardized extract three times a day (on an empty stomach).

Note: Because nettle has a diuretic effect make sure you drink plenty of liquids while taking the medication.

Olive Leaf

Overview: Extract from the olive leaf seems effective on a whole slew of viruses and bacteria. It contains a host of phytochemicals, including the active ingredient, "oleuropein," and is high in calcium. It is good for nearly any infectious disease.

Benefits: Its clinically proven effectiveness lies in its ability to lower blood pressure in patients with hypertension. Elsewhere, reports suggest that olive leaf somehow interferes with a viral infection that wants to spread, either by inhibiting that virus from invading cells or preventing it from reproducing. In this way, it may show effectiveness with the flu, herpes, and even HIV. It also could be useful for pneumonia, sore throat, sinusitis, and infections and rashes on the skin. None of these, though, have been proven

Considerations: Olive leaf is very safe, but people taking warfarin should probably avoid or limit amounts. The extract relaxes blood vessels and capillaries, and carries a mild risk of increased bleeding in those susceptible. It may also act against antibiotics, so it shouldn't be taken with them.

Side Effects: High doses can possibly lead to flu-like symptoms or allergic reactions when too many pathogens are killed off too quickly. This is also known as "Herxheimer's reaction." Orally, the herb hasn't been linked to any bad side effects specifically.

Dosage: Each pill should have between 15% and 20% of oleuropein, which is fairly potent in small amounts. How much you should take daily hasn't been completely established, but try 500 mg. This may mean one pill.

Oregon Grape

Overview: A relative of the barberry, this shrub that grows in the American Northwest, centering on Oregon of course, is a bit of a misnomer because the fruit that hangs from it is not a grape at all. It goes by a few other names too: holly-leaved berberis, holly mahonia, mountaingrape, Oregon barberry, trailing mahonia, and water holly. The root of this plant is used medicinally. It is filled with various kinds of alkaloids, including berberine.

Benefits: A few studies have found Oregon Grape, when applied to the skin, helps treat patients with the skin condition psoriasis. Oregon grape is known for its ability to aid digestion and help the gastrointestinal tract. The berberine helps it treat diarrhea in people who have contracted E. coli, as it prevents bacteria from attaching to the cells – mainly in the throat, urinary tract, and intestines. Thus, in these spots, it helps prevent infection from striking.

Considerations: Those taking the antibiotic "tetracycline" (used for infections and bad acne) should avoid Oregon grape. When used as a tea or tincture, the root may not be powerful enough to work its magic on major infections. This is because berberine is not the easiest substance to absorb. A doctor should be consulted in this case.

Side Effects: Oregon grape and berberine is safe when used in proper amounts. Other than possibly causing or worsening jaundice in infants (breast-feeding or pregnant women should be careful), and possibly worsening any existing kidney condition, it has no known side effects.

Dosage: As a tea, use one to three teaspoons of chopped-up root in boiled water for 15 minutes. It's safe to take about three cups a day. A tincture of three ml, three times daily, is also okay. For psoriasis, a cream of 10% extract can be used three times a day or more. It shouldn't be used for a prolonged period of time – no more than three weeks.

Parsley

Overview: This common herb is no secret (and certainly not in Middle Eastern cuisine) – it's the bright green small-leafed plant whose varieties are distinguished by their leaves. The flat-leafed kind is most often used in medicine. It was originally cultivated in the Mediterranean region by ancient Greeks.

Benefits: Germans are known to take parsley for treatment of urinary tract infections and to aid their intestinal tract – parsley, a bit of a diuretic, can help control gas and indigestion. It may be beneficial in helping treat gallstones and kidney stones as well. It's important to note that parsley has no reliable, scientific evidence to back up any of its medicinal claims.

Considerations: Parsley is extremely safe, and is not known to interact negatively with any drug or supplement. Some recommend that pregnant women avoid taking concentrated doses of parsley (a little with dinner won't hurt), because it may disrupt the womb. Parsley oil, refined, is too toxic for humans.

Side Effects: There are none, except if you eat very large amounts of parsley for a long period of time. Such consumption runs the risk of irritating the stomach and kidneys because of the essential oil found in the herb's seeds.

Dosage: As a tea, use ¼ teaspoon of fresh, pressed parsley (or crushed root or leaves) in boiling water and let steep for 10 minutes. You can drink two or three cups daily. For oral supplements, follow package directions.

Peppermint

Overview: Peppermint has a host of uses in the medicine world, much to do with its main ingredient, menthol. It is known as a soothing, numbing, calming agent. Commercially it's used in tea, toothpaste, gum, and other products because of these effects. The plant grows two feet tall and blooms in the height of summer, sprouting small purple flower heads. It's found all over the world.

Benefits: Peppermint can soothe upset stomachs and aid digestion. For tension headaches, it can be applied to the head to reduce symptoms. It helps soothe and relieve itching and irritations on the skin – things such as hives and poison ivy. For the intestinal tract and the stomach, its calming effect relaxes muscles, helping the flow of bile. This means it may be effective for irritable bowel syndrome. It can help relieve indigestion, gas, and bloating too. The decongestant effect produced by menthol can thin mucous and help with the common cold and flu. For sore throats and coughs, it can soothe and calm the area.

Considerations: Because it relaxes the sphincter muscle, it shouldn't be used by those who have been diagnosed with gastroesophageal reflux disease (it may worsen heartburn and indigestion). It's a good idea to avoid using peppermint on the skin if you are using other topical ointments for cancer.

Side Effects: Side effects are rare for the most part. If taking pills with peppermint oil, you may get skin rashes or muscle tremors. The oil needs to be taken in small amounts – and always diluted or taken in capsule form, because it can cause (but rarely) slowed heart rate, cramping, diarrhea, and drowsiness.

Dosage: Peppermint tea is prepared from dried leaves of the plant. Such teas are widely available commercially. A tincture that contains one part peppermint oil and nine parts pure grain alcohol (ethanol) can be made and applied lightly to the forehead for headaches. Any creams should have between one percent and 16% menthol. Use cream no more than three times a day. For irritable bowel, stomach problems, or gallstones take one to two "enteric-coated" pills three times a day (between meals). There should be 0.2 ml of oil per pill.

Phyllanthus

Overview: It seems the Phyllanthus species of plant has an age-old history of helping treat hepatitis, kidney problems, and diabetes. It is part of the Ayurvedic school of traditional medicine. The most studied member is *Phyllanthus amarus*, whose traditional use is actually for jaundice. The herb is known to grow mostly in India, to a height of 20 inches. It is as yet unknown how this herb actually works medicinally.

Benefits: Phyllanthus amarus is known mostly for its relevance to both chronic and acute hepatitis B. One double-blind study did find that it improved the speed of recovery in patients with acute hepatitis B. It has had both promising and conflicting results overall, so more research is needed into whether it can actually work or not.

Considerations: It has no known interactions with drugs or supplements. There is, though, not a great deal of research into phyllanthus. For this reason it shouldn't be taken by young children and pregnant or lactating women.

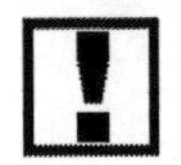

Side Effects: None reported as yet.

Dosage: The typical, recommended dose is about 600 to 900 mg a day. Because hepatitis and liver or kidney problems are of critical nature, phyllanthus should only be taken under a doctor's supervision.

Plantain

Overview: Don't confuse it with the banana-like vegetable that shares the same name. This plantain is actually a green, weedy plant that grows anywhere there is enough water. Its leaves are the source of its medicinal qualities. Its ingredients, which include tannins, make the herb a bit of an anti-inflammatory, antihemorrhagic, antimicrobial, and an expectorant.

Benefits: Its main benefit is in relieving the respiratory symptoms of cold and flu. Germany has approved plantain in soothing coughs and irritation caused by respiratory infections. Clinically, it's been found to help people who have cases of chronic bronchitis. It is also traditionally known to help skin irritations such as insect bites and dermatitis. There is a lack of scientific evidence into this herb.

Considerations: It is considered safe for anyone to take, and there is no evidence of any interactions with drugs or supplements.

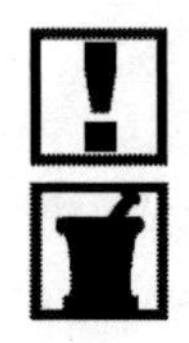

Side Effects: None reported.

Dosage: Use no more than a ½ teaspoon of the leaf in one cup of boiling water for 10 minutes. Drink no more than three cups a day. Fresh plantain leaves can actually be applied straight on skin irritations, use no more than three times daily. In a syrup or tincture, you can take a ½ teaspoon three times a day to relieve a nagging cough. Taken orally, you can juice about one teaspoon of fresh plantain.

Psyllium

Overview: Psyllium is the main ingredient of such commercial laxatives as Metamucil. It is a potent source of fiber. The seeds are used in traditional medicine and the seed *husks* are used for constipation. It's sometimes referred to as "Ispaghula."

Benefits: Psyllium is a superior laxative because the gel inside psyllium seeds is not digested. Instead it swells up and provides lubrication when combined with water. It is highly effective for chronic constipation, simple constipation, relieving diarrhea, hemorrhoids, and even abdominal pain. It might also help with weight loss, as eating psyllium makes you feel "full" and therefore stops you from overeating. What else? It may reduce cholesterol levels in patients who have mild to moderate hypercholesterolemia, ulcerative colitis, and hypertension.

Considerations: If you have been prescribed drugs to treat a condition, it might be wise to avoid psyllium because soluble fibers may hinder your body's ability to absorb drugs – these include antibiotics, antidiabetes drugs, carbamazepine, digoxin, lithium, warfarin, and possibly *every drug that is taken orally*. Pregnant women, diabetics, and people with symptoms of an obstructed bowel should consult a doctor before taking psyllium.

Side Effects: Psyllium may cause temporary bloating and gas. To avoid this, increase your dose of psyllium slowly over a week's time. You must drink plenty of water, because psyllium absorbs it and thus can cause mild dehydration. Occasionally it can cause an allergic reaction – in this case, visit your doctor immediately.

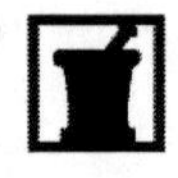

Dosage: The typical dose of psyllium for constipation and diarrhea is one to three teaspoons of powder dissolved in water. For irritable bowel syndrome, gallstones, or hemorrhoids take only one teaspoon. These are all just once a day.

Pygeum

Overview: Pygeum is derived from the bark of the tall African plum tree. Various chemicals are found within: phytosterols and triterpenes. It is part of traditional African medicine that says sipping tea made from this tree controls male urinary disorders.

Benefits: Exhibiting anti-inflammatory effects, pygeum is used to treat infections of the urinary tract in men and most often the condition benign prostate hyperplasia (BPH). It has consistently been better than placebo in improving urologic symptoms and urine flow. In Europe, pygeum has been approved for treating BPH since the 1970s. The herb contains compounds that have a diuretic action, anti-inflammatory activity, and a unique ability to dispose of any built-up cholesterol deposits.

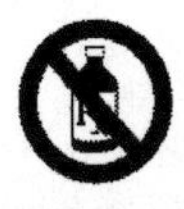

Considerations: No reported interactions with drugs. Prostate conditions, however, should be brought to a doctor's attention before any self-administered herbal therapy is initiated.

Side Effects: It can cause nausea and temporary stomach pain, but only rarely.

Dosage: Pygeum is normally taken as a pill or in a tincture. A typical dose is between 50 and 100 mg a day. For liquid extract, take 30 drops twice a day. But this herb is commonly sold along with others (such as nettle and saw palmetto) that help the prostate. Try and find a pygeum extract with 13% sterols.

Red Peony

Overview: It's a small flower that grows wild in China whose roots may be useful in medicine. Chinese researchers have performed all the research done on the herb, so it is likely to be a difficult one to acquire yet in North America. Red peony (not indicative of the flower color) is also called "chi shao." It contains a unique glycoside that is called "paeoniflorin."

Benefits: In traditional Chinese medicine it was used to treat bleeding or poor blood circulation. It may help calm nerves and relieve muscle cramps that occur because of liver cirrhosis or diabetes. One of the most recent of many preliminary studies found that an extract of red peony root helped relieve cirrhosis in patients with chronic hepatitis. It has also been found to have antioxidant properties. It needs further research before its benefits can be established.

Considerations: It should only be taken with the guidance of a doctor who is trained in traditional Chinese medicine.

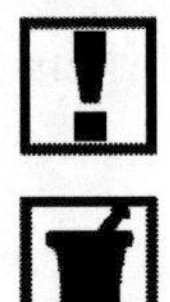

Side Effects: There are no side effects known.

Dosage: Pills of red peony are typically used in the Far East at about 1,000 to 3,000 mg, three times a day.

Rhodiola

Overview: Rhodiola is native to regions of Asia, Europe, and even the Arctic. Its history traces back to Russia and Scandinavia – some researchers believe Vikings may have regularly used the herb. It is long associated with medicine, traditionally to relieve fatigue and boost energy. The plant is a well-known "adaptogen," which means it enhances a person's endurance. (Another example is ginseng.) There are actually over 200 species of rhodiola. "*Rhodiola rosea*" is the type in question here, sometimes called "goldenroot" or "Arctic root." Sometimes it's even known as "roseroot."

Benefits: It appears to work by influencing chemicals in the nervous system that transmit signals to the brain. It is not supported by extensive studies, but preliminary ones suggest it helps fight fatigue and illnesses including: chronic fatigue syndrome, seasonal affective disorder, and fibromyalgia.

Considerations: So far, there are no known interactions. For now, it's safe to avoid taking rhodiola if you're taking another adaptogen such as ginseng. More research needs to be done into how it reacts with other supplements. It's best to check with your doctor regarding this herb.

Side Effects: High doses of rhodiola – 1,500 to 2,000 mg daily or above in an extract that contains two percent rosavin – may cause irritability and insomnia. Again, caution should be had here, as research is limited so far.

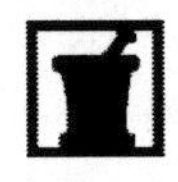

Dosage: Until more specific information is available about long-term supplementation, take a one- to two-week pause in your daily rhodiola regimen at least every three months to give your body a rest. In other words, keep repeated cycles separated by short intervals of no supplementation.

Sage

Overview: The leaves of this plant aren't just used in cooking; they also hold medicinal value. The silvery-green, fragrant leaves originated somewhere around the Mediterranean, but does grow in North America now as well. In the past it's been traditionally used to treat bleeding, ulcers, swelling, sore throats, and coughs, as well as improve memory and sharpen senses. It contains flavonoids, tannins and rosmarinic acid.

Benefits: In Germany, people use sage for mild stomach upset and excessive sweating. In the U.K. they use if for menopausal symptoms such as hot flashes. In Europe overall, they gargle sage tea to treat inflammations in the mouth, sore throat, and gingivitis. Most recently, a study found that it benefited cognition and memory in Alzheimer's patients. It may also help herpes-related cold sores.

Considerations: There are no reported interactions concerning sage. But still, patients with diabetes, hypertension, or seizure disorders should have regular check-ups if they decide to take sage. It is unsafe for pregnant or breast-feeding women.

Side Effects: An ingredient in sage is "thujone." When taken orally, thujone can lead to a higher heart rate, confusion and, if the dose is far too high, convulsions. It's best to consult a doctor before taking sage orally, and only use it for a two-week period at the most. The herb's oil should always be diluted in water. Pregnant women and those with a fever should not use sage.

Dosage: For sore throats, try three grams of chopped leaf added to 150 ml of boiling water for 10 minutes. This makes the tea, which can be drunk or used to gargle with several times a day. Also, diluted in water, use five ml of sage fluid extract a few times a day. For internal use, the same tea preparation described above may be taken three times per day.

St. John's Wort

Overview: This shrub blooms yellow flowers that when squeezed produce a red pigment. It's the flower, and the tiny black dots within the petals, that provides the medicine. It is much studied and much touted in the treatment of depression. "Hypericin" is one of its active ingredients, and is known to enhance the level of serotonin (the brain chemical that controls mood) in the bloodstream. The way it acts is similar to major drugs Prozac and Zoloft.

Benefits: As indicated, St. John's wort is an antidepressant recommended for mild to moderate depression. In 1996, an overview of 23 clinical studies dealing with 1,757 patients and published in the *British Medical Journal* found that St. John's wort was more effective than a placebo and that it caused fewer side effects than standard antidepressants. The herb may also be effective in reducing anxiety. It also may help boost the nervous system and lessen menopausal symptoms in women.

Considerations: This herb may be hazardous if combined with conventional medications. Get professional advice before mixing treatments. Also do not take St. John's wort if:

- You are epileptic or have a seizure disorder
- You are taking AIDS medication or a contraceptive pill
- You are going to do a lot of sunbathing, or are traveling to a hot country. Discontinue use if a rash develops.
- You have severe clinical depression.
- You appear to be having an allergic reaction to the herb.

Side Effects: In clinical studies, some adverse effects were noted: upset stomach, fatigue, itching, sleep disturbance, and skin rash. These were, though, less frequent than people taking antidepressants. Experts suggest protecting the skin against direct exposure to the sun as well because St. John's wort could leave it more sensitive.

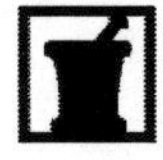

Dosage: For depression and for St. John's wort, it is very important you first consult a doctor. It's available in many forms. Common dosages include one capsule, three times a day (don't exceed 1,000 mg in a day); 10 to 15 drops of fluid extract in water three times a day, or ½ teaspoon of a herbal tincture three times a day in water. It may take two to six weeks for a visible improvement.

SAM-e

Overview: SAMe (S-adenosyl-L-methionine) is a naturally occurring compound present in the cells of the body. It's among a class of compounds that can help the body protect itself against cancer, heart disease, age-related problems, neurological disorders, and more.

Benefits: In Europe, SAMe is used to treat depression, liver disorders, osteoarthritis, and fibromyalgia; it's now available in the U.S. as a dietary supplement.

SAMe supporters claim it's as effective as tricyclic antidepressants, and there seems to be clinical evidence to demonstrate this. In 2000, researchers for the Agency for Healthcare Research and Quality (ARHQ) examined the results of 47 studies in which SAMe was used to treat depression. Among their findings:

- SAMe was already delivering a consistent improvement at three weeks – clinically acceptable as a response to treatment (and clearly superior to a placebo).
- Treatment with SAMe resulted in outcomes statistically equivalent to tricyclic antidepressants.

Considerations

- Due to weak or nonexistent regulation, the quality of brands varies. Try to find a trusted source.
- There are no medical studies that advise how to switch from prescription antidepressants to SAMe. Talk to your doctor before making this kind of change.
- Do not take SAMe until you have been off your prescription antidepressant for a week (two weeks if you are taking Nardil/phenelzine or Parnate/tranylcypromine).
- Do not drink alcohol while taking SAMe.
- Do not take while pregnant.
- Do not suddenly stop taking this medication.
- Parkinsonian symptoms have been reported with intravenous use.
- Symptoms of Parkinson's Disease may become worse with SAMe.

- Patients with bipolar depression may switch to a manic state.

Side Effects: Any side effects tend to be uncommon and temporary, but may include:

- Headache – treat with acetaminophen or aspirin.
- Diarrhea – increase fiber intake.
- Nausea – tends to disappear with higher dose and/or continued use.
- Dry mouth/thirst – temporary. Drink plenty of fluids, chew gum or suck on hard candy.
- Blurred vision – rare.
- Restlessness, anxiety, and/or elation – contact the person who prescribed your SAMe if you experience these.
- Anxiety in patients with depression and mania in those with bipolar disorder.
- Symptoms of toxicity may include disorientation, vomiting, liver damage, or shock.

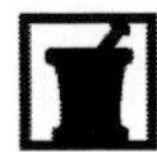

Dosage: Take SAMe on an empty stomach. Therapeutic doses range from 400 to 1600 mg daily. It should be started off at small doses and quickly increased over the span of a week or two. It may require four to eight weeks to become fully effective, so patience is mandatory. There used to be a bit of concern over whether some forms of orally-taken SAMe were stable or not, but a new technique of manufacturing has all but negated this concern.

Saw Palmetto

Overview: The berries of this plant *Serenoa repens,* are of medicinal value. The herb, a palm tree that grows in the southern United States, is also known as saw, American dwarf palm tree, and cabbage palm.

The berries have been found to have antiandrogenic and anti-inflammatory effects. A saw palmetto extract, "liposterolic," has concentrated amounts of free fatty acids and sterols, and it may reduce the levels of an active testosterone that binds in area surrounding the urethra, which could be interrupting urine flow.

Benefits: Called "the guy herb" saw palmetto has been found effective in relieving benign prostatic hyperplasia. Taking this herb will help relieve excessive urination and other symptoms of BPH, as well as possibly helping with bladder irritation. It basically functions to settle the prostate and normalize urine flow. It may help with any lower urinary tract symptoms in men.

Considerations: Palmetto may have some hormonal effects, and therefore it is not safe for women who are pregnant or lactating. If you have prostate problems, however, you should first get a medical checkup. It has no known interactions with drugs.

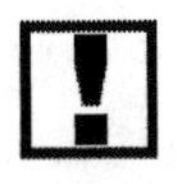

Side Effects: There have been adverse effects such as nausea, vomiting, and diarrhea – but in studies they have been mild and infrequent.

Dosage: The recommended daily dosage of saw palmetto is between one and two grams, or 320 mg of its "hexane" extract (standardized to contain approximately 85% fatty acids and sterols).

Selfheal (Prunella vulgaris)

Overview: This member of the mint family is found natively in America and it has been used for numerous treatments. It is also common in European and Asian countries for different uses. Different purposes exist for both the leaves and flowers. The leaves are generally more useful for ailments, although the flowers can be used to treat hyperactivity or headache.

Benefits: This herb has actually been found to prevent and treat herpes in a recent clinical trial. Traditionally, it is used to treat sores in the mouth and throat, as an astringent, a blood pressure reducer, and even as an anti-cancer drug. Fresh leaves are used to reduce bleeding in minor cuts, as well as to reduce the chance of infection. Without proof, it is also used for: colitis, HIV, fever, headache, liver disease, gastroenteritis, and diarrhea.

Considerations: There are no known drug interactions, but you should seek a doctor before use if you have abnormal bleeding of the mouth, uterus, or blood in stool or urine.

Side Effects: No side effects are known.

Dosage: You can brew a tea by using one oz of fresh leaves, or one teaspoon dried in a cup of boiling water. Drink several times a day to treat high blood pressure, hemorrhage, diarrhea, jaundice, convulsions, seizures, hepatitis, headache, cancer pain, and fever. For a sore throat, gargle with the tea, or to help mouth sores or bleeding gums, swish the mixture around in your mouth. For topical use, use fresh plants that are ripped up and apply with a bandage or cloth wrap.

Slippery Elm

Overview: This herb, which is the inner bark of the slippery elm tree, exerts a calming and soothing effect when it's used as a medicine. The main reason behind this is the active ingredient, "mucilage," which is a gummy substance that forms a protective layer along throat, digestive, and intestinal tract.

Benefits: Inflamed mucous membranes can be soothed with slippery elm. It has been useful in relieving coughs, sore throat, and other symptoms of a dry upper respiratory tract. It is actually used in many commercial throat lozenges. The FDA considers it an effective soothing agent for cough and cold symptoms. This soothing action may also be effective in easing heartburn, ulcers, and inflammatory bowel disease.

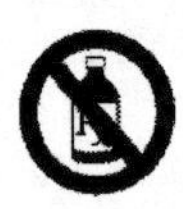

Considerations: Slippery elm is quite safe. Nevertheless, lactating women should avoid it.

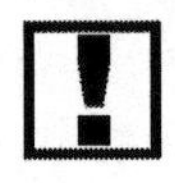

Side Effects: There are none reported (when taken at recommended doses). Slippery elm is even considered safe in pregnant women. The only thing it may do is detract the usefulness of other oral medication you might be using, so take slippery elm a few hours before other oral medication.

Dosage: For respiratory symptoms, try drinking two to three cups of tea a day, or add ½ tablespoon of slippery elm liquid extract to a cup of hot water. The extract and water can be used up to three times daily. For lozenges, simply follow package instructions. For capsules of extract, try two capsules (250 to 500 mg) a few times a day.

Soy

Overview: Soy protein has nearly as many amino acids as meat does, and amino acids are essential building blocks of protein. It has more protein and iron than beef, more calcium than milk, and is rich in "isoflavones" – powerful antioxidants that help protect against cancer and cellular damage. You can find it in tofu, miso, soy milk, soy flour, soybeans, and as supplements.

Benefits: Soy reduces total cholesterol and LDL cholesterol, while increasing the level of HDL cholesterol (the good one). Its isoflavones have been linked to a reduced risk of artherosclerosis, a condition where blood vessels that lead to the heart are restricted or tightened due to a build-up of fatty substances. The FDA says it is an acceptable way to lower the risk of heart disease. Also, soy protein is marketed as an alternative for treating menopausal symptoms such as hot flashes, osteoporosis, Type II diabetes, and even hypertension.

Considerations: There are no reported indications with drugs or supplements. But caution should still be exerted involving antibiotics, estrogen replacement therapy, and warfarin.

Side Effects: Soy is remarkably healthy. Still, it most commonly causes gastrointestinal side effects such as constipation and bloating, as well as nausea. In some people, soy can cause an allergic reaction such as a skin rash.

Dosage: The FDA has reported that it accepts soy protein, at 25 grams a day when taken within a diet low in saturated fat and cholesterol, as a legitimate way to reduce the risk of heart disease. Don't exceed 50 grams of soy protein or 150 mg of soy isoflavones a day.

Stevia

Overview: This natural agent is isolated from the plant *Stevia rebaundiana.* It is more potent than sugar as a sweetener, and has been used as such for a few decades in Japan and Brazil. The stunning fact is that, unlike sugar, it contains no calories. It hails from Paraguay.

Benefits: Preliminary studies found that this sweetener might come with a sidenote: an antihypertensive effect. Could it be? A 2003 study set out to see if stevia could be effective in 174 people. For two years they charted the course of the patients and marked their hypertension ratings. In the end, those on stevia had a far lower percentage of problems in the left ventricle than did people on placebo. Taken orally, the sugar substitute significantly decreased both systolic and diastolic blood pressure without any adverse effects.

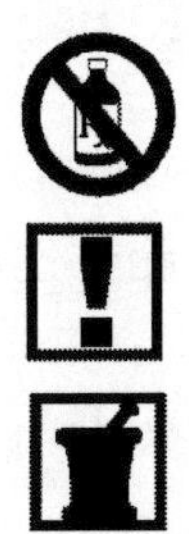

Considerations: None indicated, although it hasn't been tested too thoroughly yet.

Side Effects: At recommended doses, stevia is considered perfectly safe.

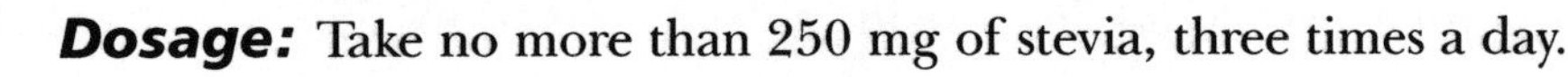

Dosage: Take no more than 250 mg of stevia, three times a day.

Tea Tree Oil

Overview: This shrub native to Australia emits an oil that can fight infections. The shrub has needle-like leaves and yellow or purple flowers. There are about 100 compounds in tea tree oil that take active action against viruses, fungi, and bacteria. The oil has antiseptic properties, which make it valuable against skin infections. The only spots in the world where it grows naturally are in Queensland and New South Wales. Most oil comes from Down Under. It smells like nutmeg.

Benefits: Tea tree oil has been found at least marginally effective in helping treat skin conditions such as acne, dermatitis, and blackheads. The oil has proven antimicrobial activities. It's very good for fungal nail infections (toe or finger), as well as athlete's foot. It can also help quell itching related to insect bites, poison ivy, chicken pox, and minor skin irritations. Tea tree oil also helps inhibit yeast organisms and thus can relieve candidiasis, a fungal/yeast infection.

Considerations: You shouldn't use a full-strength tea tree oil solution on any part of the skin because it may cause further irritation, burning, or rashes. Never swallow tea tree oil, because it's been linked to a slew of problems related to its toxicity.

Side Effects: Some people have allergic reactions, including rashes and itching, when applying tea tree oil.

Dosage: On the skin or nail, use oil at 70% or so on affected parts of the nail or skin twice a day. For athlete's foot, try a solution at 25% to 50% twice a day. Don't use too much! For use on skin that is scarred by acne, use oil diluted between five and 15%.

Turmeric

Overview: This medicine is a yellow powder that is ground from the roots of the turmeric plant, and is the common ingredient in curry (it's what turns it yellow). A member of the ginger family, it grows wild in Indonesia and India. Turmeric is a mainstay in both Chinese and Ayurvedic medicines, with the central ingredient "curcumin" holding the medicinal value. It also has bitters, a volatile oil, and other compounds that may be used for therapeutic purposes.

Benefits: The best evidence is that turmeric helps fight dyspepsia, which is a case of bad digestion. By lowering histamine levels, curcumin may reduce inflammation and for this reason is used mainly for joint pain and inflammation. The spice's antioxidant action is though to protect against liver damage. Some evidence suggests it protects the brain against the debilitating Alzheimer's disease. Animal studies show that is has the ability to stop cancerous cells from growing, again due to its antioxidant action. Even still, turmeric has been found to prevent platelets from clumping up, which guards against atherosclerosis and improves blood circulation. Its anti-inflammatory nature means it could be useful in other conditions, such as pelvic inflammatory disease, and against pain in general.

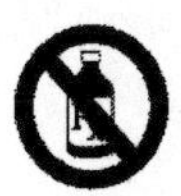

Considerations: People with gallbladder disease may experience a flare-up of symptoms if they take turmeric. People who have bleeding problems (especially those taking blood-thinning medications) shouldn't use high amounts either.

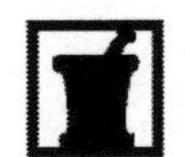

Side Effects: There are no reported side effects in regular dosage. Even in large amounts, there have been no real adverse reactions.

Dosage: In capsule form, the typical dose is between 400 mg and 1,000 mg three times a day. Look for extract that have 400 to 600 mg of curcumin. If you're taking powdered root, the dose is 500 mg to 1,000 mg up to three times a time. You may use turmeric as a tincture, with a typical dose between 0.5 and 1.5 ml a day. Finally, it's of course available as a powdered spice.

TWHF (Tripterygium wilfordii Hook F)

Overview: This ancient Chinese herb with the confounding name has both anti-inflammatory and immunosuppressive traits. Its main ingredient, triptolide, is said to have these properties and has been shown to protect neurons from injury and thus pain. To avoid rewriting it, let's appoint an acronym, TWHF. TWHF has been used for over 2,000 years in Chinese medicine. It's also referred to as "Thunder God Vine."

Benefits: Western medicine has recognized TWHF for the treatment of rheumatoid arthritis and even leprosy. In fact, as of this writing, the National Institutes of Health was recruiting participants for a new study into TWHF's effect on rheumatoid arthritis. This follows several studies in 2002 and 2003 that found it well tolerated and beneficial for patients with rheumatoid arthritis. Researchers believe it is promising and should be studied for autoimmune diseases and all kinds of inflammation. The most recent study found it to be effective in protecting against pain.

Considerations: It is still very much a new herb in terms of conventional medicine and is not yet fully understood. You should only take it under the auspices of a doctor.

Side Effects: In studies, women have experienced menstrual cessation (pregnant women should not take TWHF). The herb has also been linked to upset stomach, nausea, diarrhea, appetite loss, and dizziness.

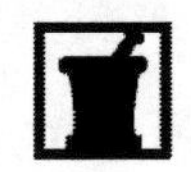

Dosage: Proper dosage needs to be worked out with a doctor. Patients should work with their doctor to get the specially prepared extracts that were found effective in clinical trials.

Tylophora

Overview: This climbing plant is native to India where it grows wild in several regions. Tylophora might exert anti-inflammatory, antiallergic, and antispasmodic actions.

Benefits: It has an age-old reputation as a treatment for asthma. Several studies have backed up this claim, but one of the best-designed trials actually found no benefit, so this herb still remains up in the air. It is occasionally used for respiratory infections, allergies, and joint pain as well.

Considerations: There aren't any comprehensive safety studies so pregnant or breast-feeding women should avoid it, as should children and people with severe renal disease. There are no drug interactions known.

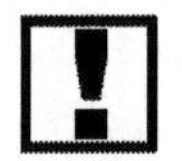

Side Effects: In a couple studies, there was reported nausea, vomiting, mouth soreness, and altered taste sensation.

Dosage: Typically, dried tylophora leaf or the herb in capsule form is used 200 mg twice a day.

Valerian

Overview: The herb, also known as heliotrope, vandal root, and all-heal, has an enormous system of roots and a collage of small pink and white flowers. The roots of this wild weed that grows in Europe and the U.K. are the parts used in medicine. Valerian has the ability to exert a soothing and calming effect on the brain, thus helping with mood-related disorders. It ingredients include "valepotriates" (relaxes muscles) as well as tannins and alkaloids. Interesting note: valerian can substitute for catnip.

Benefits: Valerian is an age-old remedy for both insomnia and anxiety – it binds itself to brain receptors and inserts its sedating, calming effects there as well as its muscle-relaxing effects. This combines for a better night's sleep, as well as calmed nerves, balanced mood swings, and less stress. It can obviously, therefore, be a possibility for conditions where insomnia is a symptom, such as chronic fatigue syndrome. Those taking it have also reported no grogginess in the morning.

Considerations: It is safe to take with any herbs known for their calming effects. In fact, it's been found to work quite well with chamomile. As with any herb, don't overuse it. Pregnant and breast feeding women should consult their doctor before taking it. It may increase the effects of any sedatives you might be taking – these include gotu kola, chamomile, cayenne, goldenseal, sage, SAMe, St. John's wort, nettle, and kava.

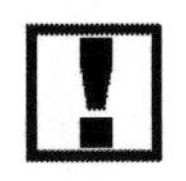

Side Effects: If taken in high doses, it can cause some cardiac disturbances, grogginess, restlessness, and headache. Like any sedative, it may lead to drowsiness if taken during the day. Occasionally it can cause gastric discomfort, dry mouth, and vivid dreams.

Dosage: For tea, use dried valerian root – one teaspoon of crushed root with 2/3 cup of hot water (drink before bed). For anxiety, you can try two to three cups. For extracts, it is widely available in pills, tinctures, and softgels: for all, follow the package directions. Hint: look for a supplement that has 0.8% valeric or valerenic acid. If taking pills, take 400 to 900 mg a day.

Vitex (Chaste Tree)

Overview: This herb is derived from the fruit of the chaste tree, which actually looks more like a tall weed. It is native to the Mediterranean, with green leaves that resemble the hemp plant and blue and white flowers. The dried fruit is used medicinally. They contain flavonoids, alkaloids, volatile oils, progesterone, and testosterone.

Benefits: Women can use vitex to control symptoms associated with PMS – the herb has been proven to help treat amenorrhea, acne, infertility, and menstrual cycle abnormalities (Vitex is one of the very few proven herbs to do so).

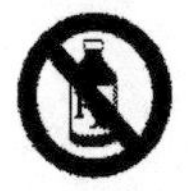

Considerations: Vitex can interact negatively with oral contraceptives, hormonal therapy, and any drugs that antagonize dopamine receptors (i.e. haloperidol). These are all because of its hormone-regulating action. Pregnant women should avoid vitex.

Side Effects: It is usually well-tolerated, but can lead to some adverse effects. These can include nausea, upset stomach, rash, itching, dry mouth, fatigue, headaches, and agitation. Changes in a woman's menstrual flow may be noticed when she first begins taking vitex.

Dosage: In Germany, the recommended dose is 30 to 40 mg a day of the dried chaste berry either in pill or liquid form. Generally, you take it in the morning with water for a few months straight. Any relief will not be immediate – it may be months before you begin to notice a difference. Vitex is a slow-acting herb. Because prolonged use will probably be needed, you should consult a doctor.

Witch Hazel

Overview: This herb, unrelated to broomsticks, is native to northeastern U.S. and eastern Canada. Its other names include: spotted alder, winterbloom, and snapping hazelnut. The oily seeds from this shrub actually burst from the tree upon ripening, and its leaves fall in autumn just like its larger neighbors in the forest. Those leaves are high in tannic, gallic acids, and some volatile oil. The bark is high in tannins, resins, and sterons, and all parts of witch hazel have astringent, sedative, and pain-relieving properties.

Benefits: The "proanthocyanidins" in witch hazel has proven antiviral activity. For this reason, it's proven to help fight the herpes simplex virus, and the cold sores that come with it. It's mainly used for skin irritations such as minor cuts, itching of insect bites, razor burns, and infection. It may even help with muscle aches. It can also help relieve (temporarily) the itching, discomfort, and burning caused by hemorrhoids.

Considerations: Although some people may experience some related skin irritation, witch hazel is safe when it's used externally. It should only be taken orally under a doctor's watchful eye. Commercial witch hazel contains a type of alcohol and should never be taken internally.

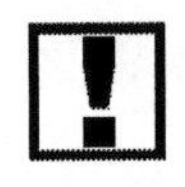

Side Effects: None besides minor irritation if taken externally. Sometimes, though, any plant with at least 10% tannins can lead to problems with the gastrointestinal system, the kidneys, and the liver. When used on the skin, witch hazel may cause contact dermatitis.

Dosage: Use topical ointment as directed on package. To make an external mixture, boil five to 10 grams of dried leaves in water, strain and compress the liquid on your skin.

Yarrow

Overview:This perennial herb grows wild, wherever it chooses: from fields, pastures, and meadows to small slopes beside railroad tracks and highways. It grows about a yard in height and blooms flower heads, yellow and white. It contains more than 120 compounds, many of which have medicinal properties. Some herbalists say if they had to choose one herb for multiple purposes, yarrow would be it.

Benefits: It's been used to halt bleeding, heal infections of the urinary tract, relieve digestive problems, and ease ailments experienced by women (menstrual bleeding, hot flashes, fibroid tumors). Azulene, one compound in yarrow, may reduce inflammation and fever. Some use yarrow to stimulate the liver and help it flush out waste – thus it is used for endometriosis.

Antiseptic and astringent properties allow yarrow to reduce inflammation and promote wound healing. It helps reduce intestinal cramps and diarrhea (antispasmodic qualities). It may be effective in lowering blood pressure as well. Fresh yarrow leaves, when chewed, may get ride of a toothache. It's important to mention that yarrow lacks clinical proof for these effects.

Considerations: This herb is generally safe when used in recommended doses. It can increase the risk of toxicity if you are taking anti-inflammatories. It also has the potential to interfere with drugs taken for hypertension, and there is some risk of hypokalemia if you're taking corticosteroids. It may also interfere with the absorption of iron and other minerals, meaning iron deficient people should probably avoid it.

Side Effects: Taking too much, as with any herb, it may lead to some minor side effects. These include drowsiness, a frequent need to urinate, and diarrhea. Since yarrow grows wild it may have some allergic similarities to ragweed, so those with seasonal allergies may react to it.

Dosage: This can be taken as a pill, juice, liquid extract, tincture, tea, or even ointment. You can take as much as 4.5 grams a day of the herb, three teaspoons of juice a day or three grams of flowers a day. In tea, yarrow can be taken along with other herbs in a 200 ml (eight fl oz) formula three times a day. As a tincture, take two to four ml three times a day in 45% alcohol. As a liquid extract, the same in 25% alcohol.

Yohimbe

Overview: Yohimbe comes from a tree native to several African countries. Indigenous peoples have used the bark for centuries to boost sexual prowess, as an aphrodisiac, and to treat angina and hypertension. The bark can be smoked as a hallucinogen as well.

Benefits: Yohimbe is used to treat erectile dysfunction, as it promotes blood flow to the genitals (it enhances sexual responsiveness in women too). Clinical studies have found it to restore potency to diabetics and heart patients. Yohimbine hydrochloride, derived from yohimbe, is approved by the FDA for the treatment of impotence.

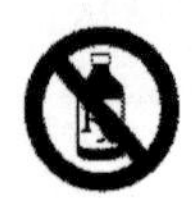

Considerations: Check with your doctor before taking this herb. Yohimbe is a MAO inhibitor and thus can adversely affect high blood pressure or any other heart conditions. Do not take it if you have kidney disease, glaucoma, or a history of ulcers. Do not take yohimbe at the same time as foods containing tyramines (cheese, chocolate, beer, nuts, deli meats) or the amino acids tyrosine or phenylalanine. Do not take yohimbe in combination with antidepressants, sedatives, amphetamines, antihistamines, or caffeine.

Side Effects: Reported side effects include increased heart rate, headache, dizziness, tremor, insomnia, anxiety, irritability, sinusitis, rash, fluid retention, nausea, and sweating. Too much can cause these symptoms plus panic attacks, hallucinations, and even heart problems. A serious overdose can cause a dangerous drop in blood pressure and may possibly cause paralysis.

Dosage: It's available in several formats including pill, capsule, drops, tincture, tea, and bark. "Yohimbine" (the active ingredient) is available only by prescription, and its typical dose is five to 10 mg, three times a day. It will take two to three weeks to really see if it's working.

Note: A recent Consumer Reports document listed yohimbe as a "supplement to avoid." It cited blood pressure change, heart arrhythmia, heart attack, and respiratory depression as related dangers. Despite this, the herb is not banned in any country.

5-HTP

Overview: This commercial product comes from the seeds of an African plant called *Griffonia simplicfolia.* The body converts 5-HTP (proper name "5-hydroxytryptophan") into serotonin. Serotonin is a neurotransmitter in the brain – part of the larger serotoninergic system which controls mood, emotion, sleep, and appetite Low levels of serotonin have been linked with a wide range of conditions – including depression, headaches, insomnia, anxiety, hyperactivity, chronic fatigue syndrome, and fibromyalgia – as well as obesity.

Benefits: 5-HTP operates as a natural appetite suppressant. In one study, participants weren't told to eat less, but after five weeks the group taking 5-HTP had lost weight – more than three pounds. Researchers found that the participants given the placebo consumed about 2,300 calories per day, while those taking 5-HTP ate only 1,800 calories daily. Other studies, in which people have been actively dieting, have yielded more dramatic results.

It has received attention in two other areas as well: 5-HTP may improve the symptoms of depression and the arthritic condition, fibromyalgia

Considerations: While 5-HTP is generally considered safe, it should not be taken by pregnant women, nursing mothers, people on low protein diets, or the extremely old. People with any of the following conditions should only use it under their doctor's supervision:

- Cardiovascular disease (including high blood pressure, post-heart attack, post-stroke)
- Parkinson's disease, cancer or autoimmune diseases (rheumatoid arthritis, multiple sclerosis, lupus, scleroderma)
- Myalgia
- Lung diseases
- Liver diseases (hepatitis or cirrhosis)
- Parasitic infection
- AIDS
- Anorexia nervosa
- Severe allergies
- Peripheral neuropathy

- Rash or flushing
- Edema
- Nausea
- Diarrhea
- Sickle cell anemia
- Hemophilia

Do not take 5-HTP if you are taking any of the following medications:

- Antidepressants
- Antibiotics
- Antihistamines and cold medications
- Anti-parkinson medications (e.g., L-dopa)
- Cancer chemotherapy
- Monoamine oxidase inhibitors
- Selective serotonin reuptake inhibitors (SSRIs, e.g., Prozac)
- Tricyclic medications
- Weight-loss medications such as dextenfluramine
- Barbituates or other tranquilizers
- Alcohol or illegal intravenous drugs

Note: Allow at least six hours between consuming alcohol and taking 5-HTP. Note: 5-HTP can magnify the effect of tranquilizers.

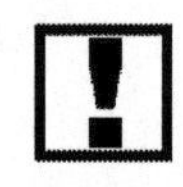

Side Effects: In one clinical trial, some participants reported mild nausea during the first six weeks, but symptoms were not severe enough to cause anyone to drop out.

Dosage: As with all nutritional supplements, individual experiences may vary. One provider of 5-HTP for weight loss recommends taking 100 mg of the supplement 20 minutes before each meal (for a total of 300 mg a day), and doubling the dose after four weeks if no results are achieved.

Note: 900 mg of 5-HTP is considered a very high dose. ***Do not exceed 900 mg per day.***

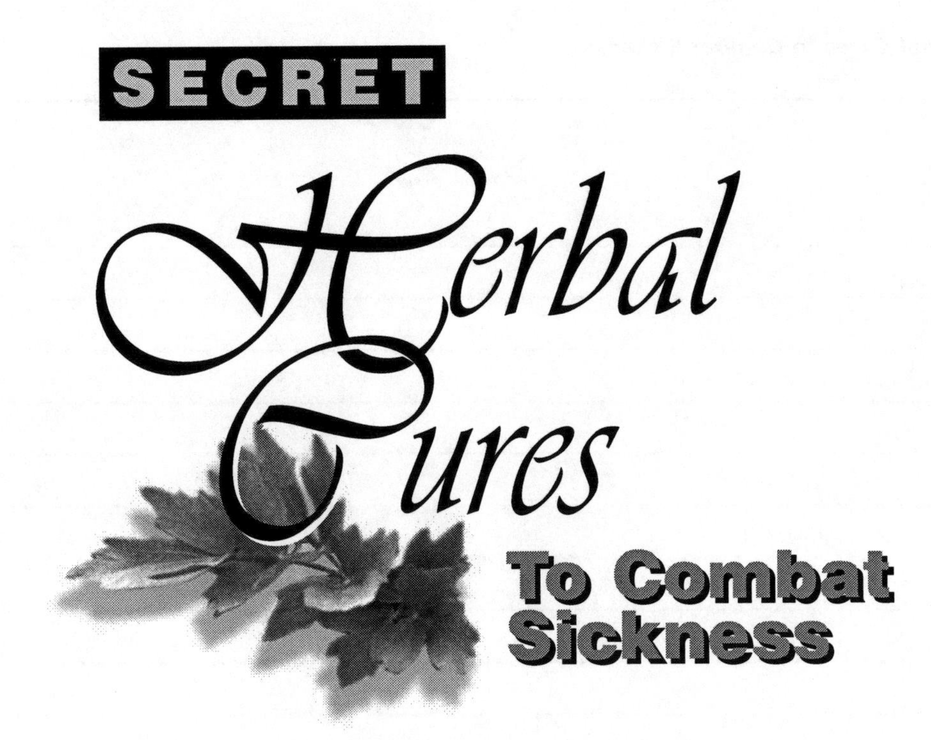

Part Four

MENTIONABLE NUTRACEUTICALS

NOTES

Throughout this book, we have highlighted "Other Nutraceuticals That May Work" and here is some accompanying information for each one not in the Index of Herbs. These are here for your reference and information, but just like the herbs in Part Three, if you are to take any therapeutic doses of any of the following, consult a doctor and make sure you know all about side effects and most importantly, any interactions these might have with drugs, supplements, or medical conditions.

Vitamins

Beta-Carotene

This is actually a natural chemical, but we'll plunk it in here because of its relationship to vitamin A: the body can transform it. It is also similar to both vitamin E and C because it is an antioxidant. Beta-carotene is the best way to get vitamin A because your body only transforms it when it needs it. The best way to get this chemical is through such yellow and orange vegetables as carrots, yams, and squash, and such dark green veggies as spinach, broccoli, and green peppers. There's conflicting research here in terms of whether beta-carotene can help slow cataracts from forming, prevent macular degeneration (eyes), protect against cancer and heart disease, boost immune function in HIV patients, protect against sunburn, and help fight Parkinson's disease, rheumatoid arthritis, and hypertension. There is no firm evidence it works in any of these.

Folic Acid

Folic Acid is also known as vitamin B-9. A deficiency of folic acid, not unlike other vitamins, can lead to anemia. Suggestions that folic acid can help prevent cognitive problems are not backed up by science, however folic acid has been associated with a smaller risk of birth defects if a woman has proper amounts before and during pregnancy. It has also been linked to helping control homocysteine levels in the blood, high amounts of which are known to be a risk factor for heart disease. Folic acid is found in leafy green vegetables (spinach, kale), organ meats such as liver, nuts and legumes, whole wheat, broccoli, and asparagus. It is also available in pills.

Lipoic acid

Not exactly a vitamin, it still fits in this category because it resembles the strong antioxidants vitamins C and E. It's a fatty acid that contains sulfur and it has grown in popularity as a dietary supplement. Lipoic acid is actually found in every cell in the body, generating the energy that keeps us going. And it has a unique mode of action. While vitamin C works in water and vitamin E works in fat, lipoic acid can function in both. Like them it is an antioxidant that battles free radicals and the damage they can cause. There's some evidence that the acid actually does the work of other antioxidants if they are not sufficient in number, making it perhaps the body's strongest antioxidant. It's found in small quantities within liver and yeast, but if you need it for a certain treatment, you'll of course need supplements.

Niacin (vitamin B-3)

This vitamin is either called niacin or nicotinic acid. Vitamin B-3 plays an active role in several important bodily functions, especially in maintaining healthy skin and a working gastrointestinal tract and nervous system. Most notably, niacin metabolizes fats, and when used medicinally it can lower the levels of LDL cholesterol while raising HDL levels. It can help widen blood vessels too, which means it's valuable as a circulatory aid. Although linked to the nervous system, it is not conclusive that niacin can help with the treatment of mental disorders (although doctors have tried). You can find vitamin B-3 in fish, beef, pork, dairy, whole wheat, potatoes, corn, broccoli, carrots, and tomatoes. It can be lost if food is boiled, though. Niacin and niacinamide are both available as supplements, mainly involved in lowering cholesterol.

Vitamin A

Everyone knows about vitamins, but perhaps not exactly what they do in the body. Vitamin A helps protect against dangerous free radicals and some other vital processes. People with diabetes tend to be deficient in vitamin A, so it has been linked to that illness. It also has been shown to benefit some skin problems such as psoriasis, acne, and rosacea. The only problem is, this vitamin runs the risk of raising toxic levels and causing some liver damage when you take too much. It is easily the most dangerous vitamin when taken in too high a dose. Experts agree that taking beta-carotene supplements is a safer way to get vitamin A, which the body can create from beta-carotene when it needs it.

Vitamin B-1

Also known as "thiamin" it was the first B vitamin ever discovered. This vitamin helps break down carbohydrates and release the needed energy within. It is also involved in the creation of cortisone and progesterone out of fatty acids. The more carbs you take in, the greater the need for enough thiamin to convert them into energy. The vitamin is best found in organ meats, pork, peas, soy products, poultry, fish, peanuts, and whole grains. It's also available as a supplement or in a B multivitamin. Unlike vitamin A, it has no known toxicity.

Vitamin B-2 (Riboflavin)

This vitamin is key to producing energy: it oxidizes fatty acids, glucose, and amino acids for this purpose. When the body needs to repair tissues, riboflavin is critical. It may also be critical for the blood in correcting cases of anemia. Interestingly, riboflavin is found in the pigment of the eye, allowing it to adapt to light. For this reason, it might delay or prevent cataracts and its deficiency could be the reason behind an oversensitivity to light, itching or burning eyes, and even tongue and mouth sores. It is available in pill form and is found naturally in foods including: cheese, organ and other meats, poultry, fish, eggs, beans, and spinach.

Vitamin B-12

The body needs vitamin B-12 in order to make red blood cells, which of course transport oxygen. It also plays a role in a healthy nervous system as it maintains the protective sheath around nerve cells. It's an important vitamin in breaking down homocysteine in the body, preventing the amino acid from building up in the arteries to toxic levels. The absorption of this vitamin depends on the "intrinsic factor" – a protein in the stomach that carries the vitamin to the digestive tract where it can be absorbed. Most people don't get adequate amounts of vitamin B-12. A deficiency can result in anemia. This vitamin is naturally found only in meats and dairy products. It can also be found in soy substitutes and fortified cereals.

Vitamin C

It's possible up to 40% of people in the U.S. don't take in enough vitamin C, an essential nutrient that fights illness and bacteria, helps maintain eyesight, and may aid asthmatics, hypertensive patients, and autistic people. It's a strong antioxidant that keeps you healthy and quickens your body's ability to shake off bacterial invasions such as the common cold. Food sources go well beyond orange juice to red chili peppers, sweet peppers, parsley, broccoli, kale, cabbage, strawberries, watercress, and citrus fruits. Eating them fresh will ensure you get the maximum effect.

Vitamin E

This vitamin is an antioxidant that roams around in the body's fat and oils to fight free radicals. It has shown some usefulness in treating pregnancy complications, side effects of antipsychotic drugs, boosting the body's immune system, improving fertility in men, slowing the progression of Alzheimer's, and even helping prevent cancer (particularly in the prostate). It may lead to blood-thinning problems if used in conjunction with a few herbs (notably garlic and ginkgo biloba). In food, you can find vitamin E in seeds, nuts, whole grains, and polyunsaturated vegetable oils. It's of course available in therapeutic doses as well.

Minerals

Calcium

There is about two-and-a-half pounds of calcium stored in our teeth and bones. It has a number of benefits in the body. First and foremost, as most people know, it keeps bones strong and healthy. Bones are actually a live tissue that are broken down and are constantly being reformed. Calcium plays a major role in that reformation, and a deficiency can lead straight to osteoporosis. There have been studies as well that linked calcium to lower blood pressure, and even a reduced risk of colon cancer. Calcium can be found in foods such as dairy products as well as soy, green leafy vegetables, and various seafood. Humans may only absorb between 20% and 40% of the calcium in food. Calcium supplements are widely taken and often recommended for people who've broken or fractured bones, have osteoporosis, or suffer from hypertension.

Magnesium

Magnesium should also be taken if you are taking calcium supplements. It is also an essential nutrient. Throughout the body it's used for relaxing muscles, blood clotting, and making energy molecules. One of the reasons it should be taken with calcium is that it prevents calcium from entering heart and muscle cells. It has been shown to help with migraine headaches, hearing loss, kidney stones, hypertension (when working with calcium and potassium), and menstrual pain. Magnesium deficiencies are actually fairly common and many people believe you should take supplements regardless of whether you need them therapeutically. Kelp is high in magnesium, as are almonds and cashews. Other sources include wheat, brewer's yeast, whole grains, and lots of common fruits and vegetables.

Chromium

You don't need much, but this mineral is still very important in our nutrition and growth. While insulin is well known for its role in regulating the movement of glucose in and out of cells, chromium plays a lesser-known supporting role; it is needed to keep the amount of blood sugar at a functional level and to allow the body to use it correctly. In fact, insulin is thought to perhaps even use chromium in this whole blood sugar regulation. For these reasons, chromium supplements may be beneficial for diabetics. Without much evidence, chromium has been suggested to have an ability to lower cholesterol, to treat acne, and to reduce the effects of migraine. It may even aid in weight loss.

Potassium

The main function of this mineral is helping your kidneys work properly. Magnesium can help ensure you have a proper balance of potassium. Things such as excessive salt, diarrhea, vomiting, sweating, and diuretics can all lead to a potassium deficiency if they continue too long. And that's not a good thing, because the mineral also plays an important role in the heart, the digestive tract, and muscle function. It's also been found to control blood pressure. High amounts of potassium result in a condition called "hyperkalemia." Too little potassium is known as "hypokalemia." For best health, potassium is found in fresh fruit and vegetables, as well as legumes. Specifically, bananas, orange juice, avocados, peaches, tomatoes, cantaloupes, and fish such as salmon and cod.

Selenium

Many enzymes that help with body functions need selenium to function properly. One of those enzymes protects against free radical damage, and thus cancer. Herein lies selenium's possible role as an antioxidant and anticancer mineral. Selenium has been linked by some clinical studies to helping prevent heart disease, treating skin disorders such as acne, blocking the toxic effects of mercury, arsenic, and copper, and helping arthritis patients respond better to conventional treatment. Selenium deficiency is rare in North America, and supplements would be used in therapeutic cases only. A lack of the mineral can cause fingernail changes, muscle weakness, and heart problems. The mineral has no accurate measurements of amounts in food, but is known to be present in organ meat, seafood, lean red meat, and grains that are grown in selenium-rich soil.

Zinc

More than 20 enzymes that play a part in the body's metabolism rely on zinc to work properly. Thus, zinc has a number of important roles. By synthesizing a couple of acids, it is critical in cell division, repair, and growth. Much zinc is found in the eye – some believe it activates vitamin A and assists night vision. It's particularly important in places that have a high turnover of cells, including the gastrointestinal system and the taste buds – in fact, an early sign of zinc deficiency is a change in your ability to taste or smell. Other signs you don't have enough zinc include wounds that don't heal quickly, a rise in infections, and poorly developed reproductive organs. You can find it in the highest quantities in meat, poultry, fish and seafood, liver, eggs, and whole grains. It is widely available as a supplement. But only a doctor should advise you to take these supplements, and never on your own should you exceed 50 mg a day. Some conditions that may require zinc supplementation include: alcoholism, burns, diabetes, Down's syndrome, eating disorders, intestinal diseases, infections, kidney or liver disease, pancreas disease, sickle cell disease, skin disorders, and continuing stress.

Natural Substances Found in Your Body (Including Amino Acids)

Adenosine Monophosphate

During normal metabolic processes, adenosine monophosphate (AMP) is created within cells. It isn't widely available as a supplement, but can be used for therapeutic purposes. It has been found to help relieve the pain of shingles and is associated with treating "postherpetic neuralgia." (AMP was injected though, not taken orally.) AMP has also been shown, when taken orally, as beneficial in helping people who have photosensitivity as a result of an adult-onset disease called "porphyria cutanea tarda." This supplement should only be taken with a doctor's approval.

Arginine

According to the Berkeley Wellness Letter, arginine is an amino acid that helps boost nitric oxide, which in turn is a compound found to relax blood vessels, keep arteries flexible, and assist with a healthy blood flow. This means that arginine may play an important role in treating cardiovascular and circulatory problems such as angina. Arginine is thought by many to treat heart diseases, lessen fatigue, stimulate the body's immune responses, and even fight cancer. This amino acid should only be taken with a doctor's permission, because its long-term effects are not well-understood. Plus, too much of one amino acid can create imbalances with others, leading to adverse effects.

Carnitine (or L-carnitine)

This naturally occurring amino acid is produced by the kidneys and liver – boosted by meat and diary products that your diet provides. Carnitine transports "long-chain fatty acids" into the mitochondria of cells, where energy is produced. People are known to have carnitine deficiencies, but the rate of such a condition in North America is not known. Genetic disorders, high-fat diets, low levels of the amino acids that make carnitine, and liver or kidney problems can all cause a deficiency – the symptoms of which include exhaustion, muscle pain, low blood pressure, chest pain, and overall weakness. It is suggested as a possible therapeutic approach to a wide range of conditions, none of which are backed up too well scientifically. You can find carnitine highest in lamb and dairy, and to a lesser, but still significant, degree in poultry, soybeans, wheat, asparagus, fish, avocados, and peanut butter. Carnitine is one of the few items not found in most common fruits and vegetables.

DHEA

This acronym says a mouthful: dehydroepiandrosterone. This is a hormone from the steroid family that is found in abundance in the bloodstream, used by the body to make testosterone and estrogen (depending on your sex). Clinical evidence has found DHEA supplements most useful for women – the best proof coming against mild or moderate lupus. Women over 70 who suffer from osteoporosis may benefit from DHEA supplements (and their libido may benefit too). Thoughts for men include enhancing performance in athletes and improving an impotent outlook. We get an unmentionable amount of DHEA through our diet; it is made instead by the body. It does not, as some would suggest, come in wild yams. The supplement is fashioned from substances found in soybeans.

Glucosamine

This is a molecule that comes from glucose. Glucosamine is a well known treatment for arthritic pain, especially when combined with chondroitin sulfate. It occurs naturally in the body, and plays a role in the creation of cartilage. Hailed as a possible "cure" for arthritis, it won't do exactly that, but it can (and has been proved to) reduce joint pain. X-rays have shown that in patients taking glucosamine, arthritis progressed slowly or not at all while others without the supplement lost cartilage at an expected rate. It is also linked to a few side effects. Once a definitive study comes out on glucosamine's arthritis-relieving effects, it will likely leap to the top of the arthritis treatment list. It's still thought by some to make it harder for the body to regulate its blood sugar levels.

Glutamine

Sometimes you see the letter L in front of this word; in either case glutamine is an amino acid that the body makes by itself to boost the immune system, and ensure a healthy digestive tract and muscle cells. Because of its apparent multi-benefits in the body, glutamine has been proposed as a treatment for many things including infections in athletes, food allergies, diseases of the digestive tract, ulcers, attention deficit disorder, and even weight loss due to HIV. This should only be used with a doctor's supervision, as safe doses have yet to be understood. Glutamine is also found in foods with lots of protein: meat, fish, dairy, and beans are the best sources.

L-tryptophan

This essential amino acid is found in animal proteins and can't be synthesized by the human body. It was first found in milk protein back in 1901. It is used in conjunction with other medications to treat depression; also, it and lithium are used for bipolar disorder. It is known to contribute to the structure of proteins. Not having enough tryptophan in the diet can enhance the negative effects of vitamin-deficiency diseases. In the recent past, the FDA has announced its concerns about supplements that contain L-tryptophan because they linked it to playing an unexplained role in the 1989 outbreak of eosinophilia-myalgia syndrome (1,500 cases, 37 deaths). Its negative effects have not, though, prevented the FDA from halting the marketing of such dietary supplements. Check with your doctor on this one.

Lecithin

The part of lecithin that is presumed to have the medicinal effect is "phosphatidylcholine" (or "PC"). Both are not essential nutrients, although PC is an important part of the membranes that surround the body's cells. When a person eats PC, it is typically broken down into "choline" – this is an essential nutrient that promotes methylation and is used to make a nerve chemical required by the brain. Evidence that lecithin works against any particular condition is not good, although preliminary studies have shown it to be useful in lowering cholesterol levels (for decades, it's been used for this purpose). It has been suggested for treatment of neurological diseases such as Alzheimer's and Tourette's because of its action on the nerve chemical.

Lysine

An essential amino acid, lysine is found in food – specifically in animal protein such as poultry and meat, but also in dairy products, eggs, and beans. Regular use of lysine supplements may help people with herpes avoid the number and intensity of flare-ups of cold sores. Scientists have found that lysine fights the herpes simplex virus by blocking another amino acid discussed above: arginine. That one is used by the virus to mutate itself. The safety of lysine supplements isn't established and thus they should not be taken without a doctor's approval.

Melatonin

This hormone is produced deep inside the brain, to a greater extent during the night than during the day. For this reason, melatonin may be the wizard behind our so-called internal body clock and our sleep cycles. Supplements of this hormone are sold as cures for insomnia. Other supposed uses include jet lag, arthritis, alcoholism, migraine, menopause, and stress. Despite what was thought previously, researchers have recently found that melatonin probably does not decrease as a person ages. Solid clinical trials are lacking into this supplement, so you should speak to a doctor before using it to cure any sleeping problems. Its effectiveness in this regard is not well-understood or definitive, and melatonin's long-term effects are to be determined.

MSM

This is also known as methylsulfonyl methane, a natural organic sulfur compound that is essential for our health. Specifically, it's thought to help relieve the pain, burning, and inflammation associated with joint diseases. MSM does so by acting to repair tissue. It has not been studied too extensively, and has actually been around for a while as a popular treatment for joint stiffness in dogs and horses. It is FDA-approved to treat "interstitial cystitis" and is used in other countries for arthritis, athletic injuries, and various muscle or skeletal problems – all because of its tissue-repairing ability. It is also thought to offset the toxic effects of mercury. It's widely available as a supplement, in pill form, crystals that are mixed with juice, creams, lotions, and gels. It is found naturally in almost all unprocessed foods, but is lost when that food is cooked or processed. The best source of MSM, in fact, is the most natural of all: mother's milk.

Phenylalanine

This is an amino acid found in "L-form" and "D-form." The L-form is an essential amino acid used in the body. It converts into "tyrosine", which is another amino acid. The D-form is a synthesized one; it is created in laboratories. L-phenylalanine is found in meat, fish, poultry, eggs, and dairy products (in short, protein-filled foods). If you get enough protein in your diet, you get enough of this amino acid and don't need a supplement. D-phenylalanine has not nutritional basis, but has been proposed to perhaps treat chronic pain because it blocks a particular enzyme that increases pain levels. Preliminary studies show that both forms of phenylalanine can help patients with depression. Other, not proven, targets include: Parkinson's disease, arthritis, vitiligo, attention deficit disorder, and multiple sclerosis.

Probiotics

Inside the gastrointestinal tract are trillions of bacteria, with hundreds of different species that outnumber the body's cell count by at least 10 times. They play a key role in digestion and immune function. Probiotics is a recently adopted medical approach that involves live bacteria in the form of supplements to boost the immune system, fight infection, and aid digestion. The idea is that having more beneficial bacteria in the intestines can help the body fight the growth of bad bacteria, those that cause disease. The bacteria in probiotics are also seen to produce natural antibiotics that then kill microorganisms harmful to the body. They may work best in relieving diarrhea, vaginitis, yeast infections, and tooth decay. There are many different kinds of probiotics available. In foods, beneficial bacteria are found most notably in yogurt (although the different kinds will vary). Supplements take the form of powder, pills, or liquid extract.

Taurine

This is yet another amino acid, found this time in the muscles and nervous system. Its main contribution to health comes in regulating heartbeat, maintaining the membranes of cells, and affecting the release of neurotransmitters that carry signals between the brain and all parts of the body where there are nerves. These are all vital functions. Therapeutically, taurine is best known in the treatment of congestive heart failure. It's also been suggested to help in viral hepatitis, cataracts, diabetes, alcoholism, hypertension, multiple sclerosis, psoriasis, and attention deficit disorder. It is found naturally in meat, poultry, eggs, fish, and dairy products. But the body can make it from vitamin B-6 and from methionine and cysteine (two other amino acids).

Enzymes

Coenzyme Q_{10}

More and more, this supplement – also known as CoQ10 – is gaining popularity as one of the most potent antioxidants available. It's alternative name, "ubiquinone" hints at its ubiquitous nature as the substance is found in every cell of the body and plays a major role in producing energy from food. It is known best as a treatment for congestive heart failure, where the cardiac muscles are weakened and maintain poor circulation. There is much clinical evidence to support facts that were widely discussed: patients with congestive heart failure seemed to have significantly lower levels of CoQ10 than healthy people. There is also some mention, although not as definitive, that this supplement could be used in other forms of heart disease, in cardiomyopathy, in hypertension, and in periodontal disease. Outside of the heart, some have proposed its effectiveness in Parkinson's disease, diabetes, infertility in males, and on athletic performance. We get trace amounts of CoQ10 in our diet (it's found in all plant and animal cells), but our body usually gets all it needs through self-manufacturing. Those who need to take therapeutic doses will need to discuss this with their doctor.

Bromelain

Widely touted in the alternative medicine world, this is the enzyme that comes in pineapple. Supplements are made from the pineapple's stem, where bromelain is concentrated. The proteolytic enzyme is a fairly strong anti-inflammatory as well as a blood-thinner. It works by breaking down "fibrin" which is a protein that can disrupt circulation, and it also blocks certain compounds that cause swelling and pain. When inflammation subsides, blood travels better and faster and can ease pain and quicken healing. Many clinical studies have identified the pineapple enzyme as useful in relieving pain and reducing swelling after surgery or if you sustain an injury. In Europe, and particularly Germany, it's often used to clear up a case of sinusitis because of its ability to reduce swelling in the nose and sinuses. Bromelain can also function as a digestive enzyme, functioning both within the stomach's acidic and the small intestine's alkaline environments.

Lipase

You come down with "steatorrhea" when your lipase levels are too low to break down dietary fats, and you can tell because you have greasy, light-colored stools. Lipase is an enzyme produced in the pancreas that breaks down fats so your body can absorb them. After the liver and bile have a go at the ingested fats, they are broken down far enough for lipase to make them absorbable. When taken in supplemental form, lipase is usually combined with other pancreatic enzymes. People who have cystic fibrosis often need these supplements, as well as those with celiac and Crohn's disease and perhaps even for indigestion. They are all probably exhibiting pancreatic insufficiency or lipase deficiency.

Papain

This digestive enzyme hails, just like bromelain, from a tropical fruit: the papaya. Papain is what's known as a "proteolytic" enzyme, meaning it digests proteins. The papaya enzyme also exerts a mild, soothing effect on the stomach. In the past, it's been used to relieve ulcers, and reduce inflammation, fever, and adhesions causes by surgery. Because of its beneficial action with digestion, it's sometimes taken orally as a supplement to treat less serious conditions such as chronic indigestion or bloating. Other, unproven, uses include decreasing pain and inflammation of rheumatoid arthritis, helping complications of diabetes, relieving chronic diarrhea, boosting immune function, and working against psoriasis when used on the skin. Interestingly, papain has been used as a meat tenderizer.

Another proteolytic enzyme often recommended is pancreatin.

Other Herbs

Blue-green Algae

This herb is also known as "spirulina" and grows in Mexican lakes and in Africa. More impoverished areas of the world use blue-green algae because of its high protein and nutrient content to fight malnutrition. Elsewhere, the herb is used as a dietary supplement. This is what it contains: B vitamins, beta-carotene, calcium, iron, magnesium, manganese, potassium, zinc, and gamma-linolenic acid. It is absolutely chalked full of protein, especially dried spirulina. In health food stores you'll find it in powder of pill form. It is used principally for nutritional support, and very preliminary evidence has suggested it could help with weight loss, fibromyalgia symptoms, HIV infection, and even cancer. Far more research needs to be done for any conclusive comments. Maximum safe doses are yet to be determined.

Cascara sagrada

You may not have heard of it, so here it is: the bark of the Californian Buckthorn tree is also known as *Cascara sagrada* or also "sacred bark." It is a shrub that grows in the northwestern United States, with bark collected and dried in spring and summer when it is easily peeled from the wood. This FDA-approved this herb because it might be effective in helping with constipation, as it is known to be a mild laxative that acts on the large intestine – in fact it is a common ingredient in over-the-counter laxatives. Its best traits may be the mildness of its laxative effect, and it is considered safe for delicate patients, the elderly, and anal or rectal-surgery patients. Occasionally using *Cascara sagrada* may also help prevent the pain of hemorrhoids. It can be taken in pill form or as a tea.

Grass Pollen

Investigated for an effect on prostatitis, prostate cancer, and cholesterol levels, grass pollen is most commonly used to help treat benign prostate hyperplasia (an enlarged prostate). There are various kinds of grass pollen extracts, and a different one altogether is used in allergy shots to combat hay fever. Its effect on an enlarged prostate has been proven clinically a couple of times. Grass pollen helps reduce the frequency of nighttime urination, and lowers the level of urine in the bladder. It might even do what few therapies can: reduce the size of the prostate. It hasn't been linked with any side effects either. It seems this may be a good herb for men to take when confronted with a large prostate.

Marshmallow Root

Ancient Greeks and Romans used marshmallow to treat bruises, blood loss, toothaches, insect bites, and generally irritated skin. Marshmallow candy was originally flavored with the marshmallow herb, however any sugared candy you see now being roasted on a campfire or added to deserts is likely not culled from the plant. Marshmallow may exert a soothing effect on mucous membranes, making it a decent treatment for colds, coughs, asthma, and other respiratory infections. This is because of its main ingredient, "mucilage," that becomes gooey when it runs into a liquid. Like peppermint, it holds the ability to soothe an irritated throat, and is even sometimes recommended to lessen the discomfort of Crohn's disease and stomach ulcers. There isn't a plethora of studies into this herb, but it is believed very safe. Steeping roots in a tea is the best way to take it. The herb is a source of both vitamin A and C, two immune boosters.

Andrographis (Indian shrub)

This bitter herb is from India and other Asian countries, so bitter in fact that it's known as the "king of bitters." The family of plants actually consists of nearly 30 species around tropical Asia – "Andrographis paniculata" is the one used medicinally (and consequently, the most popular). Interestingly, it's been credited with halting the spread of a 1919 flu epidemic that tore through India. This may explain why it is used to treat cold symptoms, backed up by reasonably good evidence. It's not exactly known why, but it can help relieve earache, lack of sleep, sore throat, and nasal drainage in particular. The herb may stimulate immunity. What it also may do is help with heart disease, liver toxicity, and gallbladder contraction. No study on humans has revealed any side effects on the liver, kidney, or blood count, but a few animal studies have raised a cautious flag regarding fertility – this link remains unclear.

Also...

Beta-Sitosterol

This is a sterol compound that is derived from plants, with a similarity to cholesterol found in our body. Beta-sitosterol is the most prevalent "phytosterol" (as they are called) that is found in the food we eat. Specifically, it is in most fruits and vegetables, as well and nuts and seeds. The best place to find these sterols is in plant oils. It's believed to help control cholesterol levels if taken as a supplement because beta-sitosterol is not well absorbed by the gastrointestinal tract and can run a kind of interference with your body's absorption of cholesterol. It's also thought to protect the body against various forms of cancer and some test-tube studies have found this possible. In addition, beta-sitosterol helps alleviate the symptoms of benign prostate hyperplasia and this has been proven. And the immune system may get a boost from this supplement as well, balancing different types of hormones and preventing the "immune suppression" that can occur following stressful physical activity.

Carotenoids

These are the substances that turn fruits and vegetables red, yellow, and orange (but are also found in dark green, leafy veggies too). The theory is that the more colorful the item, the more carotenoids it contains. Scientists have spotted over 700 carotenoids and about 50 of these are absorbable by the human body. Many, including beta-carotene, have shown vitamin A-like activity. The two we are most concerned with are "carotenes" – found predominantly in carrots, yams, squash, and other yellow and orange vegetables – and "xanthophylls" that are found in green leafy vegetables such as kale, spinach, Brussels sprouts, and broccoli. Carotenoids are natural antioxidants, protecting the plants they inhabit from any adverse damaging reactions during photosynthesis. Much conjecture about health benefits surrounds these important antioxidants (including much talk about cancer-protecting properties), but research has only validated a few, and weakly at that: these include cataracts, heart disease, macular degeneration, and sickle cell anemia.

CDP-Choline

That's better than repeating its full name: cytidinediphosphocholine. Where choline is a substance the brain needs to produce a major neurotransmitter to send impulses around the body, CDP-choline is a unique form that is almost super-charged: it passes easily through the blood-brain barrier into the brain tissue. It's spent many years in the field of medicine, and despite many uncertainties that still exist with it, several countries in Europe prescribe CDP-choline for cognitive, emotional, and behavioral deficits that are linked to cerebral disorders in elderly patients. It was recently the subject of a literature review, which found no real evidence suggesting CDP-choline had an effect on attention, but did reveal that the drug helped with memory and behavior – at least in the short and medium term. This makes it a potential therapeutic aid in Alzheimer's patients and other cognitive disorders in supplement form. Its effects over the long-term still need to be evaluated. As with any neurologic supplement, it should only be taken with a doctor's approval.

Fish Oil/Omega-3 Fatty Acids

Fish oil is becoming a tremendously popular supplement, as it is full of vitamin D and omega-3 fatty acids, both needed by the body. Cod liver oil is the most common source of fish oil, but you can also try salmon, mackerel, or halibut oils, as well as any oil that comes from cold water fish (and these may be safer than cod oil). The therapeutic possibilities of fish oil are not small. For the heart and circulatory system, there's evidence it helps prevent heart disease, lower LDL cholesterol levels, and even helps treat hypertension. To a lesser-known degree, fish oil may help with all these conditions: rheumatoid arthritis, osteoporosis, menstrual pain, lupus, psoriasis, Raynaud's phenomenon, bipolar disorder. Very preliminary, but still notable, evidence has found that it may help treat depression, kidney stones, chronic fatigue syndrome, allergies, gout, and migraines. Is it any wonder this supplement, which is safe, is gaining popularity? (Flaxseed oil is another good source of omega-3.)

O. Strepta-cantha

Also known as the nopal cactus (or "prickly pear cactus"), it goes back a long way as food and medicine. Interestingly it appears on the Mexico flag. The fruit, flowers, and stem of this cactus have been used in the treatment of diabetes, benign prostate hyperplasia, liver disease, fatigue, and shortness of breath. There isn't great evidence behind its effects, the best being diabetes. Some research points to a cholesterol-reducing effect, as well as stomach-protecting and pain-relieving traits. No dosage has been established, and people with kidney or liver disease, as well as children and pregnant women should avoid it. Despite its history it is not well known and any benefits have yet to be truly documented.

Quercetin

This flavonoid is a natural antioxidant floating around in red wine that protects the body's cells from damage done by free radicals. It was found to suppress histamines and stop them from being released by immune cells – therefore it is most popular these days as a treatment for allergic conditions: hay fever, asthma, eczema, and hives. Some preliminary evidence suggests that quercetin can help with prostatitis, heart disease, strokes, cataracts, and even cancer. For therapy, it's available as a supplement, but is also naturally found outside of red wine to the greatest degree in grapefruits, onions, apples, and black tea. Quercetin's link to cancer makes it a bit of a sketchy supplement (it's been suggested that it raises the risk of infant leukemia in pregnant women). The different forms that quercetin supplements come in are all not absorbed so easily. With doctor's permission, find the form called "quercetin chalcone."

Shark Cartilage

This is just what it says, the cartilage tissue from a shark. Dry powder, available in most health food stores, is made up of ash (calcium and phosphorus), protein, carbohydrates, water, and a minute portion of fiber. The reason this substance is of interest to scientists is that sharks are not known to get cancer and they survive for a long time. Initially it was found that shark cartilage prevents a tumor from building a network of blood vessels, meaning it will eventually recede and die. Nothing is as yet proven, but there has been a frenzy of attempted research into this cancer-shark cartilage link, even in large clinical journals. It has also been suggested that this supplement may help with arthritis and osteoporosis as well. According to the American Cancer Society, there is no proof to any claims yet beyond the fact that it appears to inhibit the growth of new blood vessels.

NOTES

NOTES

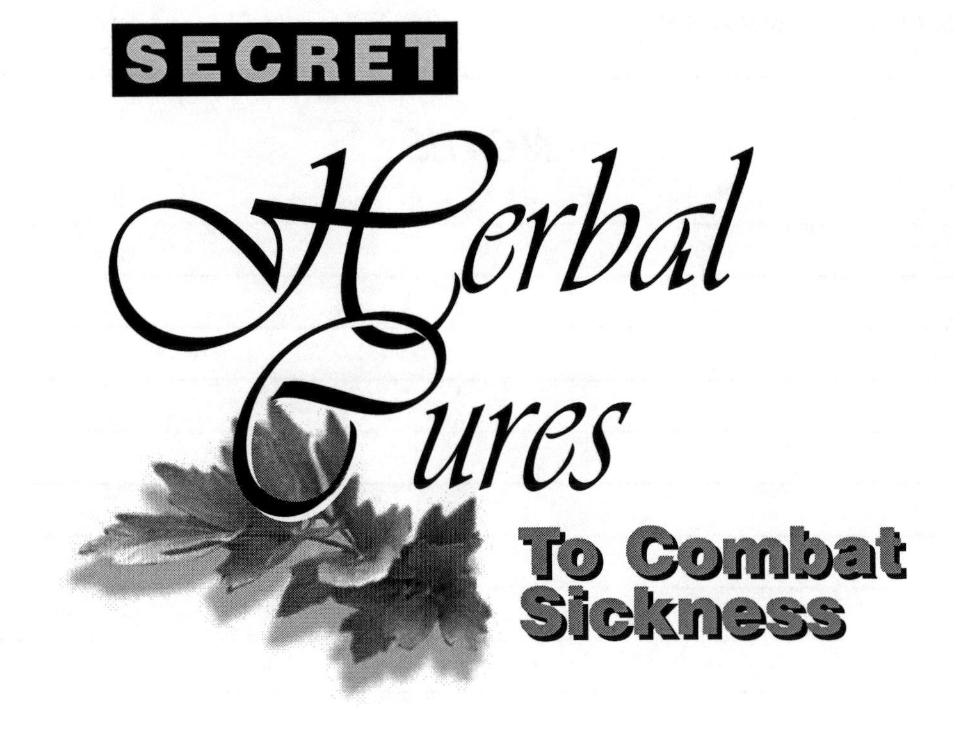

Appendix

HERBS UNAPPROVED BY GERMANY'S COMMISSION E

NOTES

For Your Knowledge:

The Commission E in Germany is frequently mentioned when discussing or researching alternative medicine. It is an official government body that resembles the Food & Drug Administration – except the Commission E focuses on herbal remedies. Germany is really at the forefront of botanical medicine, one of the most progressive and experimental countries around in this regard. It's been said that about 70% of Germany's physicians employ natural methods of treatment. The Commission was formed (back in 1978) to put some sort of stamp on how effective and safe herbs are for the public.

The Commission came back with more than 300 small articles called "monographs" that looked at the herbs considered to be most important for medicine. These write-ups were then considered the main word within the German healthcare system, written on the basis of what scientific evidence was available. The people behind Commission E are those with an expert knowledge of alternative medicine, people either practicing it or producing it. The monographs were not critical evaluations of herbal medicine, but instead summaries of their uses. They were, though, responsible for removing about 100 herbal drugs from the shelves of pharmacies.

The herbs the Commission E looked at were either approved or unapproved for use in medicine. The monographs served as an interesting research study, and are regarded in North America, not as the final word on herbal medicine, but rather the stepping stone to further thought. It may be useful to know which herbs – although all of this is not based solely on clinical evidence (thus it is not 100% trustworthy) – were found to be not useful in medicine by experts in herbal medicine, people who are not skeptical of these alternative healers, but instead are proponents of them. Specified are the parts of the plant that are unapproved, because different parts (the root, the leaf, etc) can yield different results.

The Unapproved List:

Alpine Lady's Mantle herb
Angelica seed and herb
Ash bark and leaf
Asparagus herb
Barberry
Basil herb
Bilberry leaf
Bishop's Weed fruit
Bitter Orange flower
Blackberry root
Blackthorn flower
Bladderwrack
Borage
Bryonia root
Buchu leaf
Burdock root
Calendula herb (Marigold)
Cat's Foot flower
Celery
Chamomile flower (Roman)
Chestnut leaf
Cinnamon flower
Cocoa
Colocynth
Coltsfoot
Corn Poppy flower
Cornflower
Damiana leaf and herb
Delphinium flower
Dill weed
Echinacea
Angustifolia herband root
Elecampane root
Ergot
Eyebright
Figs
Ginkgo Biloba leaf
Goat's Rue herb
Hawthorn berry, flower, and leaf
Heather herb and flower
Hibiscus
Hollyhock flower
Horse Chestnut leaf
Hound's Tongue
Hyssop
Jambolan seed
Jimsonweed leaf and seed
Kelp
Lemongrass (Citronella)
Linden
Charcoal, flower, leaf, wood
Liverwort herb
Loofa
Lungwort
Madder root
Male Fern
Marjoram
Marsh Tea
Mentzelia
Milk Thistle herb
Monkshood
Mountain Ash berry
Mugwort
Muira Puama
Night-blooming Cereus
Nutmeg
Nux Vomica
Oat herb
Oats
Oleander leaf
Olive leaf
Olive oil
Oregano
Orris root
Papain
Papaya leaf
Paprika
Parsley seed
Pasque flower
Peony flower and root
Periwinkle
Petasites leaf
Pimpinella herb
Raspberry leaf
Rhododendron
Rose Hip seed
Rue
Rupturewort
Saffron
Sandalwood (Red)
Sarsaparilla root
Senecio herb
Soapwort herb (Red)
Spinach leaf
Strawberry leaf
Sweet Woodruff
Tansy
Verbena herb
Veronica herb
Walnut hull
White Dead Nettle herb
Yohimbe bark
Zedoary rhizome

[*Source*: American Botanical Council]

"HERBS IN THIS BOOK"

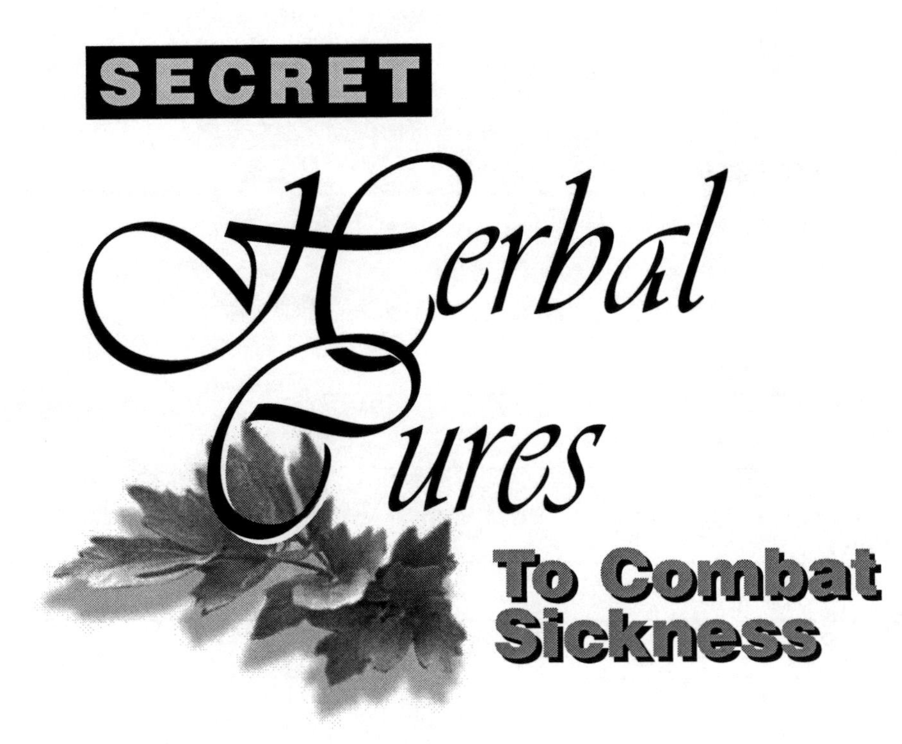

Your Herbal Medicine Diary

It is important to keep track of any and every herbal treatment you try. For one thing, you may experience side effects that you'll need to discuss with your primary health care practitioner. For another, choosing the herbal supplement or cure that's right for you is largely a process of trial and error. Use the following pages as your herbal medicine diary. Record how the treatments make you feel, make note of any side effects, and jot down questions, concerns, or ecstatic testimonials! Part of your treatment is understanding exactly how herbal medicines affect you, both positively and negatively, and this diary is the perfect way to organize that information. Feel free to photocopy the following blank diary page for your personal use. We're sure that the pages of this book contain herbal remedies that can put you on the road to recovery from your ailments, symptoms, or concerns. Your exciting journey begins today.

We wish you the best of natural health!

Herbal Remedy: ______________________

Date of First Dosage: ______________________

Source of Herb: ______________________

Dosage: ______________________

Preparation Notes: ______________________

____

____

How do you feel after one day of treatment?

____

____

____

____

How do you feel after one week of treatment with your chosen herbal cure?

____

____

____

____

How do you feel after two to four weeks of taking the herbal remedy?

____

____

____

____

____

How do you feel after trying the herbal medicine for six to eight weeks?

How do you feel after ongoing treatment?

Side Effects:

Questions to ask your primary health practitioner:

Notes:

Herbal Remedy: ______________________

Date of First Dosage: ______________________

Source of Herb: ______________________

Dosage: ______________________

Preparation Notes: ______________________

____

____

How do you feel after one day of treatment?

____

____

____

____

How do you feel after one week of treatment with your chosen herbal cure?

____

____

____

____

How do you feel after two to four weeks of taking the herbal remedy?

____

____

____

____

____

How do you feel after trying the herbal medicine for six to eight weeks?

How do you feel after ongoing treatment?

Side Effects:

Questions to ask your primary health practitioner:

Notes:

Herbal Remedy: ______________________

Date of First Dosage: ______________________

Source of Herb: ______________________

Dosage: ______________________

Preparation Notes: ______________________

How do you feel after one day of treatment?

How do you feel after one week of treatment with your chosen herbal cure?

How do you feel after two to four weeks of taking the herbal remedy?

How do you feel after trying the herbal medicine for six to eight weeks?

How do you feel after ongoing treatment?

Side Effects:

Questions to ask your primary health practitioner:

Notes:

NOTES

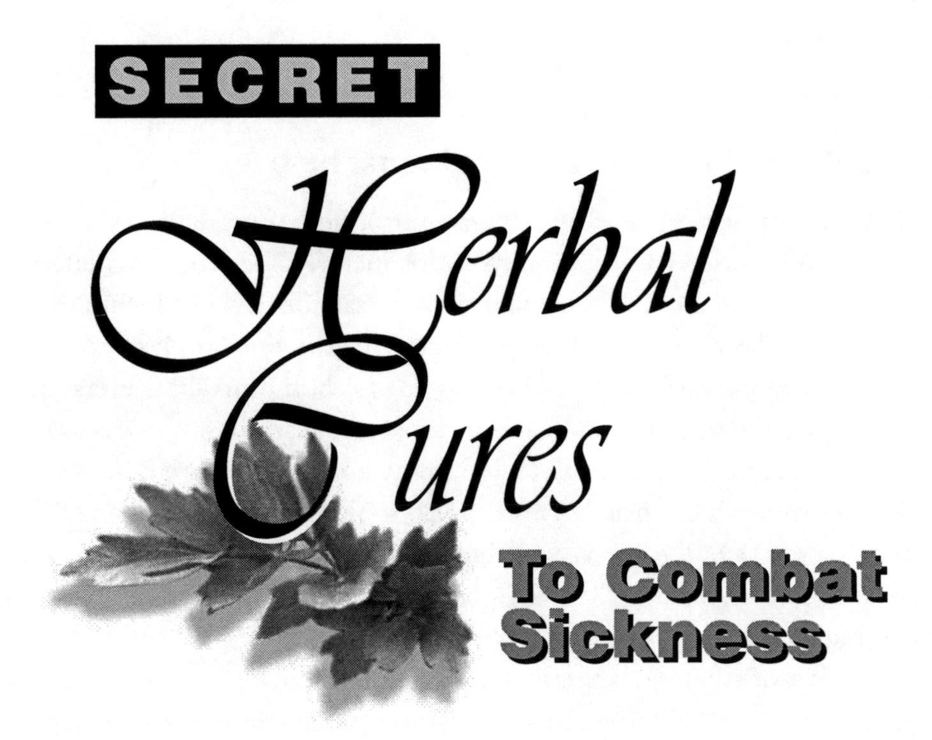

Four Common Myths

- **Myth #1: Herbs are "natural" so that they must be pure and safe.**

  Herbal preparations purchased in drug stores or health food stores may not be as pure as you think since they may contain various contaminants such as allergens, bacteria, fungi, even prescription drugs (testosterone, diazepam), or heavy metals (i.e. mercury, lead, cadmium). These contaminants may cause severe adverse reactions, including death. Besides, herbal products contain complicated mixtures of chemicals and the levels vary considerably depending upon many factors related to the growth, production and processing by the manufacturers. Speak to your doctor or pharmacist for specific advice on choosing reputable brands.

- **Myth #2: What I read on the label must be true.**

Unlike drugs (prescription or over-the-counter), herbal products are treated by the Food and Drug Administration as dietary supplements. Therefore, manufacturers of these products are not required to show that they are safe or effective before they decide to add them to the shelves of your nearest pharmacy or grocery store. It's very important to note that since there's no patent protection on any herb, the manufacturers are not willing to invest a large amount of money and a decade of research and development, including studies with thousands of patients, to determine how safe they are. That said, the three most studied herbal products include garlic (2,920 subjects), ginkgo biloba (2,326 subjects), and St. John's wort (1,851 subjects). (Reference: Blumental et al. *Herbal Medicine: Expanded Commission E Monographs* 2000.) The good news is that recently the FDA has put in place stricter requirements for dietary supplements.

A little bit of common sense and following the guidelines below will help ensure that you don't run any risk of experiencing unpleasant side effects from the herbal products you purchase:

1. Avoid use in children.
2. In general, avoid use in pregnant or breast-feeding women.
3. Be aware that the majority of herbal products in use have not been properly tested in human subjects.
4. Be aware that labels on herbal products often do not readily reveal information about possible problems, side effects, or potential interactions with drugs.
5. Be aware that the amount of the active ingredients in each herbal product may vary. product to product. This makes it impossible to know exactly how much of the active ingredient you are actually getting from any pill. If unsure, it's best to get some advice from a doctor or pharmacist.
6. Be aware of unproven claims which marketers use to advertise herbal products.
7. Inform your physician about any herbal product(s) you are currently taking. This is commonly neglected!
8. Review the potential side effects and contraindications before you start any herbal product.
9. Select only standardized herbal products from manufacturers utilizing the Good Manufacturing Practices set forth by the FDA or a similar regulatory agency.
10. Be sure to review potential herb-drug interactions with your physician or pharmacist.
11. Keep up to date with books (like this one) and newsletters on herbal medicine.

- **Myth #3: Herbs are less expensive than prescription or OTC drugs.**

  Herbal products are usually not covered by most insurance plans. In 1997, alternative treatments including vitamins, herbal products, and dietary supplements totaled $34 billion. In general, the cost of brand name herbal products are usually more expensive than generic drugs, but are generally less expensive than brand name prescription drugs.

- **Myth #4: Herbs can be taken safely without consulting a physician.**

  It is simply unwise to use any herbal product unsupervised by either your physician or your pharmacist because many of these products may have side effects or may interact with the drug(s) you are currently taking. In general, I do not recommend that you try to self-diagnose and/or self-treat because what you believe might be a minor problem may in fact turn out to be a serious one. Just to give you an example, you may choose to use saw palmetto for your urinary symptoms (i.e. urgency, frequency, dripping) thinking that these symptoms are caused by an enlarged prostate, but in fact it may be something far worse: prostate cancer.